Emotion in the Clinical Encounter

NOTICE

Medicine is an ever-changing science. As new research and clinical experience broaden our knowledge, changes in treatment and drug therapy are required. The author and the publisher of this work have checked with sources believed to be reliable in their efforts to provide information that is complete and generally in accord with the standards accepted at the time of publication. However, in view of the possibility of human error or changes in medical sciences, neither the author nor the publisher nor any other party who has been involved in the preparation or publication of this work warrants that the information contained herein is in every respect accurate or complete, and they disclaim all responsibility for any errors or omissions or for the results obtained from use of the information contained in this work. Readers are encouraged to confirm the information contained herein with other sources. For example and in particular, readers are advised to check the product information sheet included in the package of each drug they plan to administer to be certain that the information contained in this work is accurate and that changes have not been made in the recommended dose or in the contraindications for administration. This recommendation is of particular importance in connection with new or infrequently used drugs.

Emotion in the Clinical Encounter

Rachel Schwartz, PhD
Stanford University School of Medicine
Stanford, California

Judith A. Hall, PhD
Northeastern University
Boston, Massachusetts

Lars G. Osterberg, MD, MPH
Stanford University School of Medicine
Stanford, California

New York Chicago San Francisco Athens London Madrid
Mexico City New Delhi Milan Singapore Sydney Toronto

Emotion in the Clinical Encounter

1 2 3 4 5 6 7 8 9 LCR 26 25 24 23 22 21

ISBN 978-1-260-46432-0
MHID 1-260-46432-6

This book was set in Minion Pro by MPS Limited.
The editors were Karen Edmonson, Jason Malley, and Kim J. Davis.
The production supervisor was Richard Ruzycka.
Project management was provided by Jyoti Shaw of MPS Limited.
The cover designer was W2 Design.
The cover artist was Nancy Hall.

Library of Congress Cataloging-in-Publication Data

Names: Schwartz, Rachel, editor. | Hall, Judith A., editor. |
    Osterberg, Lars G., editor.
Title: Emotion in the clinical encounter / [edited by] Rachel Schwartz,
    Judith A. Hall, Lars G. Osterberg.
Description: New York : McGraw Hill, [2021] | Includes bibliographical
    references and index. | Summary: "This book provides tools for trainees and
    practicing clinicians in navigating their own and their patients' emotion,
    delivering medical education innovations to support provider wellness
    and enhance patient care."— Provided by publisher.
Identifiers: LCCN 2021004700 (print) | LCCN 2021004701 (ebook) | ISBN
    9781260464320 (paperback) | ISBN 9781260464337 (ebook)
Subjects: MESH: Physician-Patient Relations | Emotions | Clinical
    Medicine | Communication | Physician's Role—psychology
Classification: LCC R727.3 (print) | LCC R727.3 (ebook) | NLM W 62 | DDC
    610.69/6—dc23
LC record available at https://lccn.loc.gov/2021004700
LC ebook record available at https://lccn.loc.gov/2021004701

Dedicated to the countless clinicians and researchers worldwide whose experiences, efforts, and insights made this book both necessary and possible.

Contents

Contributors

Karolien Aelbrecht, PhD
Center for Medical Genetics
Ghent University Hospital
Department of Biomolecular
    Medicine
Faculty of Medicine and Health
    Sciences
Ghent University
Ghent, Belgium

Robert M. Arnold, MD
Department of General Internal
    Medicine, Section of Palliative
    Care and Medical Ethics
Institute for Doctor-Patient
    Communication
UPMC Palliative and Supportive
    Institute
University of Pittsburgh School of
    Medicine
Pittsburgh, Pennsylvania

Amber E. Barnato, MD, MPH, MS
The Dartmouth Institute for Health
    Policy & Clinical Practice
Geisel School of Medicine at
    Dartmouth
Lebanon, New Hampshire

Mary Catherine Beach, MD, MPH
School of Medicine
Berman Institute of Bioethics

Bloomberg School of Public Health
Johns Hopkins University
Baltimore, Maryland

Paula H. Bednarek, MD, MPH
Department of Obstetrics and
    Gynecology
Oregon Health & Science University
    School of Medicine
Portland, Oregon

Anely Bekbergenova, MSc
Faculty of Business and Economics
Department of Organizational
    Behavior
University of Lausanne
Lausanne, Switzerland

Danielle Blanch-Hartigan, PhD, MPH
Department of Natural and Applied
    Sciences
Bentley University
Waltham, Massachusetts

Missy Brown, MD, MPH
Department of Emergency Medicine
UCLA David Geffen School of
    Medicine
UCLA Medical Center/Olive View
    Program
Los Angeles, California

Elise C. Carey, MD
Center for Palliative Medicine
Mayo Clinic School of Medicine
Rochester, Minnesota

Valerie Carrard, PhD
Psychiatrie Liaison Service
CHUV - Lausanne University
    Hospital
Lausanne, Switzerland

Julie W. Childers, MD, MS
Section of Palliative Care and
    Medical Ethics
Division of General Internal
    Medicine
University of Pittsburgh
    School of Medicine
Pittsburgh, Pennsylvania

Calvin L. Chou, MD, PhD, FACH
Department of Medicine
University of California, San
    Francisco School of Medicine
San Francisco, California

Lidia Del Piccolo, PhD
Department of Neurosciences,
    Biomedicine and Movement
    Sciences
University of Verona
Verona, Italy

Arnstein Finset, CandPsychol, PhD
Faculty of Medicine
Department of Behavioural
    Medicine
Institute of Basic Medical Sciences
University of Oslo
Oslo, Norway

Bria Adimora Godley, MD
University of North Carolina School
    of Medicine
Chapel Hill, North Carolina

Anne-Josée Guimond, PhD
Department of Social and Behavioral
    Sciences
Lee Kum Sheung Center for Health
    and Happiness
Harvard T. H. Chan School of Public
    Health
Boston, Massachusetts

Sarah D. Gunnery, PhD
Department of Psychology
New England College
Henniker, New Hampshire

Judith A. Hall, PhD
Department of Psychology
Northeastern University
Boston, Massachusetts

Amanda R. Hemmesch, PhD
Department of Psychology
St. Cloud State University
St. Cloud, Minnesota

Martha Howell, EdD
Baylor Scott and White Health
Temple, Texas

Ben Kaplan, MD, MPH
University of North Carolina
    School of Medicine
Chapel Hill, North Carolina

Asif Khan, MD
University of North Carolina
    School of Medicine
Chapel Hill, North Carolina
Refugee Community Partnership,
    Carrboro, North Carolina

Baruch S. Krauss, MD, EdM, FAAP
Division of Emergency Medicine
Boston Children's Hospital
Department of Pediatrics
Harvard Medical School
Boston, Massachusetts

Benjamin A. Krauss, ScM, BS
Brown University
Providence, Rhode Island

Laura D. Kubzansky, PhD, MPH
Department of Social and
    Behavioral Sciences
Lee Kum Sheung Center for Health
    and Happiness
Harvard T.H. Chan School of
    Public Health
Boston, Massachusetts

Lewina O. Lee, PhD
Department of Psychiatry
Boston University School of
    Medicine
National Center for Posttraumatic
    Stress Disorder
Veterans Affairs Boston
    Healthcare System
Boston, Massachusetts

Piet L. Leroy, MD, PhD, MSc
Pediatric Intensive Care Unit &
    Pediatric Procedural
    Sedation Unit
Department of Pediatrics

Maastricht University Medical
    Centre
Faculty of Health, Medicine and
    Life Sciences
Maastricht University
Maastricht, The Netherlands

Brett Marroquín, PhD
Department of Psychology
Loyola Marymount University
Los Angeles, California

Marianne Schmid Mast, PhD
Department of Organizational
    Behavior
HEC Lausanne
University of Lausanne
Lausanne, Switzerland

Enioluwafe Ojo, MD, MPH
University of North Carolina
    School of Medicine
Durham, North Carolina

Lars G. Osterberg, MD, MPH
Department of Medicine
Stanford University School
    of Medicine
Stanford, California

Erika B. Pages, MA
Department of Psychology
Arizona State University
Tempe, Arizona

Debra L. Roter, DrPH, MPH
Department of Health, Behavior
    and Society
Bloomberg School of Public Health
Johns Hopkins University
Baltimore, Maryland

Mollie A. Ruben, PhD
Department of Psychology
University of Maine
Orono, Maine

Rachel Schwartz, PhD
Stanford University School of Medicine
Stanford, California

Michelle N. Shiota, PhD
Department of Psychology
Arizona State University
Tempe, Arizona

Caitlin Holt Siropaides, DO
Department of Internal Medicine
Section of Supportive and
    Palliative Care
University of Texas Southwestern
    Medical Center
Dallas, Texas

Stuart Slavin, MD, MEd
Accreditation Council for Graduate
    Medical Education
Chicago, Illinois

Greeshma Somashekar, MD, MBA
University of North Carolina
    School of Medicine
Chapel Hill, North Carolina

Morgan D. Stosic, MA
Department of Psychology
University of Maine
Orono, Maine

Linda Tickle-Degnen, PhD, OT,
FAOTA
Department of Occupational Therapy
Tufts University
Medford, Massachusetts

Vera Vine, PhD
Department of Psychology
Queen's University
Kingston, Ontario
Canada

Amy Weil, MD
Division of General Medicine and
    Clinical Epidemiology
University of North Carolina School
    of Medicine
The Beacon Program
Chapel Hill, North Carolina

Foreword

In the early days of HIV, that in this current pandemic of COVID-19 feels like a lifetime ago, my clinic population in rural Tennessee consisted largely of gay men facing an incurable and fatal illness. The patients were roughly my age then—mid-thirties or younger—and the experience of caring for them felt intensely personal and poignant. Each visit hammered home the notion that time was precious for us all, but especially so for them.

At that point in time, 1985, one did not expect to see HIV in a small Appalachian town; AIDS was viewed as an urban phenomenon. Yet in a few years I was seeing far more patients with HIV than predicted for the town's small population. These were hometown boys for the most part, and I sensed that their experience and mine might not be unique; that I had stumbled onto a story that held true in every small town in America. The scientific paper I wrote with my colleagues described this paradigm, a quiet yet epic journey of migration: gay men had left their rural homes for the big cities as part of the general exodus for jobs, education, opportunity, but also because they were gay and didn't want to live that lifestyle under the scrutiny of friends and relatives. In the big cities, they found themselves, came out. Now years later they were coming back home, typically because their partners whom they had nursed through illness had died, and now they themselves were ill; or else they returned hoping to escape the plague that had decimated gay communities in urban areas in America. And there I was at the tail-end of the migration, caring for them as a physician.

What I remember all these years later is not the particular infections or tumors that blossomed when their immune defenses were ravaged; instead, I remember only the emotions that our paper never quite captured: the tragic nature of this voyage, the brave escape, the search for meaning, the defeat, the return, the burden and taint that came with the disease and with their sexual preference, and the heartache of the families who for the most part cared for them with such dignity and love. The paper did not capture my own grief at witnessing this again and again, or the powerful lessons my patients taught me about manhood and courage. The emotions still live in my memory and that of their survivors.[1]

"Only connect," E.M. Forster the novelist says in *Howards End*. The experience of caring for a patient who is ill, who recovers or does not, or who has a chronic condition, is an emotional one for the patient and the doctor too. Emotions help or impede the ability to connect, they affect diagnosis, color the treatment; emotions must be recognized, must be navigated around or leveraged and their cultural roots grasped. As a young physician I doubt I understood this as clearly as I do looking back. Emotions are the substrate of our clinical encounters.

That's why this volume you hold in your hands is precious. It astonishes me that I haven't seen anything like it before, despite the importance of the topic. In short, it is overdue. I hope you will find it to be a welcome and valuable addition to the canon of books you keep on your shelf.

Abraham Verghese, MD
Professor of Medicine
Department of Medicine
Stanford University
Stanford, California

REFERENCE

1. Verghese A, Berk SL, Sarubbi F. Urbs in rure: human immunodeficiency virus infection in rural Tennessee. *J Infect Dis.* 1989;160(6):1051-1055.

Preface

Whether painful or joyous, threatening or uplifting, emotions are a constant in the work life of healthcare providers. The provider's emotional experiences, the patient's emotional experiences, and how they handle them are the dual, and intersecting, subject of this book. By combining evidence from research on emotion with the insights of experienced clinicians and medical educators, we aim to add much-needed guidance for both learners and teachers around this crucial aspect of clinical professionalism.

The idea for this book came after one of us conducted three emotion workshops among practicing clinicians, trainees, and medical educators at Stanford University. Feedback from these workshops suggested that this content was largely missing from current medical training, and participants were eager for additional evidence-based resources that could guide them in how to navigate their own and their patients' emotions more skillfully. The first workshop was on the physiological, social, and clinical function of emotion, the second was on the relationship between emotional expression and culture, gender, and specific patient populations, and the third was an interactive panel consisting of four physicians from different specialties who shared what training they did (and more notably, did not) receive in navigating emotion, and how they had handled particularly challenging patient encounters. They shared stories about situations in which their own emotional response—or lack thereof—had affected the clinician–patient relationship, and what systems-level changes they felt were necessary to support more successful clinician–patient interactions. Attendees saw the panel session as the most valuable due to how rare it is for clinicians to learn from peers about what is usually a very private endeavor. The panelists embodied the change they advocated for: namely, the need for more opportunities to talk with peers in a nonthreatening setting about challenging patient encounters, and to learn new strategies for working with patients and managing one's own reactions.

The ultimate impact of honoring, and normalizing, the emotional demands of practicing medicine has yet to be seen, though we had a hint at what it might look like at the panel. One of the panelists spoke candidly about her experience realizing she had become numb over the course of her clinical practice. She spoke of how she had learned the word "alexithymia" at a physician wellness lecture, realized she had it, and decided to seek help. After the panel, one of the younger physicians in the audience took her aside and said, "Can you tell me that word again? I think I may have it…" It may take having more senior clinician leaders bravely acknowledge the emotional costs they've paid as part of their commitment to caring for others before the next generation of clinicians can become more fully equipped with the tools necessary to engage with emotion—their own, and that of their patients.

OVERVIEW OF EMOTION IN THE CLINICAL ENCOUNTER

Emotions are ever-present in the context of illness and in the process of medical care and have an enormous impact on the well-being of patients and healthcare providers alike. However, this topic is acknowledged and taught in an inconsistent manner in medical education, and the research that should inform clinical management of emotion is scattered. In this book, we present theory and research on the broad topic of emotions in medical care, providing both basic understanding and practical insights on one of the most vital yet challenging aspects of patient care: recognizing and responding effectively to the patient's emotions as well as healthcare providers themselves recognizing and tending to their own emotions.

Healthcare providers often understand that emotions are important in the process and outcomes of care, yet frequently report feeling ill-equipped to handle their own and their patients' emotions effectively. Despite clear evidence that clinicians' responses to patients' affective cues are linked to care outcomes, instruction on how to effectively identify and manage emotion in a clinical interaction is not a systematic part of medical education curricula. While high rates of burnout, characterized by emotional exhaustion, depersonalization, and the loss of a sense of personal accomplishment, are reported for medical trainees and practicing providers, there is evidence that emotional intelligence and emotional stability may be protective against burnout. This book seeks to advance healthcare providers' knowledge of the science of emotion while providing evidence-based guidance on how to apply these principles in clinical practice. New curricular content is provided to offer pathways for developing the skill set necessary to navigate the extraordinary emotional demands of practicing medicine.

This book is organized in three sections: *Emotion's Functions, Clinical Emotional Intelligence,* and *Emotions in the Culture of Medicine.*

Emotion's Functions

The introductory chapter, *Emotions in 21st-Century Humanistic Medicine*, provides an overview of why emotions are important for patient outcomes, clinician wellness, and the clinician–patient relationship. Other chapters in the *Emotion's Functions* section provide transdisciplinary background on the evolutionary, neurobiological, and social function of emotion, the role of emotion in illness, and emotional dialogue in the medical encounter.

Clinical Emotional Intelligence

The *Clinical Emotional Intelligence* section covers the importance of identifying patients' emotional cues and provides evidence on the role this plays in the clinician–patient relationship and in clinical outcomes. This section contains chapters on nonverbal cues of emotion, strategies for emotion recognition, the role of emotion in clinical decision making, and available training tools for honing these practices. Other chapters address emotion regulation techniques, and the intersectional relationship between patient and provider background (including gender, nationality, and race/ethnicity), emotional displays, and associated bidirectional expectations and biases that shape clinical interactions and subsequent outcomes. Three chapters are devoted to specific patient populations: pediatric patient encounters, patient populations with impaired affect, and patients with a history of trauma.

Emotions in the Culture of Medicine

The *Emotions in the Culture of Medicine* section addresses the professional challenges of honoring emotion in a medical culture that praises stoicism and analytical reasoning. One chapter provides strategies for teaching about emotions in healthcare, another describes interventions that can promote emotional wellness in undergraduate and graduate medical trainees, and the concluding chapter focuses on the relationship between emotion and clinician wellness.

Taken together, this volume synthesizes concrete, actionable steps that can be taken to enhance emotional training for the well-being of clinicians and patients alike. We draw on an international cadre of experts in clinician–patient communication, clinician wellness, emotion research, and medical education. We specifically selected authors from across diverse medical specialties, research specialties, and professional perspectives outside of medicine (social psychology, clinical psychology, education, bioethics, occupational therapy, counseling, and public health) to produce a book that provides guidance for all clinicians, trainees, and medical educators, regardless of specialty, degree, or patient population. It is our hope that readers will come away with a new understanding of the importance of effective clinical management of emotion for patient and clinician wellness, new techniques for teaching emotion regulation and clinical communication strategies, an appreciation of the need for new medical education practices to support the role of emotion in the clinical encounter, and tools for beginning to effect the cultural changes necessary to honor emotions in clinical settings.

Rachel Schwartz, PhD   Judith A. Hall, PhD   Lars G. Osterberg, MD, MPH
Stanford University   *Northeastern University* *Stanford University*
Stanford, California   *Boston, Massachusetts*   *Stanford, California*

Acknowledgments

The editors would like to thank all of the authors in this volume, who came through for us with exceptional work under the most challenging of circumstances. Several were caring for ailing family members in the midst of a pandemic, or were sick themselves during the writing process. Some had to assume unexpected clinical duties, many had to transform their academic teaching practice to virtual format, and others stepped in at very late stages to create new chapters when other authors had to withdraw. All of our authors' level of professionalism was humbling and we are extraordinarily grateful to have the chance to work with these exceptional colleagues.

We are very grateful to Nancy Hall for allowing us to use her artwork on the cover.

We want to thank Christine Schirmer, the Stanford Teaching and Mentoring Academy, and all of the clinicians, researchers, and trainees who attended the workshops on emotion and provided feedback that informed the direction of this book.

We appreciate the editorial team at McGraw Hill. Finally, big thanks go to Karen Edmonson for making this book possible and for her generous advice along the way.

Author Biographies

Karolien Aelbrecht, PhD received her MA in Clinical Psychology from Ghent University in 2007, and her certificate to be a psychoanalytic therapist in 2010. She finished her PhD in Health Sciences in 2020, which focused on the patient perspective in patient-provider communication. Her dissertation is titled "Communication Through the Eyes of the Patient: The Role of Ethnicity, Language and Education." She currently works as Project Manager at the Center for Medical Genetics of the Ghent University Hospital and is affiliated as a postdoctoral researcher at the Department of Biomolecular Medicine of Ghent University. She's currently training to be a genetic counselor.

Robert M. Arnold, MD is a Professor in the Division of General Internal Medicine, Department of Medicine at the University of Pittsburgh and in the University of Pittsburgh Center for Bioethics and Health Law. He completed his medical school training at the University of Missouri-Kansas City and residency at Rhode Island Hospital. Subsequently he has been on the faculty at the University of Pittsburgh. In 2000, Dr. Arnold was named the first Leo H. Creip Chair of Patient Care. The chair emphasizes the importance of the doctor-patient relationship, particularly at the end of life. He is the Director of the Institute for Doctor-Patient Communication and the Medical Director of the UPMC Palliative and Supportive Institute. He is clinically active in palliative care. Dr. Arnold has published on end-of-life care, hospice and palliative care, doctor-patient communication and ethics education. His current research interests are focused on educational interventions to improve communication in life-limiting illnesses and better understanding how ethical precepts are operationalized in clinical practice. He also is working with the UPMC Health System to develop system-wide, integrative palliative services throughout the health system. He is the Past-President of the American Society of Bioethics and Humanities as well as the American Academy of Hospice and Palliative Medicine.

Amber E. Barnato, MD, MPH, MS is the John E. Wennberg Distinguished Professor and Director of The Dartmouth Institute for Health Policy and

Clinical Practice at the Geisel School of Medicine at Dartmouth. She is trained in two medical specialties: general preventive medicine and public health and hospice and palliative medicine. Her research focuses on understanding the causes and consequences of variation in end-of-life intensive care unit (ICU) and life-sustaining treatment use among seriously ill older adults using an array of scientific methods, including claims data analysis, participant observation and interviewing, high-fidelity simulation experiments, and randomized behavioral trials. Her work increasingly focuses on the interplay between organizational norms, provider-patient communication, and implicit cognition, and how these phenomena produce racial disparities in end-of-life treatment. This focus on implicit cognition motivates the exploration of patient and provider emotion and medical decision making described in chapter 13. In addition to her academic work, Dr. Barnato also collects and shares stories from family members regarding their experiences making life support decisions for patients in the ICU at her website www.ICUStoryWeb.org.

Mary Catherine Beach, MD, MPH is a Professor of Medicine at Johns Hopkins University. Her research focuses on clinician attitudes of respect and communication with persons from marginalized groups and has been funded by the National Institutes of Health, the Greenwall Foundation, and the Robert Wood Johnson Foundation. She has received numerous awards including the Jozien Bensing Award for Outstanding Research contributing to Effective Healthcare Communication (given by the European Association for Communication in Healthcare), the 22nd annual George L. Engel Award for Outstanding Research contributing to the Theory, Practice and Teaching of Effective Healthcare Communication and Related Skills (given by the Academy of Communication in Healthcare), and the Daniel Nathans Scientific Innovator Award from the Johns Hopkins University School of Medicine.

Paula H. Bednarek, MD, MPH is an Associate Professor of Obstetrics and Gynecology, School of Medicine, Oregon Health and Science University. Dr. Bednarek specializes in general obstetrics and gynecology with a focus in family planning, adolescent care, alternatives to hysterectomy and obstetrics. Her clinical interests range from complex contraception and public health, to international health care. Her research focuses on innovative contraceptive techniques including intrauterine devices, management of menstrual disorders, and improving pain during outpatient gynecologic procedures. Dr. Bednarek is very interested in public health and educating patients about their bodies and how to improve their health and quality of life. Her favorite part of being a doctor is helping patients through challenging situations and supporting informed decision making in health.

Anely Bekbergenova received her MSc in Finance from the University of Lausanne in 2017 and is now completing her PhD in Management in the department of Organizational Behavior at the HEC of the University of Lausanne in Switzerland. Her main research interests are in the area of gender differences, charisma, and entrepreneurship, with an additional interest in perceptions of artificial intelligence.

Danielle Blanch-Hartigan, PhD, MPH is Associate Professor of Health Studies in the Department of Natural and Applied Sciences and Director of the Health Thought Leadership Network at Bentley University in Waltham, MA. Her interdisciplinary research in psychology and public health aims to improve the patient and clinician experience and foster patient-centered care through better communication. Specifically, she studies how patients and clinicians use verbal and nonverbal behavior to form impressions and how these perceptions influence interpersonal interactions. She is currently working on an NSF-funded collaborative, panel survey project on the risk perceptions and behaviors surrounding COVID-19.

Missy Brown MD, MPH is a first-year Emergency Medicine resident at UCLA Ronald Reagan-Olive View. She completed her MPH at the UNC Gillings School of Global Public Health, where she focused on the role of the Emergency Department in mitigating health disparities, immigrant health, as well as barriers to health care access. She is interested in the role of the Emergency Department in caring for those who have experienced trauma.

Elise C. Carey, MD, FAAHPM, FACP is an Associate Professor of Medicine and a practicing palliative medicine physician at Mayo Clinic in Rochester, Minnesota. She currently serves as Education & Faculty Development Chair for the enterprise-wide Center for Palliative Medicine, supporting faculty and educational initiatives in Arizona, Florida, and the Midwest. Dr. Carey teaches communication and teaching skills to physicians across the country and has been recognized nationally for her work in education and program development, including winning the 2014 Hastings Center Cunniff-Dixon Physician Award. She has held several local and national leadership roles, including currently serving on the Board of Directors at the American Academy of Hospice and Palliative Medicine as a Partner at VitalTalk.

Valerie Carrard is a health psychologist who completed her PhD with highest distinction at the Institute of Work and Organizational Psychology of the University of Neuchâtel in Switzerland. Her research focusses on humans' ability to adapt to different medical situations and the resources facilitating this adaptation. Dr. Carrard's PhD studies investigated the facilitators and beneficial effects of physicians' behavioral adaptation to patients' preferences in general practice interactions. As a postdoc researcher, she pursues the study of physicians' interpersonal competences in the Lausanne University Hospital and supervises two PhD projects exploring patients' longitudinal psychological adaptation to the onset of chronic health conditions in the Swiss Paraplegic Research of Nottwil in Switzerland.

Julie W. Childers, MD, MS is an Associate Professor of Medicine at the University of Pittsburgh. She is board-certified in both Palliative Medicine and Addiction Medicine, and serves as a hospital consultant in palliative medicine, addiction medicine, and medical ethics. She directs end of life communication courses both locally and nationally and has served as a mentor and a trainer to new communication teachers. Her writing, research, and teaching focuses on intersecting disciplines, including conducting goals of care discussions, teaching communication, and managing addiction in patients who are nearing the end of life.

Calvin L. Chou, MD, PhD is Professor of Clinical Medicine at the University of California at San Francisco, and staff physician at the Veterans Affairs Health Care System in San Francisco. As Senior Faculty Advisor for External Education with the Academy of Communication in Healthcare (ACH), he is recognized internationally for leading workshops in relationship-centered communication, feedback, conflict, and remediation in health professions education. He has delivered communication skills curricula for providers at health systems across the country, including Mayo Clinic, Cleveland Clinic, Stanford Health, New York Presbyterian, Advent Health System, and Texas Children's Hospital. He has received numerous teaching awards at UCSF, and two of ACH's national awards, the 2019 Healthcare Communication Teaching Excellence Award, and the 2018 Lynn Payer Award for outstanding contributions to the literature on the theory, practice, and teaching of effective healthcare communication and related skills. He is co-editor of the books *Remediation in Medical Education: A Midcourse Correction*, and *Communication Rx: Transforming Healthcare Through Relationship-Centered Communication*.

Lidia Del Piccolo, PhD, Psychologist, Psychotherapist, is a Full Professor of Clinical Psychology at the Department of Neuroscience, Biomedicine and Movement Sciences, University of Verona, and Chief of the Unit of Clinical

Psychology at Verona University Hospital. After the degree cum laude in Psychology at the University of Padua, she concluded her PhD in Psychological and Psychiatric Sciences on "Doctor-patient interaction in general practice." She contributed to the creation and standardization of different measures that evaluate emotions expression and doctor-patient communication during medical consultations (the Verona Medical Interview Classification System, VR-MICS; the Verona Patient Centered Communication Evaluation Scale, VR-COPE; the Verona Coding for Emotional Sequences, VR-CODES), which she applied also in research. In 2008 Lidia won the "EACH Jozien Bensing Research Award." Since 2001 she has been teaching Clinical Psychology and Clinical Communication in Health Sciences at the Faculty of Medicine of the University of Verona and has been working as Clinical Psychologist and Cognitive Behavioural Psychotherapist at the Mental Health Department of Verona Hospital.

Arnstein Finset, PhD, Cand Psychol, is Professor Emeritus at The Department of Behavioral Medicine, Faculty of Medicine, University of Oslo and Editor-in-Chief of Patient Education and Counseling. He is accredited specialist in Clinical Psychology and Clinical Neuropsychology. His clinical experience is from the field of rehabilitation, particularly in neurorehabilitation and rheumatology. He has been active in the Norwegian Psychology Association to promote specialty accreditation of clinical neuropsychology in the 1980-ies and most recently clinical health psychology (2019). Before taking on academic positions he was Chief Psychologist at Sunnaas Rehabilitation Hospital. He has broad research experience and has published widely in the fields of clinical neuropsychology and clinical health psychology, in the last 25 years with an emphasis on clinical communication research. He has for more than 20 years taught clinical communication skills in medical school and other settings and has together with colleagues contributed to implementation of communication skills training in Norwegian hospitals based, in particular, on the Four Habits approach. In 2004-06 he served as President of the EACH – The International Association for Communication in Healthcare.

Bria Adimora Godley, MD, BS was born in Chapel Hill, North Carolina and is a fourth-year medical student at University of North Carolina School of Medicine. She graduated from Yale University in 2016 with a Bachelor of Science in Psychology. Her words have appeared in *The Atlantic*, the *Journal of the International AIDS Society*, the *Harvard Medical Student Review*, and *Current Opinion in HIV & AIDS*.

Anne-Josée Guimond, PhD is a postdoctoral research fellow at Harvard T.H. Chan School of Public Health. Her research aims to understand how positive and detrimental aspects of psychological functioning impact the incidence of age-related diseases (e.g., cardiometabolic disease, cognitive decline) and the maintenance of optimal physical health through modifiable biological and behavioral factors. Dr. Guimond received a Ph.D. in clinical psychology from Université Laval (Canada), where her doctoral thesis focused on the role of emotion regulation in psychological adjustment to breast cancer. She is also a licensed psychologist in Québec, Canada, with expertise in health psychology, anxiety, mood, and sleep disorders.

Sarah D. Gunnery, PhD is an Assistant Professor of Psychology in the Division of Science, Health, and Education at New England College. Dr. Gunnery's research focuses on stigma and quality life in people with chronic health conditions that affect nonverbal communication. She specifically studies facial masking in people with Parkinson's disease and compensatory strategies to help people with Parkinson's disease communicate emotion in their face more accurately.

Judith A. Hall, PhD is University Distinguished Professor of Psychology, Emerita, at Northeastern University in Boston, Massachusetts. She is a social psychologist who studies interpersonal interaction, with a focus on person perception and nonverbal communication. For many years, she has applied these interests in the context of provider-patient interactions. With Debra Roter, she authored *Doctors Talking with Patients/ Patients Talking with Doctors: Improving Communication in Medical Care*. Solo or co-authored nonclinical books include *Nonverbal Sex Differences: Communication Accuracy and Expressive Style*, and *Nonverbal Communication in Human Interaction*. Her edited volumes include *Interpersonal Sensitivity: Theory and Measurement* and *The Social Psychology of Perceiving Others Accurately*.

Amanda R. Hemmesch, PhD is an Associate Professor of Psychology and Co-Director of the Survey Research Center at St. Cloud State University. Dr. Hemmesch's research focuses on improving health, well-being, and quality of life for individuals with chronic conditions across the lifespan. Specifically, her research has examined stigma and social support in Parkinson's disease and Moebius syndrome, a rare congenital condition that causes facial weakness/paralysis. Her current work focuses on improving access to health care and quality of life for individuals with rare conditions.

Martha Howell, EdD leads the Relationship Centered Communication program (ART of Communication) at Baylor Scott & White Health. Her educational background includes a B.A. in Psychology, MEd in Counseling and Human Development and a doctorate in Higher Education with an emphasis in medical education. She has served as a medical educator for 16 years and has a background in simulation/standardized patient instruction, faculty development and communication skill training. Currently, she is completing the Faculty in Training program through the Academy of Communication in Healthcare. Her areas of research include communication skills assessment in graduate medical education as well as multidisciplinary team communication.

Ben Kaplan, MD, MPH is a first-year family medicine resident at the University of North Carolina Hospital. He received his BA in English from Columbia University, and his MPH from the UNC Gillings School of Global Public Health. In 2021, he will enter residency training in Family Medicine and plans to focus on mitigating health disparities through community-based participatory research and full-spectrum family care. He is a current Scholar of the Pisacano Leadership Foundation, as well as the American Academy of Family Physicians Emerging Leaders Institute. His work has been featured in the *Annals of Family Medicine*, *Academic Medicine*, and *Progress in Community Health Partnerships*.

Asif Khan, MD is a first-year psychiatry resident at the University of North Carolina Hospitals. He also received Bachelor's in Psychology from UNC and medical degree from UNC School of Medicine. Born and raised in Bangladesh, Asif moved to the United States at the age of 13. In 2012, he founded the Refugee Community Partnership (RCP), a community-based non-profit organization in North Carolina. RCP uses relationship-based accompaniment, language justice, and cultural stewardship to build vibrant, safe, and healthy communities for forcibly displaced people that center mutual aid, transformative solidarity, and community power. Rather than charity, Asif emphasized solidarity and led an interprofessional team to design trauma-informed interventions and address social determinants of health. Before medical school, he served two years as an AmeriCorps fellow for RCP and then transitioned to its Board. In medical school, he dedicated a research year to combine his interests in medical education and non-profit by offering health professional students additional skills and opportunities to meaningfully care for refugee patients in the community setting through a "healthcare hotspotting" project under guidance of Dr. Amy Weil. RCP has won multiple grants or financial support including from Robert Wood Johnson Foundation, GlaxoSmithKline, American Board of Pediatrics, and North Carolina Health Care Foundation.

Baruch S. Krauss, MD, EdM is an Associate Professor of Pediatrics and Emergency Medicine at Harvard Medical School and a pediatric emergency physician at Boston Children's Hospital. He is deeply interested in how children experience healthcare and the factors that determine the quality of their experiences. His work focuses on developing systems for managing children's pain and emotional states during medical encounters. He has developed a unique methodology for establishing trusting and cooperative relationships with children, which provides positive and rewarding healthcare experiences for them and their families. He teaches a curriculum based on the methodology to medical students and residents, and at workshops for practitioners domestically and internationally.

Benjamin A. Krauss received his ScM in Medical Sciences from Brown University in 2020 and will begin medical school in Fall 2021. He has a background in videography and video production and has, since 2014, been engaged in developing learning products for teaching medical students and health care professionals how to establish trusting relationships with children.

Laura D. Kubzansky, PhD, MPH is Lee Kum Kee Professor of Social and Behavioral Sciences at the Harvard T.H. Chan School of Public Health. Dr. Kubzansky has published extensively on the role of psychological and social factors in health, with a particular focus on the effects of stress and emotion on heart disease. She also conducts research on whether stress, emotion and other psychological factors help to explain the relationship between social status and health. Her other research projects and interests include the biological mechanisms linking emotions, social relationships, and health; relationships between early childhood environments, resilience, and healthy aging; and how interactions between psychosocial stress and environmental exposures may influence health. Dr. Kubzansky serves as Co-Director of the Lee Kum Sheung Center for Health and Happiness, as Co-Director of the JPB Environmental Health Fellowship Program, and as Director of the Society and Health Laboratory.

Lewina O. Lee, PhD is Assistant Professor of Psychiatry at the Boston University School of Medicine, and Psychologist-Clinical Investigator at the National Center for Posttraumatic Stress at the Veterans Affairs (VA) Boston Healthcare System. She received her PhD (Clinical Psychology–Aging) from the University of Southern California. She completed a Clinical Psychology internship at VA Palo Alto and a postdoctoral fellowship in Epidemiology at Boston University and VA Boston. Her research examines the role of psychosocial stress exposure – particularly early adversity – on lifespan health, and mechanisms which transmit the effects of stress on health, while adopting a lifespan developmental perspective. A related line of her research considers positive psychosocial factors which confer resilience against the effects of psychosocial stress exposure on health. She has been the Principal Investigator or Co-Investigator on multiple awards from the National Institute on Aging.

Piet L. Leroy, MD, PhD, MSc is a pediatric critical care specialist and director of the Pediatric Procedural Sedation Unit at Maastricht University Medical Centre, Maastricht, The Netherlands. He is an associate professor (domain of medical teaching) at the Faculty of Health, Life Sciences and medicine at Maastricht University and graduated in 2017 with a Master in Health Professions Education from the Maastricht School of Health Professions Education. His main research topics concern delirium in critical care and procedural sedation in children. Within these fields, he has published over 50 scientific papers, guidelines and book chapters and has presented 150 scientific lectures at international conferences. In 2013 he received the Catharina Pijls Prize for his research on improving procedural sedation quality in pediatrics. He is a board member of the International Committee for the Advancement of Procedural Sedation (www.proceduralsedation.org) and editor for the European Journal of Pediatrics. In 2018, he organized the first European Conference in Pediatric Procedural Sedation & Analgesia. Supported by the Charlie Braveheart Foundation (www.charliebraveheart.com) he set up in 2019 an interdisciplinary training program for procedural comfort in children.

Brett Marroquín, PhD is a licensed clinical psychologist and Associate Professor of Psychology at Loyola Marymount University in Los Angeles, California. His research examines interpersonal influences on emotion, emotion regulation, and cognitive processing in healthy functioning and mood disorders, particularly within the context of intimate relationships. His current work focuses on the role of social relationships in emotional and mental health outcomes of major negative events, including cancer treatment and the COVID-19 pandemic, and how effective or ineffective support between relationship partners affects physical and mental health. His private practice in Los Angeles focuses on patients with mood disorders, anxiety disorders, and couple distress.

Marianne Schmid Mast is full professor of Organizational Behavior at HEC at the University of Lausanne in Switzerland. She received her PhD in psychology from the University of Zurich. Her research addresses how individuals interact with each other in a professional context and part of her research focuses on physician-patient communication. She investigates how people perceive and communicate, verbally and nonverbally, how first impressions affect interpersonal interactions and evaluations, how people form accurate impressions of others, and how we can train social skills using new technologies such as virtual reality and computer-based automatic sensing. She is currently an Associate Editor of the Journal of Nonverbal Behavior and in the Editorial Board of the journal Leadership Quarterly. In 2018, 2019, and 2020, she has been named one of the 50 most influential living psychologists.

Enioluwafe Ojo, MD, MPH is a first-year psychiatry resident at University of North Carolina. She completed her Master of Public Health at the UNC Gillings School of Global Public Health, where she focused on ethnic variations of pathways to mental health care. Currently, she serves as a trainee member of the Gold Humanism Honor Society National Advisory Council and the UNC Psychiatry Department DEI Task Force. Her research interests include medical education, mental health policy, and diversity, equity, and inclusion work.

Lars G. Osterberg, MD, MPH, Professor of Medicine, Stanford School of Medicine is a recognized leader in medical education. He has been invited to present on medical education topics at national conferences and invited to teach bedside medicine or provide faculty development nationally and internationally on topics of medical education. In 2007 he was selected by the Senior Associate Dean of Education at the Stanford School of Medicine to direct the Educators for CARE program, a learning community of Stanford Medical School that provides a structured mentoring program for all medical students in the Stanford School of Medicine and he co-directs the Stanford Teaching and Mentoring Academy. His research interests are in areas of medical education, healthcare provider wellbeing, healthcare access and patient adherence to medications. In his clinical settings, undergraduates, medical students and house staff are enriched by his lessons in social justice and compassionate, respectful medicine. He received an undergraduate degree in bioengineering from UC Berkeley, an MD from UC Davis, and a Master's in Public Health from UC Berkeley. For more information about Lars Osterberg's teaching, research, publications, awards and service-related activities, please visit his profile on the Stanford Medical School website, http://med.stanford.edu/profiles/Lars_Osterberg.

Erika B. Pages received her MA in Social Psychology from Arizona State University and is currently working toward her PhD. Her core research interest is in humor, with studies investigating why humor is a universally desired trait in mating partners, how humor can support emotion regulation in distressing situations, and the role humor can play in social support. She is also a collaborator on research examining the implications of several emotion regulation strategies for health behavior, particularly dietary added-sugar intake.

Debra L. Roter, DrPH, MPH is a University Distinguished Professor in the Department of Health, Behavior and Society at the Johns Hopkins Bloomberg School of Public Health with joint appointments in the Schools of Medicine and Nursing. Her research focuses on interpersonal communication dynamics within medical visits and its relationship to attitudinal, behavioral and clinical outcomes. Her studies also address the influence of social factors such as implicit race and gender bias, restricted literacy and poor English language proficiency on the medical dialogue and their consequences for disparities in medical care quality. Dr. Roter is well known for development of the Roter Interaction Analysis System (RIAS) a quantitative method of medical dialogue assessment which has become the most commonly used system of its kind worldwide. She has authored over 300 articles and several books addressing issues related to these topics.

Mollie A. Ruben, PhD is an Assistant Professor of Psychology at the University of Maine and holds a joint appointment with the US Department of Veterans Affairs in the Center for Healthcare Organization and Implementation Research where she completed her postdoctoral fellowship. Dr. Ruben's research focuses on social perception and the contribution of nonverbal behaviors to how we perceive others. Dr. Ruben applies social psychological methods to the study of doctor-patient interactions with a particular interest in understanding the communication of patient pain and ameliorating health disparities especially among sexual and gender minority patients.

Rachel Schwartz, PhD is a communication scientist and health services researcher at the Stanford University School of Medicine. Her research focuses on systems-level interventions for improving clinician wellness, provider-patient communication, and developing medical education initiatives that provide clinicians with tools for navigating psychosocial aspects of the clinical encounter. She has experience leading research and quality improvement projects in pediatrics (Lucile Packard Children's Hospital), neurology (Palo Alto Medical Foundation Research Institute & Stanford School of Medicine), emergency medicine (Stanford) and primary care (Stanford and Palo Alto VA).

Michelle N. Shiota, PhD is an Associate Professor in the Department of Psychology at Arizona State University, and Director of the Substance Abuse

Translational Research Network at ASU. She is currently an Associate Editor for the Journal of Personality and Social Psychology, and a member of the Society for Affective Science Executive Committee. Her basic science research focuses on differentiating features of specific positive emotions, emotion regulation processes and outcomes, and emotional mechanisms of close relationships. Her growing body of translational/applied research examines emotional and social cognitive mechanisms of health behavior and behavior change, including implications of stress and use of particular emotion regulation strategies for healthy diet, addictive substance use, and adoption of social distancing and hygiene behaviors during the COVID-19 pandemic.

Caitlin Holt Siropaides, DO is an Associate Professor of Internal Medicine and the Director of the Vital Talk Program at the University of Texas Southwestern Medical Center. She is a practicing palliative care specialist in both inpatient and outpatient care settings at Clements University Hospital and Simmons Cancer Center, two of the key training sites for the UT Southwestern Medical School and Graduate Medical Education programs. She completed Internal Medicine Residency and Palliative Care Fellowship training at the University of Pittsburgh Medical Center, during which time she developed a significant emphasis on communication skill training and medical education. She has received national certification in leading Vital Talk communication workshops, which deliver serious illness communication training for all levels of learners in the medical field. Her research and clinical interest focus on patient-provider serious illness communication, patient experience, and medical education. She has developed and implemented communication skill longitudinal curricula at UTSW for medical students, Internal Medicine residents, various fellowship subspecialties and faculty development.

Stuart Slavin MD, MEd is Senior Scholar for Well-being at the Accreditation Council for Graduate Medical Education (ACGME). A graduate of Saint Louis University School of Medicine, Dr. Slavin completed his residency training in pediatrics at UCLA and then served as a faculty member there for seventeen years before returning to Saint Louis University as Associate Dean for Curriculum. Over the past decade, Dr. Slavin led efforts at SLU to improve the mental health of medical students that produced dramatic decreases in rates of depression and anxiety in pre-clerkship students. He joined the ACGME in 2018 and is helping to lead efforts to improve the mental health of residents and faculty across the US.

Greeshma Somashekar, MD, MBA is a first year Family Medicine resident at Swedish Medical Center/Cherry Hill in Seattle, WA. She graduated from

Stanford University in 2016, and earned her MD and MBA degrees at the University of North Carolina School of Medicine and University of North Carolina Kenan-Flagler Business School. She plans to pursue a career in health systems strategy and leadership, with a focus on bolstering high-quality primary care and social services via alternative payment models and care delivery models that center health equity. Her clinical and research interests include trauma-informed care, gender affirming care, physician advocacy, and promoting self-compassion in medical training.

Morgan D. Stosic, MA received her BS in Psychology from Oregon State University in 2019 and is now a PhD student at the University of Maine in the area of Social Psychology. Her research is driven by a nonverbal communication lens and involves the accurate perception of individuals' traits, states, and health. Within this broad area, she studies the basic processes involved in forming accurate impressions of another, as well as applied solutions that result from the inaccurate impressions of one another. Morgan actively collaborates with health professionals as well as artificial intelligence researchers in order to develop real world training and solutions to better person perception processes.

Linda Tickle-Degnen, PhD, OT is Professor of Occupational Therapy Emerita, School of Arts and Sciences, Tufts University. Dr. Tickle-Degnen is a rehabilitation scientist and experimental social psychologist. Her work aims to translate basic knowledge about social psychological processes and daily life activity into person-centered health interventions for people and their families living with chronic health conditions that are stigmatizing. She focuses in on investigating biopsychosocial and health quality of life outcomes as related to nonverbal and verbal interpersonal behavior, therapeutic rapport, and social participation. Over a forty-year period, she has led multidisciplinary lab and field experimental studies, rehabilitation trials, longitudinal studies and mixed methods (quantitative-qualitative) studies. She was an early proponent of evidence-based rehabilitation through her writings and teaching nationally and internationally.

Vera Vine, PhD is an Assistant Professor of Clinical Psychology at Queen's University, in Ontario, Canada. She completed her doctoral studies in clinical psychology at Yale University and postdoctoral studies at the University of Pittsburgh School of Medicine. Her research focuses on the costs, benefits, and bio-social foundations of emotional awareness. She is especially interested in the contributions of emotion language and nervous system activity to the construction of emotion experience, and how pressures in the social environment become embedded in the body's emotion responses over time. Dr. Vine is the recipient of multiple research fellowships and awards for teaching and leadership. Her research has been funded by the National Institute of Mental Health, and is currently supported by the American Foundation for Suicide Prevention and Canadian Foundation for Innovation John R. Evans Leaders Fund.

Amy Weil, MD, FACP is a Professor of Medicine and Social Medicine at the University of North Carolina School of Medicine at Chapel Hill. She is a general internist with a longstanding interest in caring for survivors of violence and other vulnerable populations within her primary care practice. Since 2003, she has been Medical Co-Director of UNC's hospital-based Beacon Program, a comprehensive program that cares for children, adults, and elder survivors of violence, as well as survivors of human trafficking and bullying. Dr. Weil serves as a clinician, educator, and mentor at UNC, teaching medical and other health professions students about ACES, Intimate Partner Violence, Trauma Informed Care, health care communication, reflection and narrative medicine, psychiatric care in primary care, provider wellbeing and innovative care delivery models. She advises a medical student interest group Intimate Partner Violence Awareness and Advocacy as well as the UNC Gold Humanism Honor Society chapter. Recently, she was Site Director on an Office of Women's Health Grant to re-institute IPV screening in primary care via the North Carolina Coalition on Domestic Violence. She has authored cards in UpToDate about IPV, a chapter in the Springer book Trauma Informed Healthcare Approaches: A Guide for Primary Care, focusing on addressing provider wellness as well as other articles and chapters on topics of interest.

Emotion's Functions

CHAPTER 1

Emotions in 21st-Century Humanistic Medicine

Rachel Schwartz, Judith A. Hall, and Lars G. Osterberg

> *The current state of medical education is woefully deficient in educating its learners about the role of emotions in healthcare.*
>
> —Johanna Shapiro, 2013 (p. 314)[1]

■ INTRODUCTION

Emotion is inseparable from medical care, yet its role in care delivery, healing, and the clinician experience is complex and often ignored and unaddressed by clinicians. This is in part due to how the culture of medicine has evolved; what began as a relational art has morphed into a more technical science with the rise of technology and the influence of medical forbearers who equated mastery of one's emotion with medical competence and professionalism. Ambivalence about the role of emotions, the ever-shifting tension between too much and too little emotion and uncertainty about how to make use of emotion for good ends have all, we believe, contributed to the nearly complete lack of training in emotion regulation and management that many clinicians receive. In their 2007 systematic review of emotion skills training for medical students, Satterfield and Hughes[2] concluded:

> [T]here is currently no operational definition of the superordinate construct of emotion skills in medicine, nor is there a complete developmental theory regarding the teaching and acquisition of emotion skills in medical providers. None of the studies reviewed provided a framework for understanding emotion skills development nor a discussion of how emotion skills are manifested in other areas of clinical care. (p. 939)

Despite increasing scholarship and interest in empathy and emotional socialization within the medical field,[3] scholars and medical educators have much work ahead to address this gap.

The Three Principles

Emotions are ever-present and consequential in a clinical encounter, and their importance cannot be overstated. There are three crucial, and interlocking, reasons why we say this,[4] which we call the *Three Principles*. Although these principles may seem obvious, taking them seriously has far-reaching implications. They are the basis for everything that follows in this book.

Principle 1: Both Clinicians and Patients have Emotions

Some of these emotions precede the visit and have nothing directly to do with the visit itself. The clinician might be irritable due to fatigue, worried about finances, or anxious about their competence (we will often refer interchangeably to physicians, providers, clinicians, and healthcare providers). Clinicians are not professional robots who enact a scripted role; they are people with their own issues, styles, and habits, and, consequently, the full range of emotions, both pleasant and unpleasant. Likewise, patients have their own sources of emotional experience related to work, family, society, and their health. For both parties, these emotions can have profound effects on their mental and physical well-being. Furthermore, these emotions do not vanish at the door of the examining room; they impact the transaction in both subtle and extreme ways and their impact is often outside of awareness and unacknowledged.

Other emotional experiences spring up because of words, expressions, and actions occurring within the clinical encounter. These emotions can be anger, disappointment, joy, relief, confusion, boredom, frustration, sadness, embarrassment, shame, and anxiety, to name just a few. This takes us to the next principle.

Principle 2: Both Clinicians and Patients Show Emotions

Sometimes this happens deliberately, as when the patient lets the physician know they are not happy with a diagnosis or with the way the physician has behaved. But, crucially, both parties also show emotions in spite of their best efforts at suppression or masking. These "leaked" cues can occur verbally or nonverbally, by omission or commission. Among nonverbal communication researchers, it is often said that a person cannot *not* communicate nonverbally, because whatever one does will be given meaning by the other party.

The same can be said of all behavior, not just nonverbal. This leads directly to the third principle.

Principle 3: Both the Clinician and the Patient will Interpret Each Other's Behavior

These interpretations have powerful emotional implications. A clinician who attempts "neutrality," for instance, may be seen as cold or as withholding something. A clinician who engages in more eye contact is likely to be seen as interested and warm. A clinician who keeps the patient waiting may be judged to be inconsiderate. A patient who does not say "thank you" with enthusiasm may be seen as ungrateful. Although all of these may be misinterpretations of the other's actual state or intention, they all can have serious interpersonal consequences. People's tendency to reciprocate others' behavior (as they interpret it) can lead to downward (and upward) spirals. Therefore, a corollary of Principle 3 is that, often, interpretations trump intentions. Many emotions result directly from the attributions that people make about another person's behavior.

The Need for Emotion Training

Sending a clinician into the exam room with extensive medical training but no emotional training is akin to sending a sailor to sea with only an astrolabe in an age when nautical charts and global positioning systems are readily available. These are resilient, intelligent sailors and they will do their best to navigate with what they are given, but why not arm them with tools that will make the journey safer and more successful? Jerome Groopman writes, "Cognition and emotion are inseparable. The two mix in every encounter with every patient."[5] Yet we are currently sending clinicians to practice without a full set of tools with which to connect, deduce, and heal, tools that will promote both the patient's and their own physical and psychological health. The goal of this book is to bring together theory, research, and expertise in clinical practice to provide both basic understanding and practical insights for healthcare providers and educators on one of their most vital yet challenging aspects of patient care: recognizing, expressing, regulating, and responding to patients' emotions as well as their own.

In the following chapters, we provide transdisciplinary insight from behavioral scientists, medical educators, and practicing clinicians from a range of specialties, for effectively navigating emotion in the clinical encounter. These three perspectives—from scholarship, education, and experience—dovetail, enabling us to supply an evidence base for practical advice and also legitimization of the lived clinical experience of readers of this book—who may be trainees, experienced clinicians, or scholars. The insights contained here may, in turn, inspire researchers with new ideas and new problem areas to focus on. Thus, it is our hope that this book can serve as a practical guide for medical trainees, practicing clinicians, and medical educators as we enter an era of medicine that places unprecedented demands on clinicians. By leveraging emotional skills, evidence shows that clinicians can gain opportunities for a restored sense of connection and meaning, improving patient and clinician well-being in the process.

■ WHAT IS EMOTION?

The sheer difficulty of defining emotion is often treated as its leading characteristic, for instance when in 1931 an American cardiologist described emotion as a "fluid and fleeting thing that like the wind comes and goes, one does not know how"; or when two psychologists half a century later argued that "everyone knows what an emotion is, until asked to give a definition."

—Jan Plamper, 2015 (p. 11)[6]

Emotion is defined and conceptualized in a multitude of ways; a 1981 study[7] documented 92 separate definitions from psychology alone. While theologians, philosophers, and rhetoricians have been theorizing about emotion since antiquity, experimental psychologists defined the field starting around 1860 and neuroscientists joined the debate in the late 20th century.[6] There remain at least four different emotion conceptual camps: "basic emotion" theorists, who posit that emotions are biological, physiologically distinct phenomena; "appraisal" theorists, who believe emotions are response tendencies relying on context-driven construals; "psychological constructivists," who argue that emotions emerge and are continually modified; and "social constructivists," who view emotions as social artifacts, constrained by social context and cultural practices.[8] Across theorists, there is agreement that "emotion" encompasses psychological states, expressive behavior, subjective experience, and physiological responses. Yet how these are operationalized, and the order by which this process occurs, remain subject to debate.[8]

This book approaches emotion as a metaconcept, encompassing subjective experiences, expression, physiological responses, and interpersonal sequelae. As with other ubiquitous, hard to define concepts, such as "empathy,"[9] the diversity of emotion definitions highlights its centrality in our experience of and engagement with our world. Some scholars would argue that human beings are always in some kind of emotional state, broadly defined, whether this is labeled discretely (angry, sad, and so on), with granularity (types of anger such as annoyance, rage, indignation, or irritation), or on a continuum (from not aroused to aroused, or from negative to positive). Furthermore, the ubiquity of emotion is seen in every interpersonal encounter, because—as we explained in the Three Principles—the intended or "actual" emotional state of one person is perceived, interpreted (rightly or wrongly), and acted on by the other person, producing a new round of emotional responses.

The following chapters address emotion as it pertains to the embodied, holistic experience of patient and clinician. Without taking a narrow conceptual approach to defining emotion, the authors in this volume seek to address the ways in which emotional experience manifests in medical training, in clinical settings, and as a result of medical interactions. The authors use a family of terms, including emotions, affect, feelings, and moods, to capture the world of experience that contrasts with what is typically called "cognition," although even this distinction is not always clear. Furthermore, emotions and how they are labeled are strongly shaped by how a person thinks about the circumstances and events that triggered their emotional experience. The relation of emotion to cognition is one of the topics taken up in this book.

■ OVERVIEW

Beginning with an examination of the evolutionary and social functions of emotion (Chapter 2), this book identifies how emotional processes shape interactions and human connection, health, and illness (Chapter 3). Chapters on emotional dialogue (Chapter 4) and emotion perception (Chapter 5) in the medical encounter elucidate how interpersonal cues can be used to improve patient outcomes, strengthen clinician–patient rapport, and increase clinician well-being (Chapters 15 and 16). Emotion communication strategies, tools for emotional awareness, emotion regulation (Chapter 7), and evidence for how emotion affects patients' and providers' decision making (Chapter 13) need to become standard-issue components of a medical training curriculum (Chapter 14). Understanding how gender (Chapter 11) and culture (Chapter 12) shape emotional expectations and interpretations is necessary for all training on emotion. Certain patient populations, such as pediatric patients (Chapter 8), patients with reduced expressivity (Chapter 9), and those with psychological trauma (Chapter 10), present unique challenges that require tailored strategies, including heightened attention to emotion cues (Chapter 6), for effective emotion management. Indeed, the evidence presented in the chapters suggests emotion-related skills are as essential as the stethoscope, as they are tools that enable clinicians to identify what the patient needs and are the medium through which to deliver the care necessary for healing. See Fig. 1-1 for an overview of topics addressed in the book.

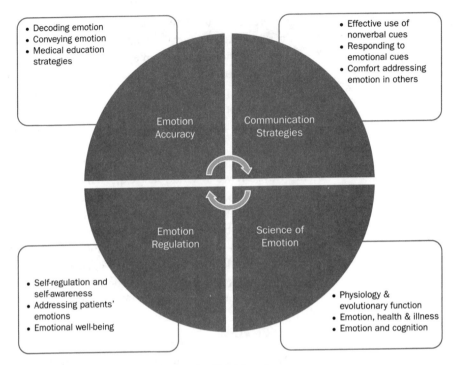

FIGURE 1-1. Overview of topics covered in this volume.

Although emotion may seem ineffable, uncontrollable, and something apart from the science and pragmatics of medicine, in fact emotion is as much a subject of scientific scrutiny, and just as relevant to healthcare training and practice, as is a correct understanding of human anatomy, physiology, and disease processes.

■ EMOTION'S FUNCTIONS

> *If emotions are, wholly or in part, biological phenomena, they must serve a purpose for survival.*

—Nico Frijda, 1986 (p. 5)[10]

At the most basic level, emotion promotes survival. Neuroscientist Antonio Damasio describes emotions as "somatic markers," a bodily response that guides actions designed to protect the organism from external threats.[11] Emotional expression and the ability to read others' emotions are critical for relational competence, allowing us to interpret others' mental states, intentions, and motivations.[12] Contradicting the Cartesian notion that emotions interfere with rationality, Damasio argues that emotions are in fact critical for rationality, and serve as cognitive representations of body states. Some definitions of what is known as "emotional intelligence" explicitly argue for the utility of emotions in guiding thought.[13]

Emotion guides cognition and decision making, shaping how people perceive and act on information.[14] Positive emotional states are conducive to global processing, allowing individuals to focus on the big picture while negative emotions direct attention locally, increasing the salience of specific details.[15] Positive emotions facilitate more flexible cognitive processing, allowing individuals to engage creatively and be more open to information, while negative emotions reduce access to more alternative solutions.[16] This has important implications for medical training and clinical practice, as both require the ability to access alternative solutions and integrate new information in order to be successful.

Emotional intelligence—the ability to identify, manage, and understand emotional interactions and experiences[17]—and emotional competencies, defined as the knowledge, abilities, skills, and attitudes necessary to appropriately regulate, understand, and express emotional phenomena,[18] are linked to a host of positive outcomes. These range from decreased stress and improved clinician well-being,[19-21] to enhanced clinical decision-making,[22,23] job satisfaction[24] and performance,[2] and increased organizational commitment and leadership abilities.[25,26] These skills translate into stronger clinician–patient relationships and care practices,[27,28] as managing patients' emotions effectively is linked to improved clinical outcomes.[29]

■ EMOTION AND ILLNESS

Emotional vomiting is just as real as the vomiting due to pyloric obstruction, and so-called "nervous headaches" may be as painful as if they were due to a brain tumor.

—Francis Peabody, 1927 (p. 880)[30]

Emotional experience affects health in a complex, interdependent manner. A study of primary care patients showed that up to 60% of patients recurrently have somatic symptoms that are an expression of psychosocial distress.[31] This echoes a book-length 1939 study of 174 patients admitted to the Johns Hopkins Hospital who were interviewed to explore the relationship between social conditions, emotional disturbances, and the presenting illness.[32] The study found that certain diseases had related social and emotional disturbances; for example, asthma attacks and gastrointestinal disorders were observed to be linked to emotional disturbance. The study noted that patients' emotional disturbance fell outside of the main objectives of the physicians and were perceived as frustrating complications. A review of the study in the *Yale Journal of Biology and Medicine*[32] concluded:

> [T]he book is a well-written and generally sound one, and shows clearly the broadening trend in the advance of medicine...the reviewer, a psychiatrist, does not hesitate to recommend that the book be read by all physicians whether in a specialty or not, but the book should not be left in the waiting room for patients if embarrassment is to be avoided. (p. 694)

Despite consistent evidence of the link between emotion and illness, over eighty years later, discussion of emotion in medicine is still embarrassing to many.

■ EMOTIONAL INTELLIGENCE

The ability to recognize emotional responses in others is a core part of emotional intelligence,[33] and an important skill to teach in medical education. Patients in a study that looked at the relationship between expressed emotion and treatment compliance found compliant patients had lower panic-fear scores than those who were noncompliant, suggesting that addressing patients' anxiety may be key to treatment success.[34] However, research shows that clinicians delivering medical care frequently do not accurately identify and appropriately respond to patients' emotional cues, causing patients to reiterate the emotional concerns, resulting in longer visits and withdrawal of patient–physician trust.[35] A 2020 review of emotional intelligence in surgeons reported that elevated levels of emotional intelligence facilitate patient examinations, mitigate communication barriers, and allow surgeons to tailor their treatment approach more effectively, resulting in more satisfied patients.[27] Integrating training for, and assessment of, emotional intelligence as a standard part of the medical education curriculum will benefit clinicians and patients alike; in addition to increasing patient satisfaction and adherence, there is evidence that emotional intelligence and emotional stability may be protective against burnout in students of medicine, surgery, physiotherapy, and nursing.[20,36]

■ CLINICIAN FEARS AROUND EMOTION

At the Stanford School of Medicine, thanks to a Teaching and Mentoring Academy Award, one of us (RS) had the opportunity to pilot test a series of workshops for clinicians on navigating emotion in medical encounters. The

25 attendees who attended the first two workshops came from a variety of fields and consisted of healthcare researchers, medical residents, physicians, medical educators, physical therapists, and veterinarians. After each session, attendees completed a survey asking them to list the most difficult part of managing emotion in a professional setting. They had a choice of four options ("inadequate time to address what comes up," "fear that I will make things worse," "don't know the right words to say," and "fear I will be emotionally affected/traumatized") as well as an open-response option.

I assumed that time constraints would consistently be ranked as the top concern, but was surprised to find "don't know the right words to say" came up as frequently as time concerns. Two of the write-in answers were also illuminating: one person described a fear of "taking on/in the other person's energy, getting 'toxic' or 'contaminated' and unable to process it through," while another highlighted the perceived danger and destructiveness of patients' emotions for colleagues, writing, "concern about what angry patients may do to other staff that would harm them."

At the end of the survey, I asked participants to share what additional information could be helpful to them. Multiple people asked for specific word choices and phrases to use with patients. One person succinctly summarized, "What are things you can say if you aren't sure what patients are experiencing? How deeply should you explore a patient's emotion, and how?" Another asked for "more content into tools that can help with different clinical situations, including family dynamics/emotions that arise in a clinical setting." Others asked for "more tips about how to recognize others' emotions." This book aims to address all of these questions using data from the literature and drawing on the clinical expertise of our chapter authors. Two of the top concerns are the perceived conflict between time constraints and exploring emotion, and fear of being unable to accurately read a patient's emotion. However, as we present below, the evidence suggests that addressing emotion *saves* time and even inaccurate attempts at addressing emotion may be beneficial.

Myth #1: Addressing Emotion Takes Longer

Time pressure in medical and surgical practices is a big source of stress for clinicians,[37] and there is a general perception that attending to patients' (or clinicians') emotions in clinic takes time that is unavailable. However, multiple studies have shown that addressing patients' emotion not only improves patient satisfaction, patient adherence,[38] and patient retention of information[39] but can also substantially *shorten* the visit. In a study of 54 primary care visits and 62 surgical consults, emotional cues were found to be present in more than half of visits and were often raised indirectly.[35] The cues were missed 79% of the time in primary care visits and 62% of the time in surgical consults. Addressing emotion shortened the visit because when emotional opportunities were missed, patients raised the issue two to three more times over the course of the visit, averaging 3 min longer per visit.[35] Other studies have echoed this finding, noting that when their emotional statements are deflected or missed, patients attempt to raise the topic again, often multiple times and with increasing intensity.[40] However, when physicians made even one positive response to patients' emotions, visits were shortened.[35]

Myth #2: "I'm Not Trained for That; I'll Just Make Things Worse"

There is a common misperception that talking about emotion without psychological training could be akin to opening Pandora's Box: fears of eliciting uncontrollable emotion and feeling helpless to address patients' needs (particularly in institutions where access to social worker, clinical psychologist, or chaplain support may be limited). However, the evidence suggests that it is the opposite—ignoring or failing to address the present emotion—that is more detrimental than even poorly navigated attempts at acknowledging emotion. One study found that analogue patient satisfaction increased when physicians misidentified the emotion or even detected a nonexistent cue compared to when physicians failed to detect a cue that was present.[41]

Clinician attempts at addressing emotion improve patient satisfaction because those attempts open the door for greater alignment. A study of hospitalist admission encounters examined how physicians responded to patients' negative emotion.[29] When the physicians responded to patients' emotion with clinical questions or directed the discussion away from the emotion, it led to interpersonal distance and in some instances created an antagonistic relationship. Acknowledgment of the emotional statement allowed the patient to direct further conversation, elucidating social factors that affected care decisions. In situations where physicians provided emotional support or attempted to explore the emotion, there was increased alignment on treatment decisions and greater clarity on patients' goals of care.

Beyond strengthening the clinician–patient relationship and facilitating elicitation of important information, clinicians' response to patients' emotion has been shown to affect patients' informational recall. When nurses responded to cancer patients by giving minimal encouragement (similar to the neutral acknowledgments described in the study above), patients remembered more information that was discussed in the visit.[39] This may be due to the fact that giving voice to emotion serves to downregulate the physiological response; putting feelings into words is associated with reductions in self-reported distress, decreased heart rate and skin conductance response, and decreased amygdala activation in functional MRI studies.[42]

It is important to acknowledge that emotional response is frequently bidirectional; emotion, and the purpose it serves in social interactions, are critical for the maintenance of social relationships. This is true, too, for the clinician–patient relationship. Much of what routinely takes place in medical encounters is stressful for patients and clinicians alike.[43] Studies of medical trainees have shown elevated cardiovascular stress and cortisol levels during history-taking and bad news consultations.[44,45] There are emotional costs to practicing medicine, but the emotional intimacy of the clinician–patient relationship is unparalleled and affords privileged opportunity to connect deeply with another human.[46] The goal is to identify and develop the support and training infrastructure that can allow clinicians to be wholly present for, and engaged in, the emotional exchange.

■ EMOTION AND THE CLINICIAN–PATIENT RELATIONSHIP

Receiving our patients' most intense fears and hopes requires that we be willing to confront our own. We must have adequate personal strength and support to cope with the additional fears and losses we will encounter through our patients, and we must be willing to relinquish the illusions of personal power, mastery, and control that are afforded us by the narrower, traditional medical model.

—Anthony L. Suchman and Dale A. Matthews, 1988 (p. 129)[46]

Nearly 30 years ago, Suchman and colleagues described the risks and rewards associated with establishing patient–clinician relationships that focused on attending to patients' emotional experiences.[46,47] They cite the limitations imposed on medicine by the rise of empirical science and its insistence that only verifiable data be considered valid in medicine, "effectively barring transpersonal phenomena from the consideration of scientific clinicians" (p. 127).[46] However, in recent years, teams of clinician researchers have gone to great lengths to prove the value of emotion and other relational elements in the clinician–patient relationship. Zulman and colleagues conducted a systematic literature review of 20,000+ articles,[48] convened a Delphi panel of healthcare communication experts,[49] and led qualitative studies on connecting effectively with patients and clients[50,51] to identify core elements of the clinician–patient interaction that could improve population health, reduce healthcare costs, and improve both the patient's and provider's experience. They concluded that addressing emotion in the clinical encounter (specifically noticing, naming, and validating patients' emotion) was a core strategic behavior that should be practiced to improve care delivery and foster patient–clinician connection.

The centrality of the patient–clinician relationship to healing is frequently acknowledged in medical education, but support for how to foster it, within the day-to-day reality of clinical practice, is often missing. There are multiple clinical communication models designed to facilitate connection; "patient-centered care," perhaps the most widely adopted framework, is an approach to care delivery that requires integrating patient preferences, values, and needs; interacting with the patient as a whole person according to a biopsychosocial framework; and involving patients in the clinical decision process.[52,53] Patient-centered care has been a predominant framework that requires attention to the patient experience, including the patient's emotions as central to a whole-person perspective. A related model, Relationship Centered Care (RCC),[54] emphasizes the bidirectional nature of the clinical encounter and places the relationship between clinician and patient as central, thereby striking a balance in valuing both the patient and the provider as crucial components of the healing exchange that takes place. Within the definition of RCC includes the two important principles that affect and emotion are important components to the healthcare provider and patient relationship, and that all healthcare relationships occur in the context of reciprocal influence.[54]

Regardless of which prevailing communication model is employed, addressing emotional aspects of the interpersonal connection requires a more nuanced approach than is currently detailed in any of the existing clinical communication models. However, the interpersonal connection that is fostered in the clinical encounter is critical, and directly impacts both the patient and provider experience; studies by Hall and colleagues[55,56] showed that patients are more well-liked by their physicians when they are in better health, and both patients and physicians were able to judge with statistically significant accuracy how well-liked they were by the other. Mutual liking predicted patient satisfaction and intention to continue seeing the same physician one year later.[55] This has important ramifications for clinical practice, since patients were significantly able to accurately judge how well-liked they are by their clinician, yet those who are sicker (and thus even more dependent on this relationship) were less well-liked. Addressing this disparity in liking will require clinician acknowledgment of the negative emotions that sicker patients engender, training in emotion regulation, and identification of support infrastructure, such as peer support groups[57–59] or Schwartz Rounds,[60–62] interprofessional medical rounds that focus on human aspects of the medical interaction,[63] that can allow clinicians to process and normalize their own emotional experience.

■ EMOTIONAL SOCIALIZATION IN THE CULTURE OF MEDICINE

Several studies have explored how emotional socialization occurs in the development of professional identity in medical trainees.[64–66] These studies reveal that the culture of medicine holds a deep-seated conflict between displaying emotions to demonstrate caring and maintaining mastery over emotional responses.[64] The explicit and implicit modeling of emotion management in clinical settings further perpetuates the culture; a recent survey of emergency medicine, internal medicine, family medicine physicians, and neurologists showed that only 10% reported receiving any emotion management training as part of their education.[67] A study exploring physicians' attitudes toward crying found that attending physicians who wept in front of trainees rarely discussed it, choosing instead to physically withdraw or ignore the tears.[6] This type of modeling conveys the message that emotion is detrimental and distracting, rather than an essential part of the care delivery process.

The Emotional Demands of Medicine

Crying may be a response of a student who is emotionally raw and fighting for a sense of equilibrium and control. It may also be the response of an emotionally mature student experiencing the poignancy of the extraordinary human drama that characterizes the practice of medicine. By ignoring or suppressing crying that springs from feelings of care, physicians risk suppressing those feelings of care.

—Nancy Angoff, 2001 (p. 1018)[69]

Clinicians are essentially pain brokers; mastery over suffering and delivery of relief are the crux of medicine. Experiencing intense positive and negative emotions is part of clinical care,[70] yet the costs of metabolizing so much distress are rarely discussed; as one physician summarized in response to a survey on emotion in medicine, "The cumulative effect on physicians of listening to so much tragedy is underrated and infrequently discussed let alone addressed."[67]

Emotional exhaustion is one of the defining features of burnout[71]; however, trainees and experienced clinicians are routinely exposed to distressing events and patient deaths without receiving much, if any, training for the emotional work required to process such daily events.[57] Undesirable emotions such as disgust, embarrassment, shame, and anger are frequently evoked in the clinician in the process of delivering care.[72,73] When guidance around handling these emotions is not made explicit, trainees and experienced clinicians alike report challenges managing them[57,66] and may develop costly coping strategies.[70,74]

One such side-effect of practicing medicine may include developing alexithymia, a term coined by Sifneos[75] in 1973 to describe people who had significant trouble describing their feelings, or difficulty recognizing, processing, and regulating emotions.[74] As trainees become inculcated into the medical culture, they are taught to keep emotional distance from patients and blunt their own emotional response.[64,66,74] In her treatise on the need for doctors to be able to modulate and manage emotions as a critical element of good patient care, Shapiro argues that much of medical training promotes the development of alexithymia.[74] As one medical student summarized, "I think the thing that frightens me is the capacity to squelch these feelings. Sometimes I think, why aren't I feeling this more?" (p. 1018).[69] Alexithymia in healthcare professionals is associated with the negative side-effects of depersonalization, emotional exhaustion, and depression.[76] A recent study of nursing assistants found that alexithymia contributed to burnout symptoms.[77] The authors argued that training these clinicians to identify and describe emotions must become a standard part of training in order to prevent clinician burnout and improve patient care.

However, training in emotion management will first require acknowledgment of the emotional distress incurred as a routine part of practicing medicine. Studies that have asked medical students and interns about crying during or in response to clinical rotations found over 71% reported crying,[68,69] with an additional 15% reporting experiences of being on the verge of tears.[2] More than 80% felt their evaluation would suffer if an attending observed them crying due to stress, explaining it was universally seen as a sign of weakness or even "a sign that you're in the wrong profession" (p. 183).[68] Dismantling a medical culture of stoicism begins by understanding its historical roots, the clinical and personal utility of emotion, and then developing concrete guidance for updating medical training to provide clinicians with the necessary tools with which to navigate today's complex healthcare environment.

History of Emotional Socialization in Medicine

The disparagement of emotion as an illegitimate form of knowledge (seen as both gendered and unscientific) in clinical training has also led to a paucity of contributions within medical education from perspectives beyond the biosciences and psychology, thereby further diminishing its visibility and viability in educational and professional contexts.

—Nancy McNaughton, 2013 (p. 72)[78]

While medicine's professional standards are continually evolving, the influence of past leaders has significantly shaped the field's approach to, and conceptualization of, emotion. Sir William Osler is known as "the father of cool detachment," due to his 1889 "Aequanimitas" address to graduating medical students at the University of Pennsylvania. In it, he advised the next generation of doctors on the importance of separating emotional experience from expression while practicing medicine, saying:

> The first essential is to have your nerves well in hand. Even under the most serious circumstances, the physician or surgeon who allows "his outward action to demonstrate the native act and figure of his heart in complement extern," who shows in his face the slightest alteration, expressive of anxiety or fear, has not his medullary centres under the highest control, and is liable to disaster at any moment. I have spoken of this to you on many occasions, and have urged you to educate your nerve centres so that not the slightest dilator or contractor influence shall pass to the vessels of your face under any professional trial. (as cited by Bryan, 2006, p. 385)[79]

This statement perpetuates a false dichotomy between emotion and reason, promoting the idea that the clinician must evacuate or titrate their emotion in order to be a competent professional.

Another articulation of emotional culture in medicine can be seen in cadaver stories,[7] narratives describing jokes played by medical students on emotionally vulnerable victims. Cadaver stories illustrate the complex relationship between medicine and emotion. The stories are told as accounts of true events, with the expectation that medical peers will view them as humorous. The stories both illustrate, and serve to perpetuate, the emotional socialization of medical students. Cadaver stories focus on the boundary between lay and medical cultures, making explicit normative expectation around the need to distance oneself from former lay emotions in order to adopt a medical professional identity. In these stories, expression of anxiety, fear, and revulsion are characterized as inappropriate. Protagonists in the stories embody "the triumph of the medical gaze over baser laylike emotions" (p. 351)[80]; medical students who violate these behavioral norms in the stories are the source of ridicule and risk further torment from peers.

Recognizing the important role that behavioral and social factors play in health and disease, in 2004 the Institute of Medicine published the report, "Improving Medical Education" outlining six important domains that should be included in medical education, including mind–body interactions in health and disease, patient behavior, physician role and behavior, physician–patient interactions, social and cultural issues in healthcare, and health policy and economics.[81] Since this report, a number of changes have occurred in medical education and assessment that emphasize the importance of social and emotional skills in physicians. The introduction of the Step 2 clinical skills section of the United States Medical Licensing Examination in 2004 included doctor–patient communication, shifting focus to more interpersonal aspects of training.[82] In 2015, the Medical College Admissions Test (MCAT) introduced major sections on behavioral and social sciences that emphasize the need for future doctors to understand the impact of behavior on health and the need for physicians to be adept at dealing with the human and social issues of medicine. Learning communities seek to improve healthcare education through the centrality of relationships among learners and teachers,[83] and provide support for students for attending to the emotional challenges of medical training and practicing medicine.[84] These groups are sustained by conveying a sense of membership, influence, and shared emotional connection while also fulfilling individual needs,[85] and foster medical student–faculty longitudinal connections and medical student wellness.[86,87]

McNaughton, in her survey of emotion within medical education,[78] identifies three prevailing discourses:

1. Emotion as physiology, a biological process with predictable outcomes delineated by neuro- and cognitive scientists who examine the neurochemical bases for behavioral affects
2. Emotions as skills that can be learned, that are psychological as well as physiological, and that can be assessed as performances
3. Emotion as a sociocultural mediator, a set of practices constructed by social, cultural, and political forces; emotion as a valuable form of knowledge for use in analysis and problem solving; emotion as collaboratively constructed through social and cultural contexts

As Nancy Angoff summarizes in her 2001 article on medical students "crying in the curriculum,"

> There is much to be learned from stories of crying and much to be taught in response to them. First, in order to hear them, educators need to acknowledge that it is not only okay to cry, but it is understandable, appropriate, and sometimes desirable given the work that we do. (p. 1018)[69]

Emotion Management by Professional Role and Medical Specialty

Medical specialties and professional roles, due to their different acculturation processes and professional expectations, bring different challenges in navigating emotion. Across roles, there is evidence that when clinicians experience emotions at odds with their perceived role expectations, for example, feeling unable to suppress negative emotions induced by a patient interaction, they feel inadequate.[57,88] This perceived disjunction between commonly experienced emotions and professional expectations does a disservice to clinicians and perpetuates a medical culture in which the humanity of the clinician is extracted from the equation, at a high personal and professional cost.

Orri and colleagues, in a metasynthesis of qualitative studies of surgeons, found that emotional dimensions consistently emerged in surgeons' narratives, and this emotion was at odds with surgeons' idealized image of being nonintrospective, tactical, individualistic, isolated, and overconfident technicians.[89] A follow-up study that asked surgeons merely to describe their past two working days demonstrated that emotions are ubiquitous before, during, and after surgery, "and invade life outside the hospital" (p. 11).[90] Throughout the article, in keeping with the depicted surgical culture, emotions are described as "burdensome" intrusions that increase the risk of surgeons being "less scientific" and doing poor quality work.[90] Furthermore, the emotional costs of upholding this stoic professional appearance may be self-perpetuating; as one of our surgical colleagues explained, "The stereotype of being curt, mean, and condescending as a surgeon is the result of actions or words that mask a surgeon's fear, anxiety, and isolation."

In nursing, emotional labor is recognized as "part and parcel of the normal routine of nursing" (p. 44) according to a qualitative study of nurses in hospital and primary care settings.[91] As one nurse described, "Part of what we do is just acting as a long-term emotional buttress for everyone and helping people get over the difficult times. That's what's expected" (p. 47).[91] The role of nurses in accompanying patients through the daily tasks of healing requires a unique set of emotional skills and engagement. Studies of emotion socialization in nursing students found that interactions with staff and patients frequently elicited negative emotions, yet guidance for emotion management was scarce.[92] While first-year students in some nursing schools report being exposed to emotion management content, in-depth interviews with those students demonstrate that this theoretical learning was inadequate for creating a repertoire of strategies which could be utilized in clinical practice.[92] Integrating targeted emotion training and time for emotional reflection as part of nursing training is needed.[93]

■ CONCLUSION

The medical encounter is a social psychological event to which both parties bring their own background, stereotypes, personalities, beliefs, values, expectations, and past and recent experiences—all of which produce emotions and emotional communication, whether they like it or not and whether they intend it or not. The production and active mutual processing of nonverbal and verbal affective cues in a dyadic interaction is constant and irresistible, and subtly reinforcing and reciprocated in ways that are intimately connected to upward and downward spirals in human interactions. Research on the unconscious communication of interpersonal expectations in every kind of human interaction shows that even very subtle emotional reactions have communicative impact. The entire process of medical care is infused with emotional experience; emotion is inseparable from the instrumental acts that define being a competent healthcare provider.

REFERENCES

1. Shapiro J. The feeling physician: educating the emotions in medical training. *Eur J Pers Cent Healthc*. 2013;1(2):310-316.

2. Satterfield JM, Hughes E. Emotion skills training for medical students: a systematic review. *Med Educ*. 2007;41(10):935-941.

3. Pedersen R. Empirical research on empathy in medicine: a critical review. *Patient Educ Couns*. 2009;76(3):307-322.

4. Roter DL, Frankel RM, Hall JA, Sluyter D. The expression of emotion through nonverbal behavior in medical visits. *J Gen Intern Med*. 2006;21:S28-34.

5. Groopman J. *How Doctors Think*. New York, NY: Houghton Mifflin; 2007:39.

6. Plamper J. *The History of Emotions: An Introduction*. New York, NY: Oxford University Press; 2015.

7. Kleinginna PR, Kleinginna AM. A categorized list of emotion definitions, with suggestions for a consensual definition. *Motiv Emot*. 1981;5(4):345-379.

8. Gross JJ, Feldman Barrett L. Emotion generation and emotion regulation: one or two depends on your point of view. *Emot Rev*. 2011;3(1):8-16.

9. Hall JA, Schwartz R. Empathy present and future. *J Soc Psychol*. 2019;159(3):225-243.

10. Frijda NH. *The Emotions*. Cambridge, UK: Cambridge University Press; 1986.

11. Damasio A. *Descartes' Error: Emotion, Reason, and the Human Brain*. New York, NY: Putnam; 1994.

12. Damasio A. *Looking for Spinoza: Joy, Sorrow, and the Feeling Brain*. New York, NY: Houghton Mifflin Harcourt; 2003.

13. Caruso DR, Mayer JD, Bryan V, Phillips KG, Salovey P. Measuring emotional and personal intelligence. In: Gallagher MW, Lopez SJ, eds. *Positive Psychological Assessment: A Handbook of Models and Measures*. Washington, D.C.: American Psychological Association; 2019:233-245.

14. Ingram R. Emotions, social work practice and supervision: an uneasy alliance? *J Soc Work Pract*. 2013;27(1):5-19.

15. McConnell MM, Eva KW. The role of emotion in the learning and transfer of clinical skills and knowledge. *Acad Med*. 2012;87(10):1316-1322.

16. Bolte A, Goschke T. Thinking and emotion: affective modulation of cognitive processing modes. In: Glatzeder B, Goel V, von Muller A, eds. *Towards a Theory of Thinking*. Berlin, Germany: Springer; 2010: 261-277.

17. Goleman D. *Emotional Intelligence*. New York, NY: Bantam Books; 1995.

18. Pérez-Fuentes MC, Herrera-Peco I, Molero M, et al. A cross-sectional study of empathy and emotion management: key to a work environment for humanized care in nursing. *Front Psychol*. 2020;11(May):1-10.

19. Molero Jurado M, Perez-Fuentes M del C, Ruiz NFO, Marquez MMS, Linares JJG. Self-efficacy and emotional intelligence as predictors of perceived stress in nursing professionals. *Medicina*. 2019;55(237):1-14.

20. Carvalho VS, Guerrero E, José M. Emotional intelligence and health students' well-being: a two-wave study with students of medicine, physiotherapy and nursing. *Nurse Educ Today*. 2018;63:35-42.

21. Lin DT, Liebert CA, Tran J, Lau JN, Salles A. Emotional intelligence as a predictor of resident well-being. *J Am Coll Surg*. 2016;223(2):352-358.

22. Bulmer Smith K, Profetto-McGrath J, Cummings GG. Emotional intelligence and nursing: an integrative literature review. *Int J Nurs Stud*. 2009;46:1624-1636.

23. Kozlowski D, Hutchinson M, Hurley J, Rowley J, Sutherland J. The role of emotion in clinical decision making: an integrative literature review. *BMC Med Educ*. 2017;17(255):1-13.

24. Tagoe T, Quarshie ENB. The relationship between emotional intelligence and job satisfaction among nurses in Accra. *Nurs Open*. 2017;4:84-89.

25. Por J, Barriball L, Fitzpatrick JRJ. Emotional intelligence: its relationship to stress, coping, well-being and professional performance in nursing students. *Nurse Educ Today*. 2011;31(8):855-860.

26. Arora S, Ashrafian H, Davis R, Athanasiou T, Darzi A, Sevdalis N. Emotional intelligence in medicine: a systematic review through the context of the ACGME competencies. *Med Educ*. 2010;44:749-764.

27. Sharp G, Bourke L, Rickard MJFX. Review of emotional intelligence in health care: an introduction to emotional intelligence for surgeons. *ANZ J Surg*. 2020;90:433-440.

28. Kaur D, Sambasivan M, Kumar N. Effect of spiritual intelligence, emotional intelligence, psychological ownership and burnout on caring behaviour of nurses: a cross-sectional study. *J Clin Nurs*. 2013;22:3192-3202.

29. Adams K, Cimino JEW, Arnold RM, Anderson WG. Why should I talk about emotion? Communication patterns associated with physician discussion of patient expressions of negative emotion in hospital admission encounters. *Patient Educ Couns*. 2012;89(1):44-50.

30. Peabody FW. The care of the patient. *JAMA*. 1927;88(12):877-882.

31. Katon W, Ries RK, Kleinman A. The prevalence of somatization in primary care. *Compr Psychiatry*. 1984;25(2):208-215.

32. Canby Robinson G. *The Patient as a Person: A Study of the Social Aspects of Illness*. New York, NY: The Commonwealth Fund; 1939.

33. Mayer JD, DiPaolo M, Salovey P. Perceiving affective content in ambiguous visual stimuli: a component of emotional intelligence. *J Pers Assess*. 1990;54(3&4):772-781.

34. Flanagan DAJ, Wagner HL. Expressed emotion and panic-fear in the prediction of diet treatment compliance. *Br J Clin Psychol*. 1991;30: 231-240.

35. Levinson W, Gorawara-Bhat R, Lamb J. A study of patient clues and physician responses in primary care. *JAMA*. 2000;284(8):1021-7102.

36. Cofer KD, Hollis RH, Goss L, Morris MS, Porter JR, Chu DI. Burnout is associated with emotional intelligence but not traditional job performance measurements in surgical residents. *J Surg Educ.* 2018;75(5): 1171-1179.

37. Prasad K, Poplau S, Brown R, et al.. Time pressure during primary care office visits: a prospective evaluation of data from the healthy work place study. *J Gen Intern Med.* 2019;35(2):465-472.

38. Espinosa A, Kadi S. The role of health consciousness, patient–physician trust, and perceived physician's emotional appraisal on medical adherence. *Heal Educ Behav.* 2019;46(6): 991-1000.

39. Jansen J, Van Weert JCM, De Groot J, Van Dulmen S, Heeren TJ, Bensing JM. Emotional and informational patient cues: the impact of nurses' responses on recall. *Patient Educ Couns.* 2010;79(2):218-224.

40. Suchman AL, Markakis K, Beckman HB, Frankel R. A model of empathic communication in the medical interview. *JAMA.* 1997; 277(8):678-682.

41. Blanch-Hartigan D. Patient satisfaction with physician errors in detecting and identifying patient emotion cues. *Patient Educ Couns.* 2013;93(1):56-62.

42. Torre JB, Lieberman MD. Putting feelings into words: affect labeling as implicit emotion regulation. *Emot Rev.* 2018;10(2):116-124.

43. Hulsman RL, Smets EMA, Karemaker JM, De Haes HJCJM. The psychophysiology of medical communication: linking two worlds of research. *Patient Educ Couns.* 2011;84(3):417-424.

44. Hulsman RL, Pranger S, Koot S, Fabriek M, Karemaker JM, Smets EMA. How stressful is doctor–patient communication? Physiological and psychological stress of medical students in simulated history taking and bad-news consultations. *Int J Psychophysiol.* 2010;77(1):26-34.

45. van Dulmen S, Tromp F, Grosfeld F, Bensing J. The impact of assessing simulated bad news consultations on medical students' stress response and communication performance. *Psychoneuroendocrinology.* 2007;32:943-950.

46. Suchman AL, Matthews DA. What makes the patient-doctor relationship therapeutic? Exploring the connexional dimension of medical care. *Ann Intern Med.* 1988;108:125-130.

47. Matthews DA, Suchman AL, Branch WT. Making "connexions": enhancing the therapeutic potential of patient-clinician relationships. *Ann Intern Med.* 1993;118(12): 973-977.

48. Haverfield MC, Tierney A, Schwartz R, et al.. Can patient–provider interpersonal interventions achieve the quadruple aim of healthcare? A systematic review. *J Gen Intern Med.* 2020; 36(7): 2107-2117.

49. Zulman D, Haverfield MC, Shaw JG, et al. Practices to foster physician presence and connection with patients in the clinical encounter. *JAMA.* 2020;94305(1):70-81.

50. Schwartz R, Haverfield MC, Brown-Johnson C, et al.. Transdisciplinary strategies for physician wellness: qualitative insights from diverse fields. *J Gen Intern Med.* 2019;34(7):1251-1257.

51. Brown-Johnson C, Schwartz R, Maitra A, et al. What is clinician presence? A qualitative interview study comparing physician and non-physician insights about practices of human connection. *BMJ Open.* 2019;9:e030831.

52. Constand MK, Macdermid JC, Bello-haas VD, Law M. Scoping review of patient-centered care approaches in healthcare. *BMC Health Serv Res.* 2014;14(271):1-9.

53. Mead N, Bower P. Patient-centredness: a conceptual framework and review of the empirical literature. *Soc Sci Med.* 2000;51:1087-1110.

54. Beach MC, Inui T. Relationship-centered care: a constructive reframing. *J Gen Intern Med.* 2005;21:S3-8.

55. Hall JA, Horgan TG, Stein TS, Roter DL. Liking in the physician-patient relationship. *Patient Educ Couns.* 2002;48:69-77.

56. Hall JA, Epstein AM, DeCiantis ML, McNeil BJ. Physicians' liking for their patients: more evidence for the role of affect in medical care. *Health Psychol.* 1993;12(2):140-146.

57. Schwartz R, Shanafelt TD, Gimmler C, Osterberg L. Developing institutional infrastructure for physician wellness: qualitative insights from VA physicians. *BMC Health Serv Res.* 2020;9:1-9.

58. Omer S, McCarthy G. Reflective practice in psychiatric training: Balint groups. *Ir J Psychol Med.* 2010;27(3):115-116.

59. Kjeldmand D, Holmström I. Balint groups as a means to increase job satisfaction and prevent burnout among general practitioners. *Ann Fam Med.* 2008;6(2):138-145.

60. Pepper JR, Jaggar SI, Mason MJ, Finney SJ, Dusmet M. Schwartz rounds: reviving compassion in modern healthcare. *J R Soc Med.* 2012;105(3):94-95.

61. Saniasiaya J, Ramasamy K. Schwartz rounds for healthcare personnel in coping with COVID-19 pandemic. *Postgr Med J.* 2020 96:425.

62. Barker R, Cornwell J, Gishen F. Introducing compassion into the education of health care professionals: can Schwartz Rounds help? *J Compassionate Health Care.* 2016;3(1):3.

63. The Schwartz Center. Schwartz Rounds. https://www.theschwartzcenter.org/programs/schwartz-rounds. Published 2020. Accessed July 27, 2020.

64. Dornan T, Pearson E, Carson P, Helmich E, Bundy C. Emotions and identity in the figured world of becoming a doctor. *Med Educ.* 2015;49:174-185.

65. Underman K, Hirsh LE. Detached concern?: emotional socialization in twenty-first century medical education. *Soc Sci Med.* 2016; 160:94-101.

66. Bolier M, Doulougeri K, Vries J De, Helmich E. "You put up a certain attitude": a 6-year qualitative study of emotional socialisation. *Med Educ.* 2018; 52:1041-1051.

67. Schwartz R, Osterberg LG, Hall JA. Physicians, emotion, and the clinical encounter: a survey of physicians' experiences. Manuscript in Preparation.

68. Sung AD, Collins ME, Smith AK, et al. Crying: experiences and attitudes of third-year medical students and interns. *Teach Learn Med.* 2009;1334.

69. Angoff N. Crying in the curriculum. *JAMA.* 2001;286(9):1017-1018.

70. Vilela da Silva J, Carvalho I. Physicians experiencing intense emotions while seeing their patients: what happens? *Perm J.* 2016;20(3):31-37.

71. Maslach C, Jackson SE. The measurement of experienced burnout. *J Occup Behav.* 1981;2:99-113.

72. Smith AC, Kleinman S. Managing emotions in medical school: students' contacts with the living and the dead. *Soc Psychol Q.* 1989;52(1):56-69.

73. Miles S. Addressing shame: what role does shame play in the formation of a modern medical professional identity? *Br J Psych Bull.* 2020;44:1-5.

74. Shapiro J. Does medical education promote professional alexithymia? A call for attending to the emotions of patients and self in medical training. *Acad Med.* 2011;86(3).

75. Sifneos PE. The prevalence of "alexithymic" characteristics in psychosomatic patients. *Psychother Psychosom.* 1973; 22:255-262.

76. Bratis D, Tselebis A, Sikaras C, et al. Alexithymia and its association with burnout, depression and family support among Greek nursing staff. *Hum Resour Health.* 2009; 7:72.

77. Aldaz E, Aritzeta A. The association between alexithymia, emotional intelligence and burnout among nursing assistants working in nursing home settings: a cross-sectional study. *J Adv Nurs.* 2019;75:2786-2796.

78. McNaughton N. Discourse(s) of emotion within medical education: the ever-present absence. *Med Educ.* 2013;47:71-79.

79. Bryan CS. "Aequanimitas" Redux: William Osler on detached concern versus humanistic empathy. *Perspect Biol Med.* 2006;49(3):384-392.

80. Hafferty FW. Cadaver stories and the emotional socialization of medical students. *J Health Soc Behav.* 1988;29(4):344-356.

81. Institute of Medicine of the National Academies, Cuff PA, Vanselow NA, eds. *Improving Medical Education: Enhancing the Behavioral and Social Science Content of Medical School Curricula.* Curricula Committee on Behavioral and Social Sciences in Medical School Curricula, and Board on Neuroscience and Behavioral Health. Washington, D.C.: National Academies Press; 2004.

82. Gilliland WR, Rochelle J La, Hawkins R, et al. Changes in clinical skills education resulting from the introduction of the USMLE TM step 2 clinical skills (CS) examination. *Med Teach.* 2009;30(3):325-327.

83. Learning Communities Institute: Learning Communities. http://learningcommunities-institute.org/. Published 2020. Accessed July 27, 2020.

84. Smith S, Shochet R, Keeley M, Fleming A. The growth of learning communities in undergraduate medical education. *Acad Med.* 2014;89(6):1-6.

85. McMillan DW, Chavis DM. Sense of community: a definition and theory. *J Community Psychol.* 1986;14:6-23.

86. Fleming A, Cutrer W, Moutsios S, et al. Building learning communities: evolution of the colleges at Vanderbilt University School of Medicine. *Acad Med.* 2013;88(9):1246-1251.

87. Hillard PJA, Basaviah P, Osterberg L. Medical student wellness: an essential role for mentors. *Med Sci Educ.* 2011;21(4):382-384.

88. Arieli D. Emotional work and diversity in clinical placements of nursing students. *J Nurs Scholarsh.* 2013;45(2):192-201.

89. Orri M, Farges O, Clavien P, Barkun J, Revah-Levy A. Being a surgeon—the myth and the reality: a meta-synthesis of surgeons' perspectives about factors affecting their practice and well-being. *Ann Surg.* 2014;260(5):721-728.

90. Orri M, Revah-lévy A, Farges O. Surgeons' emotional experience of their everyday practice: a qualitative study. *PLoS One.* 2015;10(11):1-15.

91. Smith P, Gray B. Emotional labour of nursing revisited: caring and learning 2000. *Nurse Educ Pract*. 2001;1:42-49.

92. Mccloughen A, Levy D, Johnson A, Nguyen H, McKenzie H. Nursing students' socialisation to emotion management during early clinical placement experiences: a qualitative study. *J Clin Nurs*. 2020;29:2508-2520.

93. Santo LD, Ambrosi E, Maragna M, Marognolli O, Canzan F. Nursing students' emotions evoked by the first contact with patient' s body: a qualitative study. *Nurse Educ Today*. 2020;85:104299.

The Functions of Emotion: Evolutionary and Social Perspectives

Michelle N. Shiota, Erika B. Pages, and Paula H. Bednarek

It is midnight, and you are on a labor and delivery shift that will last until 7:00 am. During one labor the baby's heart rate suddenly drops, and stays low. The mother is pushing as hard as she can, but the baby is still too high to reach with forceps or a vacuum. Anesthesia and neonatology teams are called, and the patient is moved to an operating room for an emergency cesarean section. The baby is delivered, but appears limp, and is soon taken by the neonatology team to another room while the obstetrics team manages the mother's bleeding and closes the uterine incision. Just as the surgery is completed, the neonatology team returns to tell the other providers that the baby could not be resuscitated, and did not survive. After the mother wakes and has had some time to recover, the parents are informed of their baby's death. After talking with both the obstetrics and neonatology teams, the heartbroken parents request an autopsy investigating why the baby could not be resuscitated.

> It is now 1:00 in the morning, with six more hours left in the shift. The teams meet briefly to debrief on procedural issues, but there is little time to address the emotions team members are feeling about this unexpected loss. Three other patients are still in labor, and will need care in the hours ahead.

Medical care often presents a dilemma to providers and patients alike. On one hand, the potential for intense emotions to arise is high. In office visits, deeply personal issues can emerge around patients' physical and psychological vulnerabilities, feelings of embarrassment and shame, reverberations of relationships and lifestyles, histories of traumatic experience, and dreams for the future. Such clinical encounters can quickly and unexpectedly reach a level of intimacy usually reserved for our close personal relationships.

In hospital settings the likelihood of intense emotions can be even higher as people face matters of literal life and death, evoking emotions of fear and hope, the joy and relief of successful treatment, and the grief of profound loss. On the other hand, medical practice presents a need for clear thinking, rational decision-making, and expert performance, sometimes under tight time pressure. Given these demands, "irrational" emotions can seem like a distraction at best, or even a destructive influence to be suppressed as much as possible.

The aims of this chapter are twofold. First, we articulate the "deep rationality" of human emotions, reviewing theories that emphasize emotions' evolutionary origins and explaining how emotions help us address challenges faced time and again by our ancestors.[1-5] We highlight the widespread interconnections among emotional and cognitive processes, as documented by both neuroscience and behavioral research, showing that emotion, information processing, and decision-making are intertwined for a reason.[6-8] Second, we offer evidence-based guidance in managing emotions in a healthy and constructive way within clinical settings, using them strategically to support decisions people can live with while regulating their potentially detrimental effects.[9-11] Throughout the chapter, we include real-life examples to ground the analysis and illustrate our approach. We hope readers will leave this chapter with an open mind about the value of acknowledging and dealing with emotions in clinical practice.

■ WHAT IS EMOTION?

When asked to describe an emotional experience, laypeople may mention a variety of distinct features. People often explain the situation in which the emotion occurred, such that the emotion seems like a natural or at least understandable response.[4] As William James noted more than a century ago, emotion often involves visceral sensations, and people may include a pounding heart, icy fingers, sweating, flushing, or churning stomach in their account.[12] The description may include a facial expression, gesture, or tone of voice that communicates the emotion without words. Emotional experiences commonly involve an impulse to act in a particular way, although one may not always follow through with this action.[13] And of course, emotions involve subjective feelings, which may be described simply as "good" or "crummy," or with a more specific emotion label such as "amused" or "furious."[14,15]

Although there is controversy as to how emotion should be defined for scientific purposes, many researchers endorse a definition that includes all these elements, and adopt theories that explain why these elements are likely to co-occur during emotional episodes. Many agree that emotions are typically responses to an eliciting situation, requiring what philosophers call an "intentional object." One may wake up in a grumpy or energetic mood, but we are typically angry *at* someone; we are proud *of* ourselves or another person; we are excited or sad *about* something.[16] Because we tend to localize the cause of emotion in events outside ourselves, we experience emotion as "unbidden"—something that happens to us regardless of our intent or consent.[17] A rich body of research now documents real physiological responses during emotion that may range from full-blown, sympathetically mediated fight-flight arousal to soothing, parasympathetic-driven relaxation, as well as a variety of more complex visceral profiles.[18,19] Evidence is equally strong that people around the world readily produce nonverbal signals of emotion such as facial expressions and vocalizations, and can associate such expressions with emotional labels, even agreeing to a fair extent on the expressions' specific emotional meanings.[20,21]

These diverse aspects of emotion are thought to "hang together" for a reason—because they helped our mammalian ancestors solve certain kinds of problems that occurred often and had important consequences for reproductive fitness. James Gross has offered what he calls the "modal model of emotion," capturing the core definition and process presumed by many modern emotion theorists.[9,22] In this model, an emotional episode begins with an event in the environment, but the event does not directly cause the emotion. Rather, it is one's *appraisal* of the event—an evaluation of the event's implications for one's own goals, needs, and concerns—that drives the emotional response.[4,23] A patient responds to a proposed cancer treatment with fear if they expect that treatment to cause significant pain, damage, conflict, or distress—perhaps more than they can currently imagine from the cancer itself. A colleague will react to your comment about their clinical opinion with anger if they interpret that comment as a criticism or insult. A young patient's parents will respond to a diagnosis of serious disease with hope if their attention is focused on the possibility of a cure, and they can see a pathway to that outcome. Appraisal is inherently subjective, emphasizing the perceived relationship between the person and their situation rather than the objective features of the situation itself. Thus, emotions are responses to what we believe a situation *means for us*.

While the examples above may seem fairly obvious, appraisal also explains why different people can have such divergent emotional reactions to the same situation. Consider the scenario described at the beginning of this chapter, involving the unexpected death of a baby during a labor and delivery shift. The obvious appraisal may be one of profound loss, evoking sadness or grief. However, the neonatology resident who becomes uncharacteristically withdrawn after the debriefing may be blaming himself for the failure to resuscitate the baby, perhaps having made some error along the way—an appraisal that will drive shame or guilt whether that assessment is objectively accurate or not. In contrast, a member of the labor and delivery team may focus on having excelled at a particularly difficult technique that helped save the mother's life, resulting in pride—again, whether objectively reasonable or not. The baby's father, searching for an explanation and focusing his attention on the doctors with whom he is speaking, may move from grief to blame and anger with little warning. A nurse whose attention is focused primarily on the mother's distress may primarily be feeling compassion, whereas an intern may be traumatized after seeing her first death, and feeling sudden panic about working with the next patient. These appraisals and the associated emotions are not mutually exclusive; they can co-occur, and individuals can shift unpredictably from one to another.

None of these emotional reactions is "wrong," given where the individual's attention is focused, what they believe to be happening, and the appraised meaning of that event. This is why simply telling ourselves or someone else to feel/not feel a certain way rarely works—there is no objective ground truth against which to assess an emotion's validity. We may disagree with the *understanding of the situation* at the root of someone's emotional response, but that is a different conversation. Moreover, it's a conversation in which the emotion itself offers valuable clues. The neonatology resident's shame, the father's anger, and the intern's suppressed panic all provide information about what they are thinking and how they understand the situation. These individuals may even be unaware of their own appraisals, which can be automatic and implicit as well as consciously recognized.[23] Analyzing situational appraisals—what exactly they are, the extent to which they are objectively reasonable, alternative ways of understanding the situation—can be highly constructive in working through one's own emotions and helping others process theirs. Consistent with this, cognitive-behavioral talk therapy seems to be effective in treating anxiety and depression in part because it helps people identify maladaptive appraisal biases (e.g., overappraising threat, insult, failure, and loss; underappraising opportunity, achievement, availability of social support, and personal control), and develop appraisal profiles that are more aligned with the objective environment and conducive to emotional well-being.[24-26]

If appraisals elicit emotions, what are the emotions themselves? A long-standing perspective in emotion theory posits the existence of evolved, species-typical neural "affect programs"[27] or "superordinate neural programs"[1] whose activation is triggered automatically by the relevant appraisal, and serves to initiate and coordinate the myriad physiological, expressive, cognitive, motivational, and behavioral aspects of emotional responding.[2,5,28,29] The automaticity of neural emotion program activation accounts for the "unbidden" quality emotions seem to have—the feeling that they are beyond one's control.[17]

Indeed, many theories emphasize the inevitability of an emotional response once the corresponding appraisal occurs.[2,9,23,30] Trying to stop the emotion after appraisal is as effective as closing the barn door after the horses have escaped; all you can do is go retrieve one horse at a time, and bring it back to the barn. In other words, once an emotion has begun, inhibiting the elements of the response is going to be piecemeal and highly effortful.[9]

If appraisal identifies a problem or challenge in the environment, the complex response initiated by the emotion program is geared toward solving that problem. For example, Tooby and Cosmides[31] propose that the superordinate neural program for "fear" is activated by appraisal of possible predator threat, triggering changes in attention and perception such as heightened attunement to external auditory and visual cues; information processing geared toward threat assessment (e.g., whether the threat is close or farther away[32]); enhanced memory encoding for threats[33]; autonomic nervous system responses that release glucose into the blood stream, increase overall blood flow, direct blood toward the large skeletal muscles, heart, and brain, while inhibiting energy-demanding processes such as digestion that will not help facilitate escape[18]; nonverbal facial and vocal signals that warn others of the danger and summon help[34]; and heightened motivation to protect one's self and one's kin.[35] This suite of responses is thought to serve a very clear adaptive function: to support a behavioral response that helps the organism escape the threat with life and limb intact.

There is evidence that different aspects of emotional responding cohere in a way consistent with this theoretical proposal. In one particularly strong test of this hypothesis, Mauss and colleagues[36] asked healthy young adults to watch a 5-min film clip that had a comic beginning, transitioned to a sad scene, and then back to humor. Participants' facial expressions were video recorded and coded for amusement and sadness expressions; their sweat gland and cardiac reactivity were monitored throughout the clip; and they used a handheld dial to continuously rate their subjective feelings of amusement/humor and sadness. Analyses examining average within-individual correlations over time between these aspects of emotional responding revealed quite strong correlations (*rs* in the .70s) between feelings and facial expressions, and moderate but significant correlations of feelings and expressions with sweat gland activity, though correlations involving cardiac activity were not as strong. In other words, participants tended to show facial, physiological, and self-report signs of the expected emotions at the same time, consistent with the proposal that the disparate elements of emotional responding might be coordinated by a single neural program.

The account above focuses on the evolved core of emotion episodes,. linking appraisals to activation of neural programs that initiate complex emotional responses. Evolutionary origin implies that the appraisal-emotion program activation link should be universal among humans. However, modern theories also recognize that emotions are powerfully shaped by individual experience and cultural context, from which we learn how to appraise the meaning of events around us, and what specific actions are most likely to achieve our goals.[2,5,28] For example, the traumatized intern in the scenario above may experience heightened amygdala and hippocampal activation that will generate a vivid, readily activated episodic memory linking the stimuli, people, and events immediately preceding the baby's death with danger,[37] resulting in negative future appraisals of those stimuli. We learn from our local culture as well as personal experience what events and aspects of events are worthy of notice, whose perspectives and needs are valid, what is valuable, and the implications an event has for what happens next.[38,39] For example, the team member's pride in his successful technical procedure may reflect having grown up in a highly individualistic cultural environment in which one's own actions and outcomes are more salient than those of the group.[40,41] Someone raised in a more collectivist cultural context might be more attuned to group-level outcomes, and respond emotionally to those instead.

Similarly, there is plenty of room on the back end of an emotion episode for learning, culture, and pressures of the current context to shape our emotional behavior. For example, not every emotion will be readily apparent on a person's face; people can and often do conceal, feign, or otherwise modulate their nonverbal expressions of emotion intentionally, as appropriate for the situation (e.g., pretending to be happy about a birthday gift you don't actually like).[2] In our scenario, the parents' expressions of anger will be influenced by the expressions they saw modeled growing up, and how their own expressions have previously been rewarded versus punished. Although men and women report feeling similar amounts of anger in their daily lives, open, vocal expression of men's anger is often socially accepted and rewarded, and is considerably more common, whereas women's anger is more likely to be suppressed or expressed in a subtler, tight-lipped form (see Chapter 11, Emotion and Gender, for more details on gender-based differences in emotion).[42-44] Thus, the father's anger may be more easily detected, the mother's relatively concealed. The physicians themselves may be feeling tremendous distress, but regulating its expression in order to support the parents and their clinical teams.

Again, it is crucial to emphasize that the various emotional responses of the people in this scenario are all valid in light of each person's individual history and cultural training. Each emotion reflects the person's understanding of what is happening, and what it means for their needs, goals, and concerns.

Given this interpretation, their emotional response includes elements geared toward shaping future events in a direction that is best for accomplishing their goals, reflecting the "deep rationality" of emotion to which we now turn.

■ DEEP RATIONALITY: THE EVOLUTIONARY ORIGINS AND FUNCTIONS OF EMOTION

We have described human emotion as a series of adaptations, part of our mammalian evolutionary heritage. What evidence is there for this proposal, and what specific functions do emotions serve? It was Charles Darwin himself who first suggested evolutionary origins of emotion. In fact, his third major treatise on evolution was his book *The Expression of the Emotions in Man and Animals*—a detailed comparative exploration of the nonverbal expressions of nonhuman animals, infants, and adult humans around the world in situations we think of as evoking strong emotions.[45] Darwin's analysis was a direct counter to the claim by his contemporary and teacher Sir Charles Bell, a foremost facial anatomist, that God had designed human facial musculature to express uniquely human emotions. Although Darwin did not describe emotions per se as adaptations, a central principle of this book is that the particular muscle movements in emotional expressions reflect "serviceable associated habits"— behavioral responses that served some reliable adaptive utility in particular situations faced by mammalian ancestors. For example, the piloerection response commonly seen in threatened animals as well as humans makes animals covered with hair (or feathers) appear larger and more intimidating; the nose wrinkle of disgust would reduce the amount of pathogen one might inhale while breathing near a contaminated object. This was the first major application of Darwin's theory of natural selection to human behavior.

Since Darwin's initial proposal, the question of cross-cultural "universality," not only of nonverbal emotional expressions but other aspects of emotion as well, has been one major focus of emotion research. In the late 1960s, Paul Ekman and Carroll Izard independently collected data from several cultures around the world, including some indigenous tribes with little or no prior exposure to people from the Western world, investigating the extent to which participants chose the predicted emotion labels (or an emotion-eliciting situation) for strong Western expressions of fear, anger, sadness, disgust, happiness, and surprise.[2,46] In a typical study with six or seven response options, correct responses would be expected 14–17% of the time if participants were choosing their responses at random (i.e., guessing); in studies with indigenous tribes fewer options were offered, but chance would still be about one in three. The rates at which participants agreed with the researcher's predictions were consistently in the 50–80% range, and in some cases exceeded 90%—far above the threshold for statistical significance relative to chance. These findings kicked off the modern era of emotion research. Since then, studies have documented striking cross-cultural similarities in facial and postural expressions of other emotions, nonverbal vocal expressions, emotion-antecedent appraisals, and peripheral physiological responses.[21,47-52]

As noted earlier in this chapter, these findings of cross-cultural similarity do not preclude some individual and cultural differences, which are prominent in nonverbal expressions[48,53] and in emotion concepts, vocabulary, and subjective descriptions of emotional experience.[54-58] There is no question that the human mind forms emotion concepts based on learning and experience, and that these concepts vary from person to person and across languages and cultures.[59] Even theories emphasizing emotions' evolutionary origins increasingly recognize that inherited neural templates are shaped by experience, particularly during the early years of life, such that no complex psychological mechanism is likely to be identical across individuals and cultures.[5,60] However, evidence of strong cross-cultural similarity in these various aspects of emotion indicates the existence of *some* evolved mechanisms producing this similarity, which in turn strongly suggests that our emotions serve valuable functions.

The nature of these functions is most clearly articulated in terms of Richard Lazarus's *core relational themes*.[4] Core relational themes convey both our appraisal of the personal significance of some event in the environment and our goals in responding to that event, with the emotion itself aimed at transforming the person–environment relationship. Not all situations faced by mammalian ancestors would have led to the evolution of an emotional response. According to John Tooby, situations likely to produce emotional responses were those that recurred often ancestrally, were clearly and reliably structured, were easily recognizable, required coordination across cognitive, physiological, motivational, and behavioral systems, and presented significant costs to adaptive fitness if an error occurred.[61] Examples of such situations include both threats, such as predators and pathogens; and opportunities, such as a valuable food supply, potential mates, and offspring and kin requiring care.[31,62]

In some situations, the emotional response will address the situation in a way that would have, on average, tended to directly increase the individual's fitness. An example is the fear response described earlier; all of the response components, when coordinated, should increase the individual's chance of escaping the situation and surviving to leave an ample contribution to future generations. The disgust response appears geared toward preventing exposure to pathogens or diseases that might limit reproductive fitness, or even cause an early demise.[63,64] The cognitive, physiological, and motivational elements of our response to potential rewards, such as high-calorie foods and (for humans) money, appear to promote focused attention on the reward, as well as heightened approach/appetitive motivation and physiological arousal facilitating rapid movement to acquire the reward.[18,65–67] Interestingly, anger when we are blocked from pursuing a goal also involves heightened approach motivation, promoting actions aimed at getting what we want.[68] These are all examples of *intrapersonal functions of emotion*, that is, ways in which the emotional response directly benefits the fitness of the individual experiencing the emotion.[28] Much of 20th-century emotion theory emphasized these sorts of functions, as the value of these emotional responses for survival and reproductive fitness was fairly easy to articulate.

In recent decades, however, emotion theorists have paid greater attention to the interpersonal or *social functions of emotions*.[3] Humans are "ultrasocial," depending more than almost any other animal on interdependent relationships within large groups.[69] Unlike other ultrasocial species in which group members are nearly genetically identical, such as ants and bees, humans form astoundingly complex, extended, cooperative communities of loosely related individuals in which we perform almost every major function of life. Ultrasociality presents both opportunities (division of labor, food sharing, cooperation) and challenges (competition for resources, navigating the social hierarchy) for individual reproductive fitness. A rapidly growing body of research is documenting the complex ways in which our emotions shape the relationships on which humans depend.

Some emotions serve to initiate relationships, to identify promising partners for various kinds of relationships, or to bind us to others in the long term. Sexual attraction draws our attention to promising potential sexual partners, promotes flirtatious behavior that attracts their attention and communicates our interest, and prepares the body for mating.[70–72] When someone shows us kindness, providing us with unexpected support or aid, we feel gratitude.[73] An expression of gratitude for someone else's prosocial action not only communicates the beneficiary's appreciation and willingness to reciprocate, but also tends to elicit commitment from the benefactor to help the beneficiary again in the future.[74,75] When someone is consistently there for us, supporting us in good times and bad, we form emotional attachments to them that motivate us to maintain that connection. Such attachments can provide a "secure base" that supports healthy exploration and risk-taking.[76] Shared laughter and amusement can promote social bonding, even among strangers.[77] Compassion and nurturant love motivate us to provide caregiving to others who are vulnerable, hurt, or helpless, including our own children and young kin as well as others who we believe depend on us.[78,79]

Other emotions communicate our needs, expectations, and evaluations of relationship partners' behavior, giving them a chance to respond. Expression of sadness after a loss—whether of an important relationship partner or a valued resource—can evoke others' support and assistance.[80] According to the recalibration theory of anger, anger lets a relationship partner know that they have failed to value our welfare at the level we expect of them, giving us less respect and consideration than we deserve.[81] Although uncontrolled or unfair expression of anger can have negative consequences, when perceived as justified it can evoke concessions from others.[82] Jealousy communicates that one believes a relationship is threatened, and motivates individuals to ward off potential competitors.[83] Guilt occurs when one has violated a relationship partner's trust, and motivates behavior aimed at repairing the relationship.[84]

Navigating the complex social hierarchy of human relationships requires skill, and emotions play important roles here as well. When we accomplish some socially valued task, like mastering a skill or achieving a promotion or award, we experience pride.[85] Pride has a distinct and cross-culturally recognized expression including expanded posture, head lift, and arms raised or akimbo[86] that not only radiates achievement but raises others' perceptions of one's status and worth as a social partner.[87,88] Conversely, embarrassment occurs in response to a social faux pas or other action that draws others' unexpected attention to the self.[89] Display of an embarrassed expression, which often involves blushing, gaze aversion, and a face touch as well as a controlled smile, has been found to appease others, reducing the likelihood of punishment or retaliation and helping to restore one's social status.[90,91]

In Western culture, when we talk about "rationality," we often approach it from a purely economic perspective, as though facts alone should ideally be the sole basis for making decisions and guiding our behavior. Increasingly, however, evidence shows that without emotion we may make poor decisions, especially when risk assessments and subjective preferences are involved.[6,92] Real-life good decisions—including decisions in the medical domain—depend on both the probabilities of various outcomes and the relative valuation of those outcomes. While the probabilities fall in the domain of factual information, they may involve a great deal of uncertainty and require more complicated calculations than the logical mind can manage. Personal values are beyond the domain of facts, but crucial for being able to live with one's decision. The notion that the mind includes numerous evolved mechanisms for dealing with such situations has been called "deep rationality."[93] Emotional mechanisms encode many millions of years' worth of ancient data on the success or failure of our ancestors' responses to crucial situations. These mechanisms' calculations nudge us automatically and without effortful, time-consuming logical analysis toward responses that will give the best shot at success. The ability of these mechanisms to learn and adapt to experiences along the way should enhance their predictive value, as long as the situational contingencies we face in the future map closely to those we and our ancestors faced in the past.

■ EMOTION, COGNITION, AND DECISION-MAKING

We hope that the examples above seem relatable and real. One might ask, however: if emotions serve the ancient adaptive functions we have proposed, why do they often seem messy, irrational, and destructive? We offer two answers to this. First, as noted above, people subjectively experience emotions as effortless, automatic, and compelled from us rather than under our control. This experience is so different from the effortful, deliberate cognition associated with logical decision-making that it can feel uncomfortable. Although we may subjectively experience emotion and cognition as dichotomous, opposing mental processes, both neuroscience evidence and behavioral research show that they are deeply intertwined. It is true that certain aspects of effortful cognitive control are supported by activity in highly developed regions of the human prefrontal cortex that have reciprocal negative connections with regions supporting emotion-related processes, such as the amygdala and ventral striatum.[94,95] A more fine-grained look at the brain's circuitry reveals, however, that the psychological processes of attention, perceptual filtering, information processing, memory for emotional events, valuation, inhibition, motivation, and decision-making are supported by complex networks connecting various structures in the prefrontal cortex, other cortical regions, and the subcortex.[96,97] Within the brain, emotion and cognition are not so clearly separated.

Behavioral studies also indicate that emotion exerts wide-ranging influence on attention, cognition, judgment, and decision-making, often without our awareness (see Chapter 13, Emotion and Decision Making in the Clinical Encounter).[8] Experimental studies in which emotions are manipulated prior to some cognitive task have consistently found effects on risk assessment, memory, reliance on heuristics in judgment and decision-making, and valuation/evaluation of targets unrelated to the emotion, among other effects.[33,98–103] Different emotions have different implications for cognitive processing. Appetitive enthusiasm, desire, anger, and fear tend to focus one's attention narrowly, whereas sadness and awe may lead to more distributed attention.[65,104,105] Many positive-valence emotions increase reliance on cognitive shortcuts, but awe seems to reduce this reliance.[106]

One particularly pervasive influence of current emotional experience is the tendency to bias our appraisal of subsequent events.[8] For example, much research documents people's tendency to wear "rose-colored glasses" when evaluating consumer products and other targets while in a positive mood; the opposite occurs in a negative mood.[102,107] In one series of studies, experimentally evoked anger was found to promote blaming other people for a hypothetical awkward but accidental interpersonal situation, whereas sadness increased the tendency to attribute the event to bad luck.[108] Appraisal carryover effects are likely to be functional in situations that do not change too rapidly. However, they may create a problematic bias when the decision-making target is not closely related to the event eliciting the original emotion. For example, a patient who just learned that they received a promotion at work is likely in a very good mood, but the optimistic bias that tends to accompany positive mood could lead them to underestimate their risk of contracting hepatitis. This may affect their decision about whether the three time-consuming rounds of vaccination, recommended by the provider, are worth their time.

The second reason why emotions can feel problematic is highly relevant to medical settings. From an evolutionary perspective, our emotion mechanisms are adaptations *to the environment faced by our ancient ancestors*, calibrated to predict and influence outcomes under those conditions.[1] Although the mechanisms may be capable of learning and updating, they may still be likely to fail in situations that differ greatly from ancestral conditions. The fear/anxiety response is an excellent example. In the modern world, we are far more likely to feel threatened by excessive demands, time pressure, or the possibility of another's negative evaluation than by a predator. Literally running away is not going to help, yet it's what our mind and body prepare to do anyway, with significant long-term health consequences for those experiencing chronic stress.[109] Our emotions evolved to respond to challenges of physical threat, material resource and status acquisition, relationship formation and management, and separation from and loss of loved ones. They did not evolve to deal with decisions about medical screening, reproductive technology, or cancer treatment, none of which was available in the ancestral environment. This means that skill is required to use emotions constructively in these settings when possible, and to regulate emotions effectively when strategic use is not possible (see Chapter 7, Emotion Regulation in Patients, Providers, and the Clinical Relationship). We offer some examples in the medical setting below.

■ A FUNCTIONAL PERSPECTIVE ON EMOTION IN CLINICAL SETTINGS

When emotions run high and an important decision needs to be made, or we are under pressure to perform, we may wish to simply turn our emotions off.

Unfortunately, attempting to suppress emotions does not lower the subjective experience of distress, may not reduce the emotions' effects on cognition, and comes with negative cardiovascular costs.[8,110] On the contrary, failure to acknowledge emotions may allow their effects on cognition and behavior to run rampant. Understanding, using, and skillfully managing them are more likely to be effective. What does this look like in practice?

Managing the Provider's Own Emotions

Beginning with one's own emotions, there are benefits to recognizing them, sitting with them (even briefly), naming them, and being aware of their likely influence on thought processes. Among clinical psychologists and researchers studying emotion regulation, there is growing appreciation of the advantages of simply accepting one's emotions in a mindful and nonjudgmental way.[111] Acceptance may not reduce distress right away, but it allows one to acknowledge feelings and move on from the situation, rather than letting the feelings control one's next actions. Acceptance is less cognitively demanding than other strategies aimed primarily at reducing distress, and it has been linked to positive well-being outcomes in the long term. Naming and acknowledging one's emotions may have the additional benefit of increasing awareness of cognitive and appraisal biases they may cause, making it possible to evaluate consciously whether those biases should be allowed to influence subsequent decisions.[107,112]

A more effortful strategy, but one that can be quite effective at reducing distress in the moment, is cognitive reappraisal.[9] In this strategy one deliberately redirects one's attention to a different aspect of the situation, an aspect with positive or at least neutral implications. For example, a physician in the scenario with which we opened this chapter might reduce distress by focusing attention on the team's success in saving the mother's life, rather than the loss of the baby. A rich body of evidence indicates that this strategy is effective for managing emotional experience and the associated physiological symptoms.[9,11,113] One potential drawback to consider is the risk that reappraisal may preempt constructive action that would otherwise be motivated by negative emotions.[114]

The Emotions of Patients and Families

Dealing with the emotions of patients and their loved ones can be challenging as well. Consider this situation:

A young woman is in your office, receiving her first gynecological exam. She is clearly tense and anxious—much more so than the typical patient. Upon insertion of the speculum, she first flinches, then begins crying. She says she is not in pain and is ok, but clearly she is not. You complete the exam as quickly and efficiently as possible. Afterward the patient reveals that she has a history of sexual abuse that she has never before disclosed, and the exam revived vivid memories of that trauma.

Even during routine office visits, medical practitioners may find themselves on the receiving end of extremely personal stories and the emotions that go with them. Indeed, primary care providers may be the closest thing to a therapist many patients will encounter. It is important to treat these occurrences as opportunities to strengthen the relationship and improve care. Simply listening with full attention and concern to a patient's disclosure of their experiences can be a tremendously supportive act. Research on the various factors predicting positive client outcomes in psychotherapy has found that the most important feature is not the particular therapeutic technique used, or the amount of training received by the therapist, but the extent to which the therapist–client relationship is marked by empathic rapport, warmth, and an emphasis on collaboration.[115] Listening with concern and without judgment does not mean treating the patient's distress or trying to fix their problem, and it definitely does not include "catching" the patient's emotions; the practitioner does best to keep an even keel. It does mean taking a moment to honor the disclosure in a respectful way, and show the person they've been heard with compassion. Having done that, referral to a licensed therapist is the appropriate next step. This process can help build the patient's trust not only in you as the current practitioner, but potentially in future medical professionals as well. That trust will ease the way in eliciting honest information about symptoms, and guiding them through decisions in the future.

Here's another example, this time involving a difficult decision about medical care:

A young couple comes to the obstetrician's office to begin prenatal care, thrilled at the prospect of starting a family. During the second visit, the woman mentions casually that she has noticed a lump in her breast; she thinks it's probably nothing, but decided to mention it. After a manual exam the obstetrician orders an ultrasound, which is followed by a biopsy. This reveals cancer, for which the appropriate treatment includes chemotherapy. The woman is still in her first trimester, so if she waits until the baby is born chemotherapy will be delayed several months. The couple needs to decide whether to terminate the pregnancy and begin treatment immediately, or continue the pregnancy and risk progression of the cancer beyond where it is treatable. The woman and her partner are distraught, and do not know what to do.

This is a situation in which emotions must be part of the conversation. As with the scenario above, the first step is to acknowledge and validate the couple's emotions, and demonstrate concerned attention without becoming overwhelmed by your own distress. Finding out how they feel—are they frightened? angry? grieving?—will provide some clues about cognitive biases they may be inclined to show, as well as the aspects of the situation on which they are currently focused. For example, frightened people are more likely to be risk-averse, whereas angry people tend to show higher tolerance for risk.[99] Anger tends to narrow attentional focus and increase the tendency to rely on cognitive shortcuts in decision-making, but may also facilitate goal-directed analytic reasoning, whereas low-arousal sadness may broaden attentional scope and facilitate more cautious information processing.[116–118] Heightened physiological arousal may bias attention and subsequent memory toward the most emotionally salient aspects of the situation, while inhibiting encoding of detailed technical information the couple will need to consider in making their decision.[119]

A useful next step—after a delay to let the couple to assimilate the situation, if possible—will be to guide the couple through an assessment of the values of the different outcomes, excruciating though that may be. One useful technique may involve imagining each possible outcome, and noting the emotions that arise. This is based on research suggesting that the ability to simulate the emotional consequences of hypothetical outcomes—mediated in part by the orbitofrontal cortex—plays a valuable role in making good decisions.[92] At this point the possible courses of action can be explained in more detail, along with information about outcome probabilities in each case. If at all possible, have this conversation in a place that is calm and aesthetically pleasing—even awe inspiring. While managing her father's care during stage 4 cancer, the first author was taken to a room on a high floor at the University of California, San Francisco Medical Center, with a panoramic view of the San Francisco Bay. The physiological and cognitive effects of such stimuli may make it easier to process complex information and formulate a decision with the "big picture" in mind—in this case a difficult end-of-life decision.[67,120]

Once the decision is made, it can be helpful to assist patients in differentiating what they can control from what they cannot, and focus their attention on the former. The need for control appears to be a fundamental human characteristic, and perception of personal control is vital to psychological well-being.[121] People often feel disempowered, helpless, and out of control in medical situations, potentially leading to toxic behaviors such as treatment noncompliance or the threat of legal action. Grief, in particular, involves appraisals of low personal control.[51] Highlighting where patients and their loved ones *do* have some control can be a valuable component of medical care.

A note on the emotion of hope is useful here. Hope is driven by the ability to envision a positive outcome in the midst of a difficult time. The ability to maintain hope is associated with motivation to bring about the positive outcome, and development of concrete plans aimed at that goal. Although there is more correlational than experimental evidence regarding the implications of hope in medical settings, hopefulness has been linked to better health outcomes, higher pain tolerance, and higher rates of adherence to treatment plans.[122] There are compassionate reasons to encourage patients to "manage expectations" and be prepared for the worst outcome. However, encouraging patients and their loved ones to use the energy that hope provides in a constructive way may often be more efficacious than discouraging hope.

Emotions in the Medical Team

Emotions can play valuable roles in helping medical teams function smoothly and effectively. When team members feel like they have a consistent, reliable source of support and someone to turn to when things go wrong—referred to in the psychology literature as "secure attachment"—this provides a foundation from which they can take risks, test their own limits, and learn to excel. Attachment processes were first documented in infant-caregiver dyads, and then in the context of romantic relationships, but are now acknowledged to occur in a wide range of relationships throughout the lifespan.[123–125] Providing a safe haven and secure base is not the same as coddling or encouraging dependence. Rather, it's communicating that team members can count on each other and their leaders to behave supportively when they are vulnerable. Evidence is strong that teams in which members trust each other and their leaders in this way perform substantially better in educational and work contexts.[126]

Sometimes team members make mistakes, and in the medical setting consequences can range from trivial to lethal. Many errors cannot be overlooked, but they can be handled constructively. June Tangney differentiates guilt, which is rooted in the appraisal "I *did* something wrong," from shame, which is rooted in the appraisal "I *am* bad or worthless."[127] Tangney and colleagues' research suggests quite different consequences of these emotions. Although guilt motivates taking responsibility for one's actions, seeking to repair the damage done, and trying to avoid the error in the future, shame tends to lead to avoidance and resentment at what are perceived as unreasonable expectations. Providing healthy guidance to a trainee who has made a mistake can involve encouraging them to focus their attention on the action and how they can improve, rather than on assumptions about their dispositional ability or worth.

Finally, celebrating successes and other of life's joys also plays a role in building a strong, resilient team. In the context of interpersonal relationships, *capitalization* has been defined as a process in which one person shares a positive outcome or experience; relationship partners respond positively, vocally, and enthusiastically; and good feelings are amplified and distributed throughout the team as members continue engaging with the original positive event.[128] The second phase of the capitalization process, in which the response to good news is both positive and actively expressed, appears particularly important. Gable and colleagues have found that close relationships marked by more active-positive responses to one partner's good news are characterized by higher well-being, intimacy/trust, and relationship satisfaction among both partners.[128,129] Further studies reveal that capitalization can facilitate heightened relationship satisfaction, enjoyment, and cooperative behavior even among people who are not already close.[130]

■ CONCLUSION

In a high-pressure performance situation it can be tempting to try to shut down or ignore our emotions, and those of our patients and colleagues. It is true that such situations do not offer the leisure or bandwidth for lengthy emotional processing. However, open acknowledgment and sharing of emotions can have a wide range of benefits in terms of understanding team members' mindsets, guiding complex decision-making, and building a strong, cohesive, and resilient team. Emotions must often be managed, but this can be done in a way that validates them and makes use of their advantages, without allowing them to overcome judgment and action entirely. We hope this chapter has made a convincing case for the functional value of engaging with emotions in medical settings, as well as some concrete techniques for building that skill set.

REFERENCES

1. Cosmides L, Tooby J. Evolutionary psychology and the emotions. In: Lewis M, Haviland-Jones J, eds. *Handbook of Emotions*. 2nd ed. New York, NY: Guilford; 2000:91-115.

2. Ekman P. Universals and cultural differences in facial expressions of emotions. In: Cole J, ed. *Nebraska Symposium on Motivation*. Vol 19. Lincoln, NE: University of Nebraska Press; 1972:207-283.

3. Keltner D, Haidt J, Shiota MN. Social functionalism and the evolution of emotions. In: Schaller M, Simpson J, Kenrick D, eds. *Evolution and Social Psychology*. New York, NY: Psychological Press; 2006:115-142.

4. Lazarus RS. Progress on a cognitive-motivational-relational theory of emotion. *Am Psychol*. 1991;46(8):819-834.

5. Shiota MN. Theories of basic and discrete emotions. In: Scarantino A, ed. *Routledge Handbook of Emotion Theory*. Abingdon, UK: Routledge; 2021.

6. Damasio AR. *Descartes' Error*. New York, NY: Random House; 2006.

7. Dolcos F, Iordan AD, Dolcos S. Neural correlates of emotion-cognition interactions: a review of evidence from brain imaging investigations. *J Cogn Psychol*. 2011;23(6):669-694.

8. Lerner JS, Li Y, Valdesolo P, Kassam KS. Emotion and decision making. *Annu Rev Psychol*. 2015;66:799-823.

9. Gross JJ. Emotion regulation: current status and future prospects. *Psychol Inq*. 2015; 26(1):1-26.

10. Troy AS, Shallcross AJ, Mauss IB. A person-by-situation approach to emotion regulation: cognitive reappraisal can either help or hurt, depending on the context. *Psychol Sci*. 2013;24(12):2505-2514.

11. Webb TL, Miles E, Sheeran P. Dealing with feeling: a meta-analysis of the effectiveness of strategies derived from the process model of emotion regulation. *Psychol Bull*. 2012;138(4):775-808.

12. James W. What is an emotion? *Mind*. 1884;9:188-205.

13. Roseman IJ, Wiest C, Swartz TS. Phenomenology, behaviors, and goals differentiate discrete emotions. *J Pers Soc Psychol*. 1994;67(2):206-221.

14. Russell JA. Core affect and the psychological construction of emotion. *Psychol Rev*. 2003;110(1):145-172.

15. Tugade MM, Fredrickson BL, Feldman Barrett L. Psychological resilience and positive emotional granularity: examining the benefits of positive emotions on coping and health. *J Pers*. 2004;72(6):1161-1190.

16. Deonna JA, Scherer KR. The case of the disappearing intentional object: constraints on a definition of emotion. *Emot Rev*. 2010;2(1):44-52.

17. Ekman P. All emotions are basic. In: Ekman P, Davidson R, eds. *The Nature of Emotion: Fundamental Questions*. New York: NY: Oxford University Press; 1994.

18. Kreibig SD. Autonomic nervous system activity in emotion: a review. *Biol Psychol*. 2010;84(3):394-421.

19. Levenson RW. The autonomic nervous system and emotion. *Emot Rev*. 2014;6(2): 100-112.

20. Ekman P, Friesen WV, O'sullivan M, et al. Universals and cultural differences in the judgments of facial expressions of emotion. *J Pers Soc Psychol*. 1987;53(4):712-717.

21. Sauter DA, Eisner F, Ekman P, Scott SK. Cross-cultural recognition of basic emotions through nonverbal emotional vocalizations. *Proc Natl Acad Sci*. 2010;107(6): 2408-2412.

22. Gross JJ. The emerging field of emotion regulation: an integrative review. *Rev Gen Psychol*. 1998;2(3):271-299.

23. Moors A, Ellsworth PC, Scherer KR, Frijda NH. Appraisal theories of emotion: state of the art and future development. *Emot Rev*. 2013;5(2):119-124.

24. Clark DA, Beck AT. Cognitive theory and therapy of anxiety and depression: convergence with neurobiological findings. *Trends Cogn Sci*. 2010;14(9):418-424.

25. Goldin PR, Ziv M, Jazaieri H, et al. Cognitive reappraisal self-efficacy mediates the effects of individual cognitive-behavioral therapy for social anxiety disorder. *J Consult Clin Psychol.* 2012;80(6):1034-1040.

26. Smits JA, Julian K, Rosenfield D, Powers MB. Threat reappraisal as a mediator of symptom change in cognitive-behavioral treatment of anxiety disorders: a systematic review. *J Consult Clin Psychol.* 2012;80(4):624-635.

27. Tomkins SS. Affect theory. In: Scherer KR, Ekman P, eds. *Approaches to Emotion.* Hillsdale, NJ: Lawrence Erlbaum Associates; 1984.

28. Levenson RW. The intrapersonal functions of emotion. *Cogn Emot.* 1999;13(5):481-504.

29. Keltner D, Gross JJ. Functional accounts of emotions. *Cogn Emot.* 1999;13(5):467-480.

30. Roseman IJ. Appraisal in the emotion system: coherence in strategies for coping. *Emot Rev.* 2013;5(2):141-149.

31. Tooby J, Cosmides L. The evolutionary psychology of the emotions and their relationships to internal regulatory variables. In: Lewis M, Haviland-Jones J, Barrett L, eds. *Handbook of Emotions.* New York, NY: Guilford; 2008.

32. Lang PJ. Emotion's response patterns: the brain and the autonomic nervous system. *Emot Rev.* 2014;6(2):93-99.

33. Becker DV, Anderson US, Neuberg SL, et al. More memory bang for the attentional buck: self-protection goals enhance encoding efficiency for potentially threatening males. *Soc Psychol Pers Sci.* 2010;1(2):182-189.

34. Tracy JL, Randles D, Steckler CM. The nonverbal communication of emotions. *Curr Opin Behav Sci.* 2015;3:25-30.

35. Neuberg SL, Kenrick DT, Schaller M. Human threat management systems: self-protection and disease avoidance. *Neurosci Biobehav Rev.* 2011;35(4):1042-1051.

36. Mauss IB, Levenson RW, McCarter L, Wilhelm FH, Gross JJ. The tie that binds? Coherence among emotion experience, behavior, and physiology. *Emotion.* 2005; 5(2):175-190.

37. Phelps EA. Human emotion and memory: interactions of the amygdala and hippocampal complex. *Curr Opin Neurobiol.* 2004;14(2):198-202.

38. Graham J, Haidt J, Koleva S, et al. Moral foundations theory: the pragmatic validity of moral pluralism. In: *Advances in Experimental Social Psychology.* Vol 47. Elsevier; 2013:55-130.

39. Mesquita B, Ellsworth PC. The role of culture in appraisal. In: Scherer KR, ed. *Appraisal Processes in Emotion: Theory, Methods, Research.* Oxford, UK: Oxford University Press; 2001:233-248.

40. Chentsova-Dutton YE, Tsai JL. Self-focused attention and emotional reactivity: the role of culture. *J Pers Soc Psychol.* 2010;98(3):507-519.

41. Kitayama S, Markus HR, Matsumoto H. Culture, self, and emotion: a cultural perspective on "self-conscious" emotions. In: Tangney J, Fischer K, eds. *Self-Conscious Emotions: The Psychology of Shame, Guilt, Embarrassment, and Pride.* New York, NY: Guilford; 1995: 439-464.

42. Brescoll VL, Uhlmann EL. Can an angry woman get ahead? Status conferral, gender, and expression of emotion in the workplace. *Psychol Sci.* 2008;19(3):268-275.

43. Fischer AH, Rodriguez Mosquera PM, Van Vianen AE, Manstead AS. Gender and culture differences in emotion. *Emotion.* 2004;4(1):87-94.

44. Simon RW, Nath LE. Gender and emotion in the United States: do men and women differ in self-reports of feelings and expressive behavior? *Am J Sociol.* 2004;109(5):1137-1176.

45. Darwin C. *The Expression of the Emotions in Man and Animals.* New York, NY: Oxford University Press; 1872/1998.

46. Izard CE. *Human Emotions.* New York, NY: Plenum Press; 1977.

47. Cordaro DT, Sun R, Keltner D, Kamble S, Huddar N, McNeil G. Universals and cultural variations in 22 emotional expressions across five cultures. *Emotion.* 2018;18(1):75-93.

48. Elfenbein HA, Beaupré M, Lévesque M, Hess U. Toward a dialect theory: cultural differences in the expression and recognition of posed facial expressions. *Emotion.* 2007;7(1):131-146.

49. Cordaro DT, Keltner D, Tshering S, Wangchuk D, Flynn LM. The voice conveys emotion in ten globalized cultures and one remote village in Bhutan. *Emotion.* 2016;16(1):117-128.

50. Roseman IJ, Dhawan N, Rettek SI, Naidu R, Thapa K. Cultural differences and cross-cultural similarities in appraisals and emotional responses. *J Cross Cult Psychol.* 1995;26(1): 23-38.

51. Scherer KR. The role of culture in emotion-antecedent appraisal. *J Pers Soc Psychol.* 1997;73(5):902-922.

52. Levenson RW, Ekman P, Heider K, Friesen WV. Emotion and autonomic nervous system activity in the Minangkabau of West Sumatra. *J Pers Soc Psychol.* 1992;62(6): 972-988.

53. Laukka P, Neiberg D, Elfenbein HA. Evidence for cultural dialects in vocal emotion expression: acoustic classification within and across five nations. *Emotion.* 2014;14(3): 445-449.

54. Mesquita B, Frijda NH. Cultural variations in emotions: a review. *Psychol Bull.* 1992;112(2):179-204.

55. Russell JA. Culture and the categorization of emotions. *Psychol Bull.* 1991;110(3):426-450.

56. Shiota MN, Campos B, Gonzaga GC, Keltner D, Peng K. I love you but...: cultural differences in complexity of emotional experience during interaction with a romantic partner. *Cogn Emot.* 2010;24(5):786-799.

57. Soto JA, Levenson RW, Ebling R. Cultures of moderation and expression: emotional experience, behavior, and physiology in Chinese Americans and Mexican Americans. *Emotion.* 2005;5(2):154-165.

58. Tsai JL, Simeonova DI, Watanabe JT. Somatic and social: Chinese Americans talk about emotion. *Pers Soc Psychol Bull.* 2004;30(9):1226-1238.

59. Barrett LF. The conceptual act theory: a précis. *Emot Rev.* 2014;6(4):292-297.

60. Ekman P, Cordaro D. What is meant by calling emotions basic. *Emot Rev.* 2011;3(4): 364-370.

61. Tooby J. The emergence of evolutionary psychology. In: Pines D, ed. *Emerging Syntheses in Science.* Santa Fe, NM: Santa Fe Institute 1985.

62. Shiota MN, Campos B, Oveis C, Hertenstein MJ, Simon-Thomas E, Keltner D. Beyond happiness: building a science of discrete positive emotions. *Am Psychol.* 2017;72(7):617-643.

63. Rozin P, Haidt J, McCauley CR. Disgust: the body and soul emotion. In: Dalgliesh T, Power M, eds. *Handbook of Cognition and Emotion.* Chichester, England: John Wiley & Sons; 1999:429-445.

64. Schaller M, Park JH. The behavioral immune system (and why it matters). *Curr Dir Psychol Sci.* 2011;20(2):99-103.

65. Gable PA, Harmon-Jones E. Approach-motivated positive affect reduces breadth of attention. *Psychol Sci.* 2008;19(5):476-482.

66. Panksepp J, Moskal J. Dopamine and SEEKING: subcortical "reeard" systems and appetitive urges. In: Elliot A, ed. *Handbook of Approach and Avoidance Motivation.* New York, NY: Taylor & Francis; 2008:67-87.

67. Shiota MN, Neufeld SL, Yeung WH, Moser SE, Perea EF. Feeling good: autonomic nervous system responding in five positive emotions. *Emotion.* 2011;11(6): 1368-1378.

68. Harmon-Jones E, Peterson C, Gable PA, Harmon-Jones C. Anger and approach-avoidance motivation. In: Elliot A, ed. *Handbook of Approach and Avoidance Motivation.* New York, NY: Psychology Press; 2008:399-413.

69. Campbell DT. The two distinct routes beyond kin selection to ultrasociality: implications for the humanities and social sciences. In: Bridgeman D, ed. *The Nature of Prosocial Development: Theories and Strategies.* New York, NY: Academic Press; 1983:11-41.

70. Gonzaga GC, Turner RA, Keltner D, Campos B, Altemus M. Romantic love and sexual desire in close relationships. *Emotion.* 2006;6(2):163-179.

71. Griskevicius V, Goldstein NJ, Mortensen CR, Cialdini RB, Kenrick DT. Going along versus going alone: when fundamental motives facilitate strategic (non) conformity. *J Pers Soc Psychol.* 2006;91(2):281-294.

72. Haj-Mohamadi P, Gillath O, Rosenberg EL. Identifying a facial expression of flirtation and its effect on men. *J Sex Res.* 2020:1-9.

73. Trivers RL. The evolution of reciprocal altruism. *Q Rev Biol.* 1971;46(1):35-57.

74. Bartlett MY, DeSteno D. Gratitude and prosocial behavior: helping when it costs you. *Psychol Sci.* 2006;17(4):319-325.

75. Algoe SB, Fredrickson BL, Gable SL. The social functions of the emotion of gratitude via expression. *Emotion.* 2013;13(4):605-609.

76. Mikulincer M, Shaver PR. Boosting attachment security in adulthood: the "broaden-and-build" effects of security-enhancing mental representations and interpersonal contexts. In: Simpson J, Rholes W, eds. *Attachment Theory and Research: New Directions and Emerging Themes.* New York, NY: Guilford; 2015:124-144.

77. Graham EE. The involvement of sense of humor in the development of social relationships. *Comm Rep.* 1995;8(2):158-169.

78. Goetz JL, Keltner D, Simon-Thomas E. Compassion: an evolutionary analysis and empirical review. *Psychol Bull.* 2010;136(3):351-374.

79. O'Neil MJ, Danvers AF, Shiota MN. Nurturant love and caregiving emotions. In: Lench HC, ed. *The Function of Emotions.* New York, NY: Springer; 2018:175-193.

80. Balsters MJ, Krahmer EJ, Swerts MG, Vingerhoets AJ. Emotional tears facilitate the recognition of sadness and the perceived need for social support. *Evol Psychol.* 2013;11(1):148-158.

81. Sell A, Sznycer D, Al-Shawaf L, et al. The grammar of anger: mapping the computational architecture of a recalibrational emotion. *Cognition.* 2017;168:110-128.

82. Wang L, Northcraft GB, Van Kleef GA. Beyond negotiated outcomes: the hidden costs of anger expression in dyadic negotiation. *Organ Behav Hum Decis Process.* 2012;119(1):54-63.

83. Buss DM, Schmitt DP. Sexual strategies theory: an evolutionary perspective on human mating. *Psychol Rev.* 1993;100(2):204-232.

84. Tangney JP. Situational detenninants of shame and guilt in young adulthood. *Pers Soc Psychol Bull.* 1992;18(2):199-206.

85. Tracy JL, Robins RW. Emerging insights into the nature and function of pride. *Curr Dir Psychol Sci.* 2007;16(3):147-150.

86. Tracy JL, Robins RW. Show your pride: evidence for a discrete emotion expression. *Psychol Sci.* 2004;15(3):194-197.

87. Martens JP, Tracy JL. The emotional origins of a social learning bias: does the pride expression cue copying? *Soc Psychol Pers Sci.* 2013;4(4):492-499.

88. Tracy JL, Shariff AF, Zhao W, Henrich J. Cross-cultural evidence that the nonverbal expression of pride is an automatic status signal. *J Exp Psychol Gen.* 2013;142(1):163-180.

89. Keltner D, Buswell BN. Embarrassment: its distinct form and appeasement functions. *Psychol Bull.* 1997;122(3):250-270.

90. Keltner D. Signs of appeasement: evidence for the distinct displays of embarrassment, amusement, and shame. *J Pers Soc Psychol.* 1995;68(3):441-454.

91. Keltner D, Anderson C. Saving face for Darwin: the functions and uses of embarrassment. *Curr Dir Psychol Sci.* 2000;9(6):187-192.

92. Bechara A, Damasio H, Damasio AR. Emotion, decision making and the orbitofrontal cortex. *Cereb Cortex.* 2000;10(3):295-307.

93. Kenrick DT, Griskevicius V, Sundie JM, Li NP, Li YJ, Neuberg SL. Deep rationality: the evolutionary economics of decision making. *Soc Cogn.* 2009;27(5):764-785.

94. Kober H, Mende-Siedlecki P, Kross EF, et al. Prefrontal–striatal pathway underlies cognitive regulation of craving. *Proc Natl Acad Sci.* 2010;107(33):14811-14816.

95. Ochsner KM, Silvers J, Buhle J. Functional imaging studies of emotion regulation: a synthetic review and evolving model of the cognitive control of emotion. *Ann N Y Acad Sci.* 2012;1251:E1-24.

96. Hiser J, Koenigs M. The multifaceted role of the ventromedial prefrontal cortex in emotion, decision making, social cognition, and psychopathology. *Biol Psychiatry.* 2018;83(8):638-647.

97. Okon-Singer H, Hendler T, Pessoa L, Shackman AJ. The neurobiology of emotion–cognition interactions: fundamental questions and strategies for future research. *Front Hum Neurosci.* 2015;9:58.

98. Clore GL, Huntsinger JR. How emotions inform judgment and regulate thought. *Trends Cogn Sci.* 2007;11(9):393-399.

99. Lerner JS, Keltner D. Fear, anger, and risk. *J Pers Soc Psychol*. 2001;81(1):146-159.

100. Lerner JS, Small DA, Loewenstein G. Heart strings and purse strings: carryover effects of emotions on economic decisions. *Psychol Sci*. 2004;15(5):337-341.

101. Miller SL, Maner JK. Overperceiving disease cues: the basic cognition of the behavioral immune system. *J Pers Soc Psychol*. 2012;102(6):1198-1213.

102. Pham MT. Emotion and rationality: a critical review and interpretation of empirical evidence. *Rev Gen Psychol*. 2007;11(2):155-178.

103. Schwarz N. Emotion, cognition, and decision making. *Cogn Emot*. 2000;14(4):433-440.

104. Danvers AF, Shiota MN. Going off script: effects of awe on memory for script-typical and-irrelevant narrative detail. *Emotion*. 2017;17(6):938-952.

105. Finucane AM. The effect of fear and anger on selective attention. *Emotion*. 2011; 11(4):970-974.

106. Griskevicius V, Shiota MN, Neufeld SL. Influence of different positive emotions on persuasion processing: a functional evolutionary approach. *Emotion*. 2010;10(2):190-206.

107. Han S, Lerner JS, Keltner D. Feelings and consumer decision making: the appraisal-tendency framework. *J Consum Psychol*. 2007;17(3):158-168.

108. Keltner D, Ellsworth PC, Edwards K. Beyond simple pessimism: effects of sadness and anger on social perception. *J Pers Soc Psychol*. 1993;64(5):740-752.

109. Sapolsky RM, Freeman W. *Why Zebras Don't Get Ulcers: An Updated Guide to Stress, Stress Related Diseases, and Coping*. 2nd ed. New York, NY: WH Freeman and Company; 1998.

110. Gross JJ, Levenson RW. Hiding feelings: the acute effects of inhibiting negative and positive emotion. *J Abnorm Psychol*. 1997;106(1):95-103.

111. Troy AS, Shallcross AJ, Brunner A, Friedman R, Jones MC. Cognitive reappraisal and acceptance: effects on emotion, physiology, and perceived cognitive costs. *Emotion*. 2018;18(1):58-74.

112. Schwarz N, Clore GL. Mood, misattribution, and judgments of well-being: informative and directive functions of affective states. *J Pers Soc Psychol*. 1983;45(3):513-523.

113. Shiota MN, Levenson RW. Turn down the volume or change the channel? Emotional effects of detached versus positive reappraisal. *J Pers Soc Psychol*. 2012;103(3):416-429.

114. Ford BQ, Troy AS. Reappraisal reconsidered: a closer look at the costs of an acclaimed emotion-regulation strategy. *Curr Dir Psychol Sci*. 2019;28(2):195-203.

115. Lambert MJ, Barley DE. Research summary on the therapeutic relationship and psychotherapy outcome. *Psychother Theor Res Pract Train*. 2001;38(4):357-361.

116. Gable P, Harmon-Jones E. The blues broaden, but the nasty narrows: attentional consequences of negative affects low and high in motivational intensity. *Psychol Sci*. 2010;21(2):211-215.

117. Gable PA, Poole BD, Harmon-Jones E. Anger perceptually and conceptually narrows cognitive scope. *J Pers Soc Psychol*. 2015;109(1):163-174.

118. Moons WG, Mackie DM. Thinking straight while seeing red: the influence of anger on information processing. *Pers Soc Psychol Bull*. 2007;33(5):706-720.

119. Mather M, Sutherland MR. Arousal-biased competition in perception and memory. *Perspect Psychol Sci*. 2011;6(2):114-133.

120. Shiota M, Thrash T, Danvers A, Dombrowski J. Transcending the self: awe, elevation, and inspiration. In: Tugade MM, Shiota MN, Kirby L, eds. *Handbook of Positive Emotion*. New York, NY: Guilford; 2014:362-395.

121. Leotti LA, Iyengar SS, Ochsner KN. Born to choose: the origins and value of the need for control. *Trends Cogn Sci*. 2010;14(10):457-463.

122. Snyder CR. Hope theory: rainbows in the mind. *Psychol Inq*. 2002;13(4):249-275.

123. Ainsworth MD. Attachments across the life span. *Bull N Y Acad Med*. 1985;61(9):792-812.

124. Ainsworth MDS. The Bowlby-Ainsworth attachment theory. *Behav Brain Sci*. 1978; 1(3):436-438.

125. Mikulincer M, Shaver PR. The attachment behavioral system in adulthood: activation, psychodynamics, and interpersonal processes. In: Zanna M, ed. *Advances in Experimental Psychology*. Vol 35. Philadelphia, PA: Elsevier; 2003:53-152.

126. De Jong BA, Dirks KT, Gillespie N. Trust and team performance: a meta-analysis of main effects, moderators, and covariates. *J Appl Psychol*. 2016;101(8):1134-1150.

127. Tangney JP. Shame and guilt in interpersonal relationships. In: Tangney J, Fischer K, eds. *Self-Conscious Emotions: The Psychology of Shame, Guilt, Embarrassment, and Pride*. New York, NY: Guilford; 1995:114-139.

128. Peters BJ, Reis HT, Gable SL. Making the good even better: a review and theoretical model of interpersonal capitalization. *Soc Pers Psychol Compass*. 2018;12(7):e12407.

129. Gable SL, Reis HT, Impett EA, Asher ER. What do you do when things go right? The intrapersonal and interpersonal benefits of sharing positive events. *J Pers Soc Psychol*. 2004;87(2):228-245.

130. Reis HT, Smith SM, Carmichael CL, et al. Are you happy for me? How sharing positive events with others provides personal and interpersonal benefits. *J Pers Soc Psychol*. 2010;99(2):311-329.

Emotion and Illness

Anne-Josée Guimond, Laura D. Kubzansky, and Lewina O. Lee

■ UNDERSTANDING THE ROLE OF EMOTIONS IN HEALTH

Perspectives on Emotion and Health: An Overview

Emotions can affect health in numerous ways. Perhaps the most well-appreciated is that chronic illnesses present significant challenges in terms of psychological adjustment. Individuals not only have to navigate various physical symptoms and related emotional and social stressors in the time surrounding diagnosis and treatment, they also have to adapt to the longer-term consequences of disease and treatments (e.g., persistent pain, fatigue, cognitive impairment). Illness-related emotional experiences range from transient feelings of vulnerability, sadness, and fear, to conditions that can be long-lasting and more disabling, such as clinically significant depression and anxiety.[1] While many patients who develop chronic disease often report relatively low levels of psychological distress, prevalence of clinically relevant disorders (e.g., anxiety, depression) tends to be higher in these patients than in the general population. For example, the rate of major depressive disorder is two- to threefold higher in patients with cancer[2] or cardiovascular disease (CVD).[3,4] Psychological distress associated with illness and medical treatments is consequential for subsequent health outcomes. For instance, depression is linked to increased healthcare use,[5] poorer adherence to medical treatment,[6] and elevated risk for suicidal thoughts and actions in patients treated for cancer.[7] Depression and anxiety are related to poorer quality of life and daily functioning in cancer and CVD patients.[5,8] Conversely, indicators of psychological well-being, such as optimism and a capacity to experience positive emotions, suggest better adjustment to illness.[9]

Much has been written on emotions as a consequence of disease or as part of the disease management process (for more discussion on psychological adjustment to disease, see Hoyt and Stanton[9]), whereas the hypothesis that emotions play a role in health maintenance or disease development is more controversial.[10] However, substantial empirical evidence from the past decades has strongly suggested a causal relationship. In light of the evidence and to address the scarcity of resources for clinicians on this topic, in this chapter we focus on the role of emotions in disease development and health maintenance.

The pathways by which emotion influences health in different stages of illness (i.e., development, triggering, exacerbation, or progression of disease) are likely to differ. Thus, findings on effects of emotion on health do not necessarily generalize from the general population to patients (and vice versa). Hence, we prioritize research conducted in the general population aimed at understanding whether emotions influence the likelihood of developing disease. When relevant, we also discuss research showing how emotions influence disease progression in already-ill patients (e.g., recurrence or secondary episode of an illness, or exacerbation of symptoms). In addition, we recognize recent literature suggesting that the effects of different emotions are not uniform. In early research, investigators assumed that apparent health-beneficial effects of positive emotions were not due to unique effects of positive emotions per se, but rather because they indicated low levels of negative emotions. However, empirical evidence increasingly indicates that while negative emotions are likely to increase disease susceptibility, positive emotions appear to confer protective effects beyond simply signaling the absence of negative emotions.[11] Careful consideration of both the affective experience (i.e., valence, intensity, duration, frequency) and disease dimensions (e.g., type, stage, onset vs. progression, severity, and biological alterations) is thus needed when evaluating research in this area.

Emotions are multifaceted and involve one's subjective experience, behaviors, and physiology.[12] Specific emotions are thought to emerge as a product of the interaction between the person and the environment and to mediate between continually changing situations and the person's behavior.[12] Both positive and negative emotions are functionally necessary. For example, they can motivate adaptive behavioral responses to change problematic situations that triggered the emotion. For instance, fear motivates escape from danger, sadness motivates disengagement from loss, happiness motivates approach behaviors toward others, and so on.[12] Emotions may enhance decision making, provide information regarding the best course of action, inform us about other's intentions, and help us communicate our affective state and social behavior to others.[12] Importantly, the extent to which a specific emotion is harmful or helpful is context-dependent. Emotions are likely to be harmful when their intensity, duration, frequency, or type is inappropriate for a particular situation.[13]

Differentiating Between Stress and Emotion in the Context of Health: New Directions

Because research on emotion and health often involves "stress" as an exposure, an outcome, or a contextual factor, it is useful to distinguish between emotion and stress. The most widely adopted definition of stress comes from the stress and coping theory,[14] wherein stress occurs when individuals perceive or appraise external demands as exceeding their ability to cope. Links to health occur because the psychological appraisal triggers a cascade of physiological changes. While researchers and practitioners often agree on the potential detrimental influence of stress on health, there is tremendous ambiguity and inconsistency in definitions and measures of stress.[15] Briefly, a *stressor* refers to a stimulus that elicits a *stress response. Stressors* can be external to oneself such as life events, or internal such as memories of a traumatic event; they can occur across contexts, from socioeconomic such as neighborhood deprivation, to individual such as daily hassles. *Stress responses* can also occur across levels of experience, including emotional, behavioral, cognitive, neural, and physiological. *Perceived stress* commonly refers to a mix of emotions and thoughts in response to a stressor, such as feeling overwhelmed or anxious, and believing one has little control over the situation. Stressors and stress responses can vary temporally, from short-term (acute) to chronic. *Emotional states* are elicited when an important personal goal or value has been engaged, as these motivate adaptive action.[12] While emotional states are transient, *emotional traits* represent individual differences in the likelihood and intensity of experiencing specific emotions, which tend to generalize across a range of situations.

Research on the health sequelae of emotions has traditionally assessed emotional distress or well-being using time frames spanning months or years (see below for more detailed review). However, recent studies suggest that examining affective states and their dynamics over narrower time windows of days or hours may provide a more granular understanding of the processes by which emotional responses to events may influence subsequent health and well-being. Experience sampling methods assess participants' environments (e.g., presence of stressors), emotions, thoughts, and behaviors at random or fixed intervals over days. Daily diary and ecological momentary assessment (EMA) designs are examples of experience sampling methods. In daily diary designs, participants complete end-of-day diaries reporting on stressful events, their appraisals of these events, mood, and physical symptoms that occurred on each day. In EMA designs, participants take a short survey on a digital device (e.g., a smart phone application) at predetermined or random times throughout the day. Despite greater costs and participant burden, compared with traditional observational designs, experience sampling designs are less prone to recall bias and capture real-life experiences as they occur in daily life. Experience sampling also permits examination of temporal patterns among daily events, emotional and behavioral responses to events, and health outcomes ranging from short-term changes in glycemic control to longer-term phenomena like disease onset when such data collection strategies are embedded within longer-term follow-up studies.[16]

Increasingly, studies are leveraging experience sampling designs to examine different components of the daily stress processes, such as exposure to daily stressful events and emotional reactivity to stressors, as antecedents of downstream pathophysiological processes or adverse health outcomes. Emotional reactivity (also known as *affective reactivity*) to stressors refers to the likelihood of reacting emotionally to stressors.[17] For example, more emotionally reactive individuals tend to respond to stressors with stronger spikes in negative affect and greater reductions in positive affect. In a prospective study of older men followed for 10 years after an 8-day daily diary study, men with greater reductions in positive affect following daily stressors had higher risk of all-cause mortality, even after accounting for mean daily levels of positive and negative affect.[18] In one of the largest daily diary studies to date, higher emotional reactivity was associated with higher levels of inflammation cross-sectionally[19] and greater risk of developing one or more chronic conditions over 10 years.[20]

Technological advances have enabled researchers to incorporate ambulatory measures of objective health markers into experience sampling paradigms with relative ease and low costs. For example, physical activity can be assessed with an accelerometer embedded in popular wearable devices such as FitBit. The Pittsburgh Healthy Heart Project was among the earliest studies to bring together EMA measures of daily experiences, ambulatory biomarker measures, and objective assessment of health outcomes. It included 337 healthy older adults who completed two 3-day periods of ambulatory blood pressure monitoring and electronic diary assessments over a 4-month interval. Individuals who reported feeling their daily activities required high levels of effort had higher ambulatory blood pressure levels, which in turn explained their higher levels of atherosclerosis.[21]

Beyond the focus on stressful events, researchers have also begun to consider the association between daily positive events and physical health. For example, in one study positive events experienced in the morning were associated with steeper decline in cortisol on the same day; the association was independent of daily stressors and was not explained by daily positive affect levels.[22] As researchers explore innovative ways of leveraging the unique features of experience sampling designs and pairing these with ambulatory assessments, there are rich opportunities to learn about the more granular processes by which emotional experiences "get under the skin" to influence health.

A Model of Emotion and Health

Following prior work, we are guided by a conceptual model that illustrates how emotions influence physical health (see Fig. 3-1). This model suggests emotions can affect health directly and indirectly via different biobehavioral pathways. Emotions may directly influence health through biological alterations. For instance, hypothalamic-pituitary-adrenocortical (HPA) axis over-activity is a consequence of many negative psychological states (e.g., anger, anxiety, depression, posttraumatic stress disorder [PTSD]), and leads to dysregulation in the autonomic nervous system and a cascade of effects (e.g., endothelial dysfunction) that contribute to disease risk.[8] Emerging evidence suggests that bidirectional associations between sustained negative affect and altered gut microbiota play a role in the development of some illnesses such as irritable bowel syndrome (IBS).[23,24] More acute distress can trigger immediate

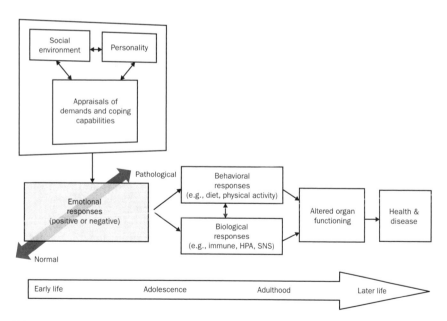

FIGURE 3-1. A model of the stress–emotion–health process. HPA: hypothalamic–pituitary–adrenal; SNS: sympathetic nervous system.

changes (e.g., elevations in catecholamines) that increase the risk of cardiac events.[25]

In contrast, accumulating research shows that positive emotions foster better physical health by enhancing the likelihood of restorative effects on biological processes (e.g., increases in anti-inflammatory processes) and/or buffering the toxic physiological effects of stressful experiences. Several indicators of positive psychological functioning (e.g., positive emotions, life satisfaction, and optimism) have been associated with healthier basal levels of cardiac function such as heart rate and heart rate variability and with healthier biological stress response.[11] Blood pressure, lipids, immune response, and inflammation are examples of other likely biological pathways. However, findings are not fully consistent, and results from larger longitudinal studies suggest that effects are small and can vary according to factors such as gender or race.[11] While some biological pathways are shared across negative and positive psychological factors,[11] negative and positive emotions may also have distinct effects on biological processes. For example, prior research showed associations of higher depression with higher concentrations of low-density and very-low-density lipoprotein cholesterol,[26] whereas higher psychological well-being levels have been linked to higher high-density lipoprotein levels only.[27]

Emotions may also affect health indirectly by influencing thoughts, decisions, and behaviors that in turn alter physiology. For example, boosts of positive affect experienced while engaging in health behaviors such as physical activity initiate unconscious or spontaneous cognitive processes (e.g., positive thoughts) that may orient individuals to repeat the previously enjoyed behaviors.[28] Emotions can change risk perception, which influences health-relevant decisions such as undergoing screenings, seeking treatment, or adhering to diet regimens, and thus shape subsequent physical health.[8] In CVD patients, psychological distress has been linked to worse medication adherence,[6] whereas positive affect has been associated with better medication and treatment adherence.[29] Effects of emotions on health can also be exerted via social processes, such as the quality and quantity of one's social relationships.[8] As highlighted in the model, all processes unfold over the life course. Further, the model recognizes that both the physical environment and social context play an important role in determining which emotions are likely to be experienced, how they are expressed, and their consequences.

A number of study design issues present challenges for research on emotion and health. First, due to feasibility issues (i.e., it is impossible to assign individuals to experience chronically one emotion or another prior to disease development), randomized controlled studies cannot be used to test if an emotion is causally associated with increased risk of developing disease. Prospective cohort studies, in which emotions are measured among initially disease-free individuals, are the most convincing design for testing this hypothesis as they preserve the temporal order of the linkage between emotion and disease onset and reduce concerns about reverse causality. However, these designs remain susceptible to concerns such as hidden sources of reverse causality (i.e., prodromal disease influencing emotions), or unmeasured variables (e.g., genetic risk) that drive the apparent emotion–health relationship. Moreover, variations in exclusion criteria for baseline health status and in covariate adjustment present challenges for comparing findings across studies. While most epidemiological studies are designed to test the unidirectional hypothesis that emotions influence health, clinicians should keep in mind that emotion–health relationships are likely to be bidirectional.

Other issues relate to the definition and measurement of emotion and health. Because psychological phenomena are not commonly the main focus of epidemiological research, measurement of emotion is less than ideal in many studies (e.g., single-item measures). Moreover, epidemiological studies often lump together depression and anxiety as if they represent a single emotion, while mental health specialists view them as distinct states that, albeit highly comorbid, can be experienced independently from one another.[30] Inconsistent definitions of emotional phenomena (e.g., psychological distress) or health outcomes (e.g., metabolic syndrome) across studies can also make comparison of findings difficult.

■ EVIDENCE FOR THE ROLE OF EMOTION IN HEALTH

In this section, we review evidence regarding the association of psychological ill-being (depression, anxiety, posttraumatic stress, and anger) and well-being (e.g., optimism, purpose in life) in relation to the etiology and progression of several disease types. Much research on the role of emotion in maintaining health or in the etiology of disease has been carried out in the context of cardiometabolic conditions which are leading causes of morbidity and mortality in the United States. Hence, we focus on these outcomes, but also consider associations with cancer, infectious and immune-mediated diseases, as well as functional somatic syndromes when the research is reasonably robust. Given the volume of work available, we focus on landmark studies and key findings and prioritize the most methodologically rigorous research. Much of this work reports either the odds of developing a given health outcome associated with the emotion under study, or the relative risk, i.e., the ratio of the probability that the disease/condition will occur in the group experiencing a given emotion versus the probability that the same endpoint will occur among individuals who did not experience that emotion.[31] Based on the totality of evidence reviewed in this section, clinical takeaways will be provided later in this chapter.

Cardiometabolic Conditions

Psychological Ill-Being and Coronary Heart Disease

Much of the research on psychological ill-being and coronary heart disease (CHD) has focused on depression as a risk factor for both disease development and progression. Six meta-analyses consistently documented that depressed individuals were 1.3 to 2.1 times[1] more likely to develop CHD than nondepressed individuals (see review by Carney and Freedland[32]). Variations in effect size estimates are attributable to differences in study selection criteria, study population, assessment method and definition of depression and CHD, follow-up duration, and importantly, covariate adjustment. Notwithstanding the limitation that not all studies include a comprehensive panel of potential confounders, the bulk of the evidence suggests depression is an independent risk factor for CHD even after accounting for demographics, traditional coronary risk factors (e.g., cholesterol, blood pressure), and lifestyle factors.

Meta-analytic findings also support anxiety as an etiologic factor in the development of CHD, with 26 prospective studies reporting on average a 1.5-fold higher risk[2] after carefully accounting for baseline health status.[33] An earlier meta-analysis, which considered studies among initially healthy individuals only, reported a 26% greater risk[3] among those with higher anxiety.[34] Recent studies have also examined the role of posttraumatic stress disorder (PTSD) in the development of CHD. PTSD is a psychiatric disorder which entails severe emotional distress in conjunction with dysregulation of the stress response system following exposure to at least one traumatic event, such as threatened or actual death, serious injury, or sexual violence. Its hallmark features include persistent re-experiencing of the traumatic event (e.g., nightmares or intrusive memories), avoidance of thoughts, feelings, and reminders of the event, trauma-related negative thoughts (e.g., exaggerated self-blame), feelings (e.g., guilt), arousal (e.g., sleep and concentration difficulties), and reactivity (e.g., constant vigilance) for at least 1 month. In a meta-analysis of six studies comprising 402,274 initially CHD-free individuals, PTSD was associated with a 55% greater risk[4] for CHD onset and

---

[1]Odds ratios (ORs) or relative risks (RRs) ranged from 1.30 (95% confidence interval [CI] 1.22–1.40) to 2.08 (95%CI 1.69–2.55).
[2]Pooled RR = 1.49, 95%CI 1.31–1.69.
[3]95% CI 1.15–1.38.
[4]95%CI 1.34–1.79.

cardiac-specific mortality.[35] More recently, Gibson et al.[36] examined PTSD and CVD using nationwide patient health records between 2008 and 2015 from the U.S. Veterans Health Administration. Among 2.7 million veterans who were initially CVD-free, PTSD, diabetes, and their comorbidity were each independently associated with higher risk of CVD onset, after adjusting for demographics and other cardiometabolic conditions.

The etiologic role of anger and hostility in CHD has its roots in research on the Type A behavior pattern, an action–emotion complex characterized by hostility, competitiveness, and a sense of urgency. Mixed evidence for its association with CHD led researchers to question its clinical utility (see review by Matthews[37]), and subsequent work has focused on anger and hostility. Anger refers to an unpleasant emotion in response to events perceived as unjust and is sometimes operationalized as comprised of related but distinct components such as trait or dispositional anger, anger expression, and anger control. Hostility refers to an attitude directed toward others, often accompanied by the emotional component of anger. A meta-analysis of 17 initially healthy cohorts comprising 71,606 individuals reported higher anger and hostility were associated with moderately greater risk of developing CHD in men, but not in women.[5,38] Of note, only four of these studies reported findings on women. Importantly, findings further suggested behavioral factors (e.g., smoking, sedentary behavior) may largely explain the relationship between anger and hostility and CHD development, suggesting that targeting changes in health behaviors could disrupt the linkages between anger and CHD-related outcomes.

A large literature has also documented the role of negative emotions in CHD progression. Important for clinicians to note, though, it is not always the case that the emotions are specifically triggered by disease development, and in fact some research suggests that effects are particularly problematic among those patients who were experiencing high levels of these negative emotions well before the disease onset.[39] As a result, different treatments for these psychological states may be more effective if clinicians can establish whether distress has been long-standing or has only recently onset in the context of the acute health events. For example, PTSD has been linked with both onset and progression of CVD; however, many studies considering incidence (i.e., newly developed disease) have been able to rule out the possibility that the PTSD was triggered by receiving a life-threatening diagnosis.

With regard to the role of emotion in disease progression, depression has received the most attention and is recognized by the American

---

[5]Hazard ratio (HR) for men = 1.22, 95%CI 1.09–1.36; HR for women = 1.07, 95%CI 0.70–1.63.

Heart Association (AHA) as a risk factor for poor prognosis among patients with acute coronary syndrome (ACS; i.e., a range of conditions associated with sudden, reduced blood flow to the heart, such as myocardial infarction[40]). Summarizing the findings of six meta-analyses on depression and CHD progression, Carney and Freedland[32] reported depression was associated with 33–171% greater risk for all-cause mortality, cardiac mortality, or cardiovascular events. Because these associations may be partially due to greater CHD severity among more severely depressed patients, to account more fully for potential confounding (or reverse causality), some studies have incorporated a composite index summarizing across a large set of cardiac risk factors that predicts short-term mortality risk among patients hospitalized for ACS. Even after adjusting for this index, depression remained predictive of cardiac event recurrence among myocardial infarct (MI) survivors,[41] further supporting depression as an independent risk factor for worse prognosis among CHD patients. Anxiety is also linked to worse clinical outcomes in this patient population. Two recent meta-analyses have found it was associated with substantially greater risk of subsequent major cardiovascular events, cardiovascular or all-cause mortality ranging from 21 to 47% excess risk depending on the endpoint and the specific patient population.[42,43] Notably, adjusting for depression consistently and strongly attenuated the association of anxiety to clinical outcomes in CHD patients, suggesting likely overlap in the pathways by which these negative emotions influence CHD progression. Such findings may suggest that clinicians working with these patient populations may want to assess patients for emotional disturbances beyond depression and consider carefully the potentially greater impact of comorbid forms of emotional disturbance.

Anger and hostility have also been consistently linked to worse cardiac outcomes in CHD patients. A meta-analysis of 19 prospective studies found anxiety and hostility were associated with a 23% greater risk[6] for CHD outcomes in patient populations.[38] Similar to findings with new onset CHD, studies generally suggested this association among CHD patients might also be largely explained by the greater likelihood of individuals with high levels of anger and hostility to engage in unhealthy behaviors, and targeting such behaviors as well as the upstream psychological distress might be one way to improve outcomes in this population. Finally, growing evidence supports a bidirectional association between PTSD and cardiac pathology.[44] A meta-analysis of three studies found that PTSD was associated with twice the risk[7]

---

[6]95%CI 1.08–1.42.
[7]95%CI 1.69–2.37.

for ACS recurrence or mortality even after adjustment for demographical, clinical, and psychosocial risk factors, including depression.[45] A nascent body of research provides suggestive evidence that PTSD can develop subsequent to life-threatening illness, including ACS (see Ref. 44).

Psychological Ill-Being and Stroke

Similar to CHD, most research on psychological risk factors for stroke has focused on depression. Meta-analytic evidence based on 24 prospective studies of initially stroke-free participants suggested a 44% greater risk[8] for incident stroke for individuals with versus without depression. Risk estimates were similar for men and women; however, individuals aged 65 or older were at greater risk than younger individuals (77% greater risk in older vs. 30% greater risk in younger individuals).[46] A recent study examined 2-year change in depressive symptoms in relation to incident stroke risk among 4,319 Medicare-eligible adults aged 65 and older.[47] Relative to stable low depressive symptoms, persistently elevated depressive symptoms conferred substantially higher risk[9] for incident stroke in the following year, independently of previous cumulative exposure to depressive symptoms. Neither new onset of depressive symptoms nor improved depressive symptoms was associated with elevated risk.

Few studies have examined anxiety in relation to stroke onset, even fewer have considered PTSD, and a limited set has evaluated anger. For anxiety, initial evidence is suggestive. In eight prospective cohort studies, three found anxiety disorders associated with a moderately increased risk for stroke.[48] For example, considering PTSD, in a sample of 987,855 users of the U.S. Veterans healthcare system without any history of stroke or transient ischemic attack (TIA), PTSD diagnosis was associated with substantial excess risk[10] for incident ischemic stroke and incident TIA over 13 years. Importantly, the risk remained significantly elevated after adjustment for lifestyle factors, comorbid depression, and generalized anxiety, indicating effects of PTSD on stroke risk above and beyond these factors.[49] Evidence is more mixed for anger and hostility as etiologic factors for stroke. In the only meta-analysis to date, anxiety and hostility were not associated with a significantly increased risk[11] for incident stroke.[50] However, these studies were heterogeneous with regard to how anger/hostility was measured and the extent to which they accounted for baseline health status. The meta-analysis further reported more robust

---

[8]95%CI 1.26-1.65.
[9]HR=1.65, 95% CI 1.06–2.56.
[10]HR for stroke=1.60, 95%CI 1.45–1.77; HR for TIA=1.84, 95%CI 1.46–2.32.
[11]HR=1.08, 95%CI 0.79–1.47.

associations evident among individuals aged ≥60 (40% greater risk), those without baseline CHD (33% greater risk[12]), and after omitting one study using an all-male sample of higher-SES health professionals.

Beyond research on the prevalence of common psychiatric disturbances such as anxiety, depression, PTSD, or difficulties controlling anger and aggression among stroke patients, the impact of negative emotions on post-stroke clinical outcomes is largely understudied. A few studies have linked depression to greater risk of cerebrovascular event recurrence and mortality.[51] A recent joint statement from the AHA and American Stroke Association provides a comprehensive review on the epidemiology, pathophysiology, outcomes, management, and prevention of poststroke depression, demonstrating explicit acknowledgment of, and intervention for, the interrelatedness of emotion and illness.[51]

Psychological Ill-Being and Diabetes

Depression and anxiety have been identified as risk factors for the development of diabetes. In a meta-analysis conducted among 424,557 adults, a 38% greater risk[13] was found for incident diabetes in depressed versus non-depressed individuals.[52] For anxiety, a meta-analysis comprising 15 studies conducted among over 1.7 million individuals reported an even more substantial risk[14] for developing diabetes in anxious versus nonanxious individuals. This association was robust to adjustment for a comprehensive range of potential confounders, though there was significant heterogeneity across studies in covariate adjustment.[53] Growing evidence also supports the etiologic role of PTSD in diabetes. In a large prospective study of U.S. military service members followed for 6 years, PTSD was associated with 38% greater odds[15] of developing diabetes, after adjusting for numerous other risk factors.[54] A recent longitudinal study reported lower diabetes incidence[16] among individuals with PTSD who did versus did not experience a clinically meaningful reduction in PTSD symptoms in a 1-year period.[55] Such findings are particularly exciting as they suggest reductions in psychological distress might translate into lower disease risk. While clinicians are often focused on mental health as an important endpoint in its own right, these data suggest successful treatment may have important sequelae for physical health as well.

---

[12]Aged ≥60: 95%CI 1.01–1.93; without baseline CHD: 95%CI 1.06–1.67.
[13]95%CI 1.23–1.55.
[14]OR=1.47, 95%CI 1.23–1.75.
[15]95%CI 1.02–1.87.
[16]HR=0.49, 95%CI 0.26–0.95.

Less is known about the role of anger in the development of diabetes. Two studies have examined trait anger and its two subscales, anger temperament (i.e., being generally quick tempered and hotheaded) and anger reaction (i.e., the degree to which one experiences anger when provoked), in relation to incident diabetes. In a biracial cohort study of 11,615 middle-aged U.S. adults, those in the highest versus lowest tertile of anger temperament had 31% elevated risk[17] of developing Type 2 diabetes over 6 years, after adjusting for demographics and lifestyle factors, although no associations with trait anger or anger reaction were evident. In a multiethnic U.S. population-based cohort of 6,814 adults, those with high versus low levels of trait anger and anger reaction (but not anger temperament) had elevated risks of incident diabetes over a median follow-up of 9 years.[56] In both studies, the effect estimates were attenuated by adjustment for metabolic factors (e.g., fasting glucose, waist-hip ratio), suggesting anger may contribute to diabetes risk via biological pathways such as insulin insensitivity and adiposity.

Given the chronic course of diabetes and the challenges of managing a highly complex regimen to control the illness and prevent complications, it is unsurprising that psychological distress is highly prevalent among diabetic patients.[57] Progression-related research has considered the role of negative emotions in relation to clinical markers, disease management, and psychological factors related to coping with the disease (see Refs. 57 and 58 for reviews). Related work has also examined psychological ill-being in relation to metabolic syndrome, the co-occurrence of cardiometabolic conditions that precede the development of diabetes and CVD, including obesity, hyperglycemia, dyslipidemia, and hypertension.

Our review indicates there is strong prospective evidence linking various forms of distress to both the onset and progression of CHD. Strong prospective evidence supports an association of depression with both the onset and progression of stroke, as well as supports a role for both depression and anxiety in the development of diabetes. As discussed later in this chapter, these findings suggest that population-level surveillance of negative emotions may help identify those at risk for developing chronic health conditions. In clinical settings working with patients with cardiometabolic conditions, routine screening of patients' emotional states may also be useful for identifying individuals who are at greater risk of poor adherence to prescribed regimens and a worse prognosis. Clinicians should also attend to and inquire about contextual factors (e.g., socioeconomic status, social support) that influence patients' emotional well-being. Referrals to and care coordination with mental health

---

[17]95%CI 1.08–1.60.

specialists (e.g., psychologists, social workers) should be incorporated as standard practice.

Psychological Well-Being and Cardiometabolic Disease

Over three decades of research has established an association between psychological well-being and reduced risks of developing cardiometabolic disease. A systematic review focusing on the most rigorous studies identified several facets of psychological well-being that were consistently associated with reduced risk of incident CVD in prospective studies.[11,59] Importantly, the associations generally withstood adjustment for psychological distress, indicating that the presence of well-being signaled more than the absence of ill-being. Across studies, prospective evidence was strongest for optimism. For example, in a prospective study of 70,021 women followed for 10 years, those scoring in the highest versus lowest quartile of optimism were associated with approximately 40% lower risk[18] of CHD and stroke mortality, after adjusting for sociodemographic factors and even after excluding women with prevalent diseases at baseline.[60] Numerous studies have also reported a prospective association of purpose in life with reduced risk of CVD onset and progression. For example, in a study drawn from a U.S. nationally representative sample of adults aged 50 and above, Kim et al.[61] reported that risk[19] of stroke incidence was reduced monotonically with each standard deviation increase in purpose in life score over 4 years. The association was maintained after adjustment for demographics, biological factors, health behaviors, negative, and other positive (optimism, social participation) psychological factors. Using data from the same panel study but focusing on a subset of 1,546 individuals with prevalent CHD at baseline, Kim et al.[62] further reported a reduced risk for MI over a 2-year follow-up among those with higher baseline levels of purpose in life.

Psychological well-being has also been associated with more favorable outcomes on other cardiometabolic endpoints, including disease progression. For example, in a study of 754 middle-aged adults, each standard deviation higher in life satisfaction at baseline was associated with a modestly lower risk[20] of developing a range of self-reported cardiometabolic conditions 9 years later, after adjusting for demographics, family history of heart disease, and depression. Moreover, in additional analyses that accounted for having a cardiometabolic condition at baseline, higher initial life satisfaction levels were also associated with having a lower cardiometabolic risk score as defined

---

[18]HR for CHD mortality = 0.62, 95%CI 0.50–0.76; HR for stroke mortality = 0.61, 95%CI 0.43–0.85.
[19]OR = 0.78, 95%CI 0.67–0.91.
[20]Prevalence ratio = 0.93, 95%CI 0.88–0.99.

according to objective assessment of eight different biomarkers at follow-up, suggesting findings are not simply an artifact of the tendency of people who have a more positive outlook to report themselves to be in better health.[63] This study further found that smoking cessation and higher physical activity were associated with both higher life satisfaction and reduced cardiometabolic risk suggesting a behavioral pathway by which life satisfaction might protect against the development and progression of metabolic dysregulation. Relatedly, a systematic review of studies conducted with diabetic patients found that positive psychological characteristics, such as higher levels of positive affect and self-efficacy, were associated with better glycemic control, fewer medical complications, and lower mortality risk.[64] While medicine has traditionally adopted a deficits approach that emphasizes negative risk factors for adverse health outcomes, these findings highlight the potential value of efforts to assess and promote psychological well-being in healthcare and community settings.

Cancer

The hypothesis that emotions can influence the development and the progression of cancer has long been controversial. In the 1980s and 1990s, this idea was mostly influenced by empirical studies that showed associations between a cancer-prone "type C personality" (i.e., poor recognition of one's emotions and needs, and feeling helpless or fatalistic about negative events)[65] and higher risk of developing cancer, considering all cancers together.[66] Spiegel's findings of associations between supportive-expressive group therapy—a psychological intervention that encourages the expression of feelings and concerns—and increased survival in women with metastatic breast cancer further fueled the hypothesis that emotions could influence the course of cancer.[67] However, many of these studies failed to replicate and some were criticized for their methodological flaws.[68] Mixed findings may be partly due to challenges in conducting methodologically rigorous studies on the contribution of emotions to cancer incidence and mortality. To avoid small samples and limited power that often occur when examining specific cancers, many studies combine cancer types. However, the term "cancer" refers to over 100 diseases with multiple etiologies and varied biological specificities; thus, combining across cancers may obscure important relationships. Moreover, for most cancers there is a long latency in their development and it can be difficult to ascertain the true date of onset. Because it may take as long as 18 years for tumor cells to develop into detectable tumors, a minimum of 18-year follow-up has been recommended for studies of cancer incidence, a significant challenge for conducting longitudinal research.[69]

These challenges notwithstanding, several high-quality studies have recently investigated the effect of negative emotions, notably depression, anxiety, and PTSD, on both incidence and progression of several types of cancer. A recent meta-analysis of cohort studies reported that depression and anxiety disorders were prospectively associated with a modestly increased risk[21] for developing cancer.[70] When considering specific cancer sites, significant associations were observed only for lung, oral cavity, prostate, and skin cancer. Associations were generally stronger in studies with follow-up $\geq$ 10 years. In one recent study, researchers reported a twofold increased risk of ovarian cancer in women with PTSD symptoms as compared to women without trauma exposure,[71] although findings in other studies examining PTSD and cancer risk have been less consistent, perhaps due in part to small case counts and limited statistical power.[72] Regarding cancer progression, studies have also demonstrated depression and anxiety are linked to a markedly greater risk[22] of cancer-specific mortality.[70] Taken together, these findings suggest that negative emotions, especially anxious and depressive symptoms, may have far-reaching effects beyond those on mental health; thus, otherwise healthy patients experiencing high levels of distress may benefit from more frequent screening for cancer (or other chronic diseases) while cancer patients may benefit from more routine screening for anxiety and depression and referrals to specialized mental healthcare such as psycho-oncology services.

Less work has considered positive psychological functioning in relation to cancer incidence and progression. The idea that positive thinking and a "fighting spirit" can slow the progression and rate of disease development has been controversial; some have argued the unrealistic pressure of feeling constantly positive when facing a life-threatening illness can encourage the suppression of negative emotions that are normal in that context, induce guilt and self-blame for the disease or its progression, and promote false hope to the patients and their families.[73] This "tyranny of positive thinking"[74] is particularly salient in the media and popular discourse surrounding cancer, perhaps more than for other illnesses. It is therefore important to consider these issues carefully while examining how positive psychological functioning may contribute to cancer onset and progression and evaluating how this knowledge can be used to inform the development of psychosocial interventions. Among the handful of prospective studies examining whether positive emotions might reduce risk of developing cancer, evidence has been mixed. For example, while in one large study of 50,358 participants followed for an

---

[21]RR=1.13, 95%CI 1.06–1.19.
[22]RR=1.21, 95%CI 1.16–1.26.

average of 8 years, higher life satisfaction was inversely related to cancer risk in women[75] other somewhat smaller studies showed no association between life satisfaction or *ikigai* (a Japanese concept referring to one's sense that life is worth living) and risk of developing cancer.[76] With regard to disease progression, findings on cancer are generally weaker than results for cardiometabolic or infectious outcomes.[73] Although a recent 6-year follow-up study of more than 70,000 women showed highest versus lowest quartile of optimism was associated with significantly lower risk[23] of cancer mortality (all types),[60] more research is needed to understand how positive emotions influence cancer progression, including recurrence.

Infectious and Immune-Mediated Diseases

Psychological distress and stressors are posited to affect susceptibility to infectious diseases via immune function downregulation.[77] For instance, a 1-year prospective study of healthy midlife adults examined bidirectional associations between levels of psychological distress and changes in markers of immune function, including natural killer (NK) cell, B-, and T-cell counts.[78] Higher levels of distress were associated with future suppression of NK cell immunity (but not the other cell types), but not the reverse, suggesting that emotions may alter cellular immunity. Other work has tested effects of distress on immune-related outcomes using a viral challenge paradigm. In these studies, emotions' levels were measured before exposing healthy participants to a common cold virus. Participants were then quarantined and monitored for the development of clinically verified illness ascertained with markers including antibody response, nasal mucociliary clearance, and nasal mucus production.[79] After controlling for various potential confounders, participants with higher levels of negative emotion were more likely to develop clinical illness,[80] while those expressing more positive emotions were at reduced risk.[79] Related work has linked psychological distress with a less robust immune response to vaccination[81] and an amplified inflammatory response after vaccination.[82] Because they evaluate real-world outcomes (i.e., common cold, vaccination response), these studies are uniquely compelling; however, relatively few such studies have been conducted due to their methodological and logistical complexities.

Only a handful of epidemiological studies have investigated the prospective associations of emotion and infectious disease onset or progression, in part because such endpoints can be challenging to track. However, findings to

---

[23]HR = 0.84, 95%CI 0.74–0.96.

date are intriguing. A population-based study of 976,398 Danish individuals reported that the risk of a wide range of infections increased substantially[24] during the first year after the onset of a depressive episode and remained elevated for up to 11 years and beyond.[83] In a recent study conducted among 144,919 individuals with stress-related disorders (i.e., PTSD, acute stress reaction, adjustment disorder, and other stress reactions) and their matched siblings during a mean follow-up of 8 years, individuals with a diagnosis of any stress-related disorder were also at marked increased risk of developing life-threatening infections. When considering PTSD alone, the risk for life-threatening infection was increased almost twofold[25] in individuals with versus without PTSD.[84] Little work to date has considered anxiety or positive emotions in relation to infectious disease onset.

Both negative and positive emotions have been associated with markers of infectious disease progression and mortality. For example, a longitudinal study of 1,494 HIV patients investigated the links between longitudinal trajectories of depression and CD4 count, a marker of immune function. Contrary to the researcher's hypothesis, patients who sustained high versus low levels of depression were not at higher risk of having a low (i.e., unhealthy) CD4 count. However, patients with moderate and ascending levels of depression across the follow-up were at higher risk of having a low CD4 count.[85] These findings suggest an increase in negative emotions may indicate a greater likelihood of having a heightened vulnerability to compromised immune function, and therefore highlight the potential value of clinicians explicitly considering changes in emotion over time. For instance, by monitoring HIV patients' emotions routinely, clinicians might have early warning of further deterioration in this already vulnerable population, and thereby may be able to intervene before more pronounced problems occur. Other work has found higher levels of positive affect are associated with subsequently having higher viral suppression in women with HIV.[86] Consistent with these findings, other studies have not only demonstrated that higher levels of depression and psychological distress predict greater risk of mortality in patients with HIV,[87] but have also shown positive psychological well-being (e.g., positive affect, optimism) is linked with lower mortality in HIV patients,[88] and with lower risk of mortality from infection in the general population.[60]

Studying other immune-mediated outcomes can present methodological challenges given the long latency, their relatively earlier onset in the life course, and the frequency of nonspecific symptoms that occur prodomally,

---

[24]Incidence rate ratio=1.61, 95%CI 1.49–1.74.
[25]Any stress-related disorder HR=1.47, 95%CI 1.37–1.58; PTSD alone HR=1.92, 95%CI 1.46–2.52.

all of which make it difficult to disentangle causes and consequences of emotional experience. That said, while prospective studies are limited, they have generally found anxiety, depression, and PTSD are associated with increased risk of incident rheumatoid arthritis[89] and asthma.[90] Prospective research also showed depressed mood preceded (as well as followed) higher levels of markers of disease activity in 545 patients with rheumatoid arthritis.[91] Most research on emotion in relation to risk of autoimmune disorders has focused on psychological distress and anxiety, but two large cohort studies have recently reported that higher levels of psychological well-being were linked with decreased risk of incident arthritis.[92,93] Taken together, these findings suggest that identifying patients' levels of negative as well as positive emotions is relevant not only to immune-mediated disease onset, but also to treatment and clinical outcomes. This highlights the importance of referring patients who experience elevated or sustained negative emotions to specialists such as health psychologists, who have expertise in the assessment and treatment of psychological disorders in patients presenting physical illnesses using evidence-based treatments such as cognitive behavioral therapy.

Functional Somatic Syndromes

Functional somatic syndromes encompass a set of conditions for which there is no known physical or biological etiology or that demonstrate inconsistent laboratory abnormalities.[94] They include, but are not limited to, IBS, fibromyalgia, and chronic fatigue syndrome. Typically complex and highly overlapping, these conditions are characterized by the predominance of psychosomatic symptoms such as pain and fatigue.[94] Comorbidity with psychiatric disorders, particularly anxiety and depression, tends to be high.[94] Because their etiology is influenced by biological, behavioral, environmental, and psychological factors, functional somatic syndromes are often conceptualized as biopsychosocial disorders.[95,96] One of the most widely used frameworks for understanding and treating functional somatic syndromes in health psychology is the cognitive-behavioral approach. According to the cognitive-behavioral therapy case conceptualization, negative emotions can be viewed as either predisposing (e.g., early-onset psychiatric disorders or trait anxiety), precipitating (e.g., acute episodes of anxiety or mood disorder), or perpetuating (e.g., hypersensitivity to anxiety-induced somatic reactions) factors for functional somatic syndromes, alongside other risk factors[95,96] (for a detailed illustration of the cognitive-behavioral model applied to IBS, see Ref. 95).

Results from several prospective studies support the idea that anxiety, depression, and trauma-related symptoms are risk factors for functional somatic syndromes. A meta-analysis of prospective and case-control studies reported a twofold risk[26] of developing IBS in individuals with versus without anxiety and depressive disorders.[96] Another meta-analysis showed that exposure to trauma was associated with an almost threefold increased risk of developing a functional somatic syndrome.[94] Other work has suggested a bidirectional relationship between anxiety and depression and functional somatic syndromes.[97] Some research has also focused on the contribution of negative emotions to symptom exacerbation in these disorders. In patients with IBS, anxiety, depression, and anger have been associated with increased abdominal pain, colonic motility, and diarrhea (for a detailed review, see Muscatello et al.[24]). Mood and anxiety disorders have also been linked with higher levels of pain and poorer health status in patients with fibromyalgia.[98]

Interpretation and increased attention to somatic symptoms can exacerbate symptoms and lead to their perpetuation.[95] Biological mechanisms are also likely at play. For instance, increasing evidence suggests that dysfunction of the gut–brain axis is involved in both the onset and exacerbation of IBS. The gut–brain axis represents the bidirectional connection between the brain and the gastrointestinal tract that involves a complex interplay between the endocrine system (e.g., HPA axis), immune system (e.g., proinflammatory cytokines), as well as the autonomic nervous system.[23] Signals from the gastrointestinal tract (e.g., visceral sensation, intestinal microbiota) influence reflex regulation, mood states, and behavioral regulation in a bottom-up relation.[23] In turn, signals from the brain can modify the motor, sensory, secretory, and immune functions of the gastrointestinal tract in a top-down relation.[23] Thus, psychosocial mechanisms such as behavioral, cognitive, and affective processes are thought to interact with the gut–brain axis in a way that amplifies intestinal symptomatology.[23]

■ SYNTHESIS OF EMPIRICAL EVIDENCE AND LESSONS LEARNED FOR CLINICIANS

Accumulating evidence supports the role of negative and positive emotions in disease etiology and health promotion. Depression has been most studied in relation to negative health outcomes, with established links to onset and progression of an array of diseases. Interestingly, research on other negative emotions, and especially anxiety, shows similar effects across adverse health outcomes, while positive emotions are generally associated with favorable health outcomes. This raises questions about whether the effects of emotions on health are shared across multiple emotions or unique to specific emotions.

---

[26]Anxiety RR=2.38, 95%CI 1.58–3.60; depression RR=2.06, 95%CI 1.44–2.96.

In the past two decades, accruing evidence from genetic, neurological, developmental, behavioral, and cognitive research has prompted a movement toward a transdiagnostic approach to psychopathology, which emphasizes shared mechanisms (e.g., cognitive and social processes, responses to adverse vs. positive contexts) that underlie psychiatric disorders.[30] Evidence on the comparable efficacy between transdiagnostic treatments that target core cognitive and behavioral components of mood and anxiety disorders (e.g., rumination, avoidance, and emotion regulation) and diagnostic-specific cognitive-behavioral therapies[99] has highlighted the relevance of the shared underlying components of emotions for understanding and treating psychiatric disorders. However, for physical health outcomes, it remains unclear whether these shared components matter more than the unique aspects of emotions, especially because most studies evaluate the effect of a single emotion in relation to a single health outcome. Moreover, some results suggest that unique effects due to the nonshared aspects might be important. For instance, in the meta-analysis by Edmondson et al.,[35] effects of PTSD on incident CHD remained significant, although attenuated, after adjusting for depression, suggesting both shared and unique effects might be at play. More research is needed to understand if specific versus shared components of emotions matter more for physical health.

Although the extant literature suggests that negative emotions may exert deleterious effects on health, it should be stressed that specific emotions are not inherently harmful or helpful. Emotions exist because they serve distinct purposes. Transitory negative feelings of sadness, anger, or fear in the face of stressful events are likely to reflect a normal reaction. On the other hand, emotions whose intensity or duration is disproportionate to the context, or that become disabling, signal the need for intervention. Besides the effects of emotions per se, the way individuals regulate emotions may also impact health. Emotion regulation, which refers to the strategies by which individuals influence the nature of emotions they experience as well as when and how they experience these emotions,[13] has been the subject of growing interest in the past two decades (see Chapter 7, Emotion Regulation in Patients, Providers, and the Clinical Relationship, for more details). Studies have mostly focused on the health-related effects of two types of emotion regulation strategies: response-focused strategies employed after an emotion has occurred (e.g., suppression), and antecedent-focused strategies used before the emotional response is fully deployed (e.g., cognitive reappraisal). Suppression consists of inhibiting behaviors relating to the expression of emotions such as facial expressions (e.g., repressing crying or laughing) or verbal expression, so as not to communicate information to others about their emotional states.[13] Research has generally suggested suppression is an ineffective emotion regulation strategy with multiple short- and long-term costs; it not only diminishes the subjective experience of positive emotions, it also has the paradoxical effect of increasing the negative emotions that individuals seek to suppress, and can lead to more sustained activation of the sympathetic nervous system.[100] In epidemiological studies, suppression has been associated with higher inflammation levels and higher CVD risk,[101] and with greater risk of all-cause and cancer mortality.[102] Cognitive reappraisal involves modifying one's assessments of a given situation to either attenuate or amplify the attendant emotional experience.[13] Unlike suppression, cognitive reappraisal does not appear to have a deleterious impact on the sympathetic nervous system activation or cognitive resources,[13] and has been associated with reduced risk of CVD.[101] Although the adaptiveness of any emotion regulation strategy is context-dependent, antecedent-focused strategies such as cognitive reappraisal generally seem to be more adaptive in relation to health.[101]

Emotions, both negative and positive, are relevant for clinicians not only because they provide information on one's psychological adjustment (or maladjustment) to physical illness, but also because emotions may impact physical health and therefore constitute risk indicators for downstream health problems. Compelling evidence shows that emotions, along with other well-established modifiable risk factors such as health behaviors, are key targets for primordial prevention (i.e., the prevention of risk factor development). Health professionals should, therefore, pay close attention to identify patients who present with higher levels of negative emotions or low levels of positive emotions, since these patients may be at increased risk of developing physical ailments. Brief self-report instruments such as the Primary Care Evaluation of Mental Disorders (PRIME-MD)[103] can quickly screen for clinically significant levels of negative emotions such as anxiety and depression, and serve as the first step toward a more in-depth conversation with the patient. Systematic screening for affective problems may help to ensure early identification of individuals in need of additional support either with a targeted intervention (e.g., psychoeducation intervention on emotions and their adaptive functions) or referral to psychosocial services for patients with more chronic or heightened levels of negative emotions (e.g., cognitive behavioral therapy, to foster better emotion regulation skills). See Chapter 5 (Perception of Emotion in the Medical Visit) and Chapter 6 (Emotion Cues as Clinical Opportunities) for additional guidance for healthcare providers on recognizing and responding to emotion in patients. Patients with affective problems may also warrant closer monitoring for the development of physical health conditions.

It is also critical to note that emotions arise in a broader social context, which must be taken into account when assessing the patient. For instance, persons with low social status are more frequently exposed to negative life events and chronic social stressors.[104] Furthermore, individuals from socially disadvantaged backgrounds (e.g., lower socioeconomic status) tend to report higher levels of distress.[104] Social disadvantage tends to cluster with higher exposure to chronic and acute stressors, which adversely affects emotional experience.[104] Clinicians should be especially vigilant to signs of emotional distress among socially disadvantaged patients, who are already at elevated risk of experiencing numerous poor health outcomes, including chronic illness and curtailed life expectancy.

Despite robust evidence supporting the role of negative emotions in the onset and progression of major diseases, clinical guidelines have lagged behind in translating these critical findings into recommendations for optimizing patient care. The 2019 American College of Cardiology/AHA Guideline on the Primary Prevention of CVD[105] recommends that clinicians address "social determinants of health," such as via routine assessments of and interventional recommendations for psychosocial stressors to prevent atherosclerotic CVD, and addressing stress and depression to improve obesity and diabetes management. Depression has also been recognized as a risk factor for poor prognosis among ACS and stroke patients.[51,106] While these are encouraging steps, beyond depression, there is considerably less attention on the role of anxiety, PTSD, anger, and hostility in major conditions. Ambiguity in differentiating between stress and emotions is evident in the language of professional guidelines. Thus, it is important to educate health professions on the distinction among psychosocial determinants in their relations to major diseases, and best practices in assessing and treating specific psychosocial factors with known associations with health conditions. The "one size fits all" approach to considering psychosocial factors ignores the differential evidence linking specific factors to disease onset and progression, as well as unique patient experiences which affect their disease predisposition, protective factors, symptom manifestation, prognosis, and management.

While medicine and public health have traditionally adopted a deficit-based approach to health, there is increasing recognition that a comprehensive understanding of health needs to consider the presence of favorable health and its determinants. The World Health Organization (WHO) has long defined health as "a state of complete physical, mental, and social well-being and not merely the absence of disease or infirmity."[107] A growing body of evidence now supports the role of a positive psychological (e.g., optimism), social (e.g., marriage), structural (e.g., education), and environmental assets (e.g., green space) in preserving good health, delaying disease onset and progression, and mitigating the harmful influences of negative exposures, with effect sizes often comparable to traditional risk factors.[108] Importantly, these health assets are often modifiable, and do not merely signal the absence of a risk factor, as studies have increasingly accounted for predisposing risks, such as depression and baseline diseases. Recently, the AHA summarized evidence for the association of psychological well-being to cardiovascular health and CVD prevention, and discussed existing interventions for psychological well-being that appear to be beneficial for cardiovascular health including mindfulness-related interventions (e.g., meditation, yoga, tai-chi) and positive psychology interventions that aim to promote optimism, gratitude, and positive affect.[59] Based on the evidence, the AHA recommended incorporating assessment and education about psychological well-being into routine care, prevention and rehabilitation programs, community resources (e.g., exercise classes in churches, hobby groups in senior centers), and existing mental health interventions. While this chapter focuses on psychosocial factors, these recommendations extend to nonpsychological health assets as well (e.g., green space). Technological advances can also be harnessed to enhance surveillance and assessment of health assets through the use of mobile health tools (e.g., mobile apps to track and summarize daily positive mood, exercise, and green space exposure), and delivery of "just-in-time" interventions during vulnerable windows when individuals are at particularly high risk for health-damaging behaviors (e.g., depressed mood leading to binge eating).[109] Such tools have the potential to facilitate the implementation of psychosocial interventions and allow clinicians to more easily monitor and intervene upon patient's health and well-being in a more comprehensive and systematic way.

ACKNOWLEDGMENT

This work was supported by salary and training support from the Canadian Institute of Health Research (postdoctoral fellowship) and the Lee Kum Sheung Center for Health and Happiness to Anne-Josée Guimond, and from the National Institute on Aging (K08 AG048221) to Lewina O. Lee. Portions of this work are based on the study by Kubzansky and Winning.[110]

REFERENCES

1. National Comprehensive Cancer Network. NCCN clinical practice guidelines in oncology: NCCN practice guidelines for the management of psychosocial distress. Available at http://www.nccn.org/professionals/physician_gls/f_guidelines.asp. Published 2012. Accessed 1 May, 2018.

2. Mitchell AJ, Chan M, Bhatti H, et al. Prevalence of depression, anxiety, and adjustment disorder in oncological, haematological, and palliative-care settings: a meta-analysis of 94 interview-based studies. *Lancet Oncol.* 2011;12(2):160-174.

3. Kuhlmann SL, Arolt V, Haverkamp W, et al. Prevalence, 12-month prognosis, and clinical management need of depression in coronary heart disease patients: a prospective cohort study. *Psychother Psychosom.* 2019;88(5):300-311.

4. Ferrari AJ, Somerville AJ, Baxter AJ, et al. Global variation in the prevalence and incidence of major depressive disorder: a systematic review of the epidemiological literature. *Psychol Med.* 2013;43(3):471-481.

5. Kroenke K, Theobald D, Wu J, Loza JK, Carpenter JS, Tu W. The association of depression and pain with health-related quality of life, disability, and health care use in cancer patients. *J Pain Symptom Manage.* 2010;40(3):327-341.

6. Goldstein CM, Gathright EC, Garcia S. Relationship between depression and medication adherence in cardiovascular disease: the perfect challenge for the integrated care team. *Patient Prefer Adherence.* 2017;11:547-559.

7. Mystakidou K, Parpa E, Katsouda E, Galanos A, Vlahos L. The role of physical and psychological symptoms in desire for death: a study of terminally ill cancer patients. *Psychooncology.* 2006;15(4):355-360.

8. Cohen BE, Edmondson D, Kronish IM. State of the art review: depression, stress, anxiety, and cardiovascular disease. *Am J Hypertens.* 2015;28(11):1295-1302.

9. Hoyt MA, Stanton AL. Adjustment to chronic illness. In: Revenson TA, Gurung RA, eds. *Handbook of Health Psychology.* 1st ed. New York, NY: Routledge; 2018:179-194.

10. Coyne JC, Tennen H. Positive psychology in cancer care: bad science, exaggerated claims, and unproven medicine. *Ann Behav Med.* 2010;39(1):16-26.

11. Boehm JK, Kubzansky LD. The heart's content: the association between positive psychological well-being and cardiovascular health. *Psychol Bull.* 2012;138(4):655-691.

12. Lazarus RS. Progress on a cognitive–motivational–relational theory of emotion. *Am Psychol.* 1991;46(8):819-834.

13. Gross JJ. Emotion regulation: current status and future prospects. *Psychol Inq.* 2015;26(1):1-26.

14. Folkman S, Lazarus RS. *Stress, Appraisal, and Coping.* New York, NY: Springer Publishing Company; 1984.

15. Epel ES, Crosswell AD, Mayer SE, et al. More than a feeling: a unified view of stress measurement for population science. *Front Neuroendocrin.* 2018;49:146-169.

16. Almeida DM, Piazza JR, Stawski RS, Klein LC. The speedometer of life: stress, health and aging. In: *Handbook of the Psychology of Aging.* Elsevier; 2011:191-206.

17. Almeida DM. Resilience and vulnerability to daily stressors assessed via diary methods. *Curr Dir Psychol Sci.* 2005;14(2):64-68.

18. Mroczek DK, Stawski RS, Turiano NA, et al. Emotional reactivity and mortality: longitudinal findings from the VA Normative Aging Study. *J Gerontol B Psychol.* 2015;70(3):398-406.

19. Sin NL, Graham-Engeland JE, Ong AD, Almeida DM. Affective reactivity to daily stressors is associated with elevated inflammation. *Health Psychol.* 2015;34(12):1154-1165.

20. Piazza JR, Charles ST, Sliwinski MJ, Mogle J, Almeida DM. Affective reactivity to daily stressors and long-term risk of reporting a chronic physical health condition. *Ann Behav Med.* 2013;45(1):110-120.

21. Kamarck TW, Schwartz JE, Shiffman S, Muldoon MF, Sutton-Tyrrell K, Janicki DL. Psychosocial stress and cardiovascular risk: what is the role of daily experience? *J Pers.* 2005;73(6):1749-1774.

22. Sin NL, Ong AD, Stawski RS, Almeida DM. Daily positive events and diurnal cortisol rhythms: examination of between-person differences and within-person variation. *Psychoneuroendocrinology.* 2017;83:91-100.

23. Pellissier S, Bonaz B. The place of stress and emotions in the irritable bowel syndrome. *Vitamins and Hormones.* 2017;103:327-354.

24. Muscatello MR, Bruno A, Scimeca G, Pandolfo G, Zoccali RA. Role of negative affects in pathophysiology and clinical expression of irritable bowel syndrome. *World J Gastroenterol.* 2014;20(24):7570-7586.

25. Medina de Chazal H, Del Buono MG, Keyser-Marcus L, et al. Stress cardiomyopathy diagnosis and treatment: JACC state-of-the-art review. *J Am Coll Cardiol.* 2018;72(16):1955-1971.

26. Tsuboi H, Tatsumi A, Yamamoto K, Kobayashi F, Shimoi K, Kinae N. Possible connections among job stress, depressive symptoms, lipid modulation and antioxidants. *J Affect Disord.* 2006;91(1):63-70.

27. Soo J, Kubzansky LD, Chen Y, Zevon ES, Boehm JK. Psychological well-being and restorative biological processes: HDL-C in older English adults. *Soc Sci Med.* 2018;209:59-66.

28. Van Cappellen P, Rice EL, Catalino LI, Fredrickson BL. Positive affective processes underlie positive health behaviour change. *Psychol Health.* 2018;33(1):77-97.

29. Sin NL, Moskowitz JT, Whooley MA. Positive affect and health behaviors across five years in patients with coronary heart disease: the Heart and Soul Study. *Psychosom Med.* 2015;77(9):1058-1066.

30. Norton PJP, Roberge PP. Transdiagnostic therapy. *Psychiatr Clin North Am.* 2017;40(4):675-687.

31. Rothman KJ, Greenland S, Lash TL. *Modern Epidemiology.* 3rd ed. Philadelphia, PA: Wolters Kluwer Health; 2015.

32. Carney RM, Freedland KE. Depression and coronary heart disease. *Nat Rev Cardiol.* 2017;14(3):145.

33. Batelaan NM, Seldenrijk A, Bot M, van Balkom AJ, Penninx BW. Anxiety and new onset of cardiovascular disease: critical review and meta-analysis. *Br J Psychiat.* 2016;208(3):223-231.

34. Roest AM, Martens EJ, de Jonge P, Denollet J. Anxiety and risk of incident coronary heart disease: a meta-analysis. *J Am Coll Cardiol.* 2010;56(1):38-46.

35. Edmondson D, Kronish IM, Shaffer JA, Falzon L, Burg MM. Posttraumatic stress disorder and risk for coronary heart disease: a meta-analytic review. *Am Heart J.* 2013;166(5):806-814.

36. Gibson CJ, Li Y, Inslicht SS, Seal KH, Byers AL. Gender differences in cardiovascular risk related to diabetes and posttraumatic stress disorder. *Am J Geriat Psychiat.* 2018;26(12):1268-1272.

37. Matthews KA. Coronary heart disease and Type A behaviors: update on and alternative to the Booth-Kewley and Friedman (1987) quantitative review. *Psychol Bull.* 1988;104(3):373-380.

38. Chida Y, Steptoe A. The association of anger and hostility with future coronary heart disease: a meta-analytic review of prospective evidence. *J Am Coll Cardiol.* 2009;53(11):936-946.

39. Glassman AH, Bigger JT, Gaffney M, Shapiro PA, Swenson JR. Onset of major depression associated with acute coronary syndromes: relationship of onset, major depressive disorder history, and episode severity to sertraline benefit. *Arch Gen Psychiatry.* 2006;63(3):283-288.

40. American Heart Association. Acute coronary syndrome. Available at https://www.heart.org/en/health-topics/heart-attack/about-heart-attacks/acute-coronary-syndrome. Accessed 29 September, 2020.

41. Meurs M, Zuidersma M, Dickens C, de Jonge P. Examining the relation between post myocardial infarction depression and cardiovascular prognosis using a validated prediction model for post myocardial mortality. *Int J Cardiol.* 2013;167(6):2533-2538.

42. Celano CM, Millstein RA, Bedoya CA, Healy BC, Roest AM, Huffman JC. Association between anxiety and mortality in patients with coronary artery disease: a meta-analysis. *Am Heart J.* 2015;170(6):1105-1115.

43. Li J, Ji F, Song J, et al. Anxiety and clinical outcomes of patients with acute coronary syndrome: a meta-analysis. *BMJ open.* 2020;10(7):e034135.

44. Edmondson D, von Känel R. Post-traumatic stress disorder and cardiovascular disease. *Lancet Psychiat.* 2017;4(4):320-329.

45. Edmondson D, Richardson S, Falzon L, Davidson KW, Mills MA, Neria Y. Posttraumatic stress disorder prevalence and risk of recurrence in acute coronary syndrome patients: a meta-analytic review. *PloS one.* 2012;7(6):e38915.

46. Pan A, Sun Q, Okereke OI, Rexrode KM, Hu FB. Depression and risk of stroke morbidity and mortality: a meta-analysis and systematic review. *JAMA.* 2011;306(11):1241-1249.

47. Gilsanz P, Kubzansky L, Tchetgen EJT, et al. Changes in depressive symptoms and subsequent risk of stroke in the Cardiovascular Health Study. *Stroke.* 2017;48(1):43-48.

48. Pérez-Piñar M, Ayerbe L, González E, Mathur R, Foguet-Boreu Q, Ayis S. Anxiety disorders and risk of stroke: a systematic review and meta-analysis. *Eur Psychiat.* 2017;41:102-108.

49. Rosman L, Sico JJ, Lampert R, et al. Posttraumatic stress disorder and risk for stroke in young and middle-aged adults: a 13-year cohort study. *Stroke.* 2019;50(11):2996-3003.

50. Chen H, Zhang B, Xue W, et al. Anger, hostility and risk of stroke: a meta-analysis of cohort studies. *J Neurol.* 2019;266(4):1016-1026.

51. Towfighi A, Ovbiagele B, El Husseini N, et al. Poststroke depression: a scientific statement for healthcare professionals from the American Heart Association/American Stroke Association. *Stroke.* 2017;48(2):e30-e43.

52. Rotella F, Mannucci E. Diabetes mellitus as a risk factor for depression. A meta-analysis of longitudinal studies. *Diab Res Clin.* 2012;99(2):98-104.

53. Smith KJ, Deschênes SS, Schmitz N. Investigating the longitudinal association between diabetes and anxiety: a systematic review and meta-analysis. *Diab Med.* 2018;35(6):677-693.

54. Boyko EJ, Seelig AD, Jacobson IG, et al. Sleep characteristics, mental health, and diabetes risk: a prospective study of U.S. military service members in the Millennium Cohort Study. *Diabetes Care.* 2013;36(10):3154-3161.

55. Scherrer JF, Salas J, Norman SB, et al. Association between clinically meaningful posttraumatic stress disorder improvement and risk of type 2 diabetes. *JAMA Psychiatry.* 2019;76(11):1159-1166.

56. Abraham S, Shah NG, Roux AD, et al. Trait anger but not anxiety predicts incident type 2 diabetes: the Multi-Ethnic Study of Atherosclerosis (MESA). *Psychoneuroendocrinology*. 2015;60:105-113.

57. de Groot M, Golden SH, Wagner J. Psychological conditions in adults with diabetes. *Am Psychol*. 2016;71(7):552-562.

58. Gonzalez JS, Tanenbaum ML, Commissariat PV. Psychosocial factors in medication adherence and diabetes self-management: implications for research and practice. *Am Psychol*. 2016;71(7):539-551.

59. Kubzansky LD, Huffman JC, Boehm JK, et al. Positive psychological well-being and cardiovascular disease. *J Am Coll Cardiol*. 2018;72(12):1382-1396.

60. Kim ES, Hagan KA, Grodstein F, DeMeo DL, De Vivo I, Kubzansky LD. Optimism and cause-specific mortality: a prospective cohort study. *Am J Epidemiol*. 2017;185(1):21-29.

61. Kim ES, Sun JK, Park N, Peterson C. Purpose in life and reduced incidence of stroke in older adults: 'The Health and Retirement Study'. *J Psychosom Res*. 2013;74(5):427-432.

62. Kim E, Sun J, Park N, Kubzansky L, Peterson C. Purpose in life and reduced risk of myocardial infarction among older U.S. adults with coronary heart disease: a two-year follow-up. *J Behav Med*. 2013;36(2):124-133.

63. Boehm JK, Chen Y, Williams DR, Ryff CD, Kubzansky LD. Subjective well-being and cardiometabolic health: an 8–11 year study of midlife adults. *J Psychosom Res*. 2016;85:1-8.

64. Celano CM, Beale EE, Moore SV, Wexler DJ, Huffman JC. Positive psychological characteristics in diabetes: a review. *Current Diabetes Reports*. 2013;13(6):917-929.

65. Temoshok L. Personality, coping style, emotion and cancer: towards an integrative model. *Cancer Surveys*. 1987;6(3):545-567.

66. Grossarth-Maticek R, Kanazir DT, Schmidt P, Vetter H. Psychosocial and organic variables as predictors of lung cancer, cardiac infarct and apoplexy: some differential predictors. *Pers Individ Differ*. 1985;6(3):313-321.

67. Spiegel D, Bloom JR, Kraemer HC, Gottheil E. Effect of psychosocial treatment on survival of patients with metastatic breast cancer. *The Lancet*. 1989;334(8668):888-891.

68. Ranchor AV, Sanderman R, Coyne JC. Invited commentary: Personality as a causal factor in cancer risk and mortality—time to retire a hypothesis? *Am J Epidemiol*. 2010;172(4):386-388.

69. Pössel P, Adams E, Valentine J. Depression as a risk factor for breast cancer: investigating methodological limitations in the literature. *Cancer Causes Control*. 2012;23(8):1223-1229.

70. Wang YH, Li JQ, Shi JF, et al. Depression and anxiety in relation to cancer incidence and mortality: a systematic review and meta-analysis of cohort studies. *Mol Psychiatry*. 2020;25:1487-1499.

71. Roberts AL, Huang T, Koenen KC, Kim Y, Kubzansky LD, Tworoger SS. Posttraumatic stress disorder is associated with increased risk of ovarian cancer: a prospective and retrospective longitudinal cohort study. *Cancer Res*. 2019;79(19):5113-5120.

72. Gradus JL, Farkas DK, Svensson E, et al. Posttraumatic stress disorder and cancer risk: a nationwide cohort study. *Eur J Epidemiol*. 2015;30(7):563-568.

73. Aspinwall LG, Tedeschi RG. The value of positive psychology for health psychology: progress and pitfalls in examining the relation of positive phenomena to health. *Ann Behav Med.* 2010;39(1):4-15.

74. Holland JC, Lewis S. *The Human Side of Cancer: Living with Hope, Coping with Uncertainty.* New York, NY: HarperCollins; 2000.

75. Feller S, Teucher B, Kaaks R, Boeing H, Vigl M. Life satisfaction and risk of chronic diseases in the European prospective investigation into cancer and nutrition (EPIC)-Germany study. *PLoS One.* 2013;8(8):e73462.

76. Folker AP, Hegelund ER, Mortensen EL, Wimmelmann CL, Flensborg-Madsen T. The association between life satisfaction, vitality, self-rated health, and risk of cancer. *Qual Life Res.* 2019;28(4):947-954.

77. Cohen S, Doyle WJ, Skoner DP, Fireman P, Gwaltney JM, Newsom JT. State and trait negative affect as predictors of objective and subjective symptoms of respiratory viral infections. *J Pers Soc Psychol.* 1995;68(1):159-169.

78. Nakata A, Irie M, Takahashi M. Psychological distress, depressive symptoms, and cellular immunity among healthy individuals: a 1-year prospective study. *Int J Psychophysiol.* 2011;81(3):191-197.

79. Cohen MS, Alper JC, Doyle JW, Treanor BJ, Turner BR. Positive emotional style predicts resistance to illness after experimental exposure to rhinovirus or influenza A virus. *Psychosom Med.* 2006;68(6):809-815.

80. Cohen S, Tyrrell DAJ, Smith AP. Negative life events, perceived stress, negative affect, and susceptibility to the common cold. *J Pers Soc Psychol.* 1993;64(1):131-140.

81. Segerstrom SC, Hardy JK, Evans DR, Greenberg RN. Vulnerability, distress, and immune response to vaccination in older adults. *Brain Behav Immun.* 2012;26(5):747-753.

82. Glaser R, Robles TF, Sheridan J, Malarkey WB, Kiecolt-Glaser JK. Mild depressive symptoms are associated with amplified and prolonged inflammatory responses after influenza virus vaccination in older adults. *Arch Gen Psychiatry.* 2003;60(10):1009-1014.

83. Andersson NW, Goodwin RD, Okkels N, et al. Depression and the risk of severe infections: prospective analyses on a nationwide representative sample. *Int J Epidemiol.* 2016;45(1):131-139.

84. Song H, Fall K, Fang F, et al. Stress related disorders and subsequent risk of life threatening infections: population based sibling controlled cohort study. *BMJ.* 2019;367:l5784.

85. Owora AH. Major depression disorder trajectories and HIV disease progression: results from a 6-year outpatient clinic cohort. *Medicine.* 2018;97(12):e0252.

86. Wilson TE, Weedon J, Cohen MH, et al. Positive affect and its association with viral control among women with HIV infection. *Health Psychol.* 2017;36(1):91-100.

87. Ironson G, Fitch C, Stuetzle R. Depression and survival in a 17-year longitudinal study of people with HIV: moderating effects of race and education. *Psychosom Med.* 2017;79(7):749-756.

88. Moskowitz TJ. Positive affect predicts lower risk of AIDS mortality. *Psychosom Med.* 2003;65(4):620-626.

89. Lee YC, Agnew-Blais J, Malspeis S, et al. Post-traumatic stress disorder and risk for incident rheumatoid arthritis. *Arthritis Care Res.* 2016;68(3):292-298.

90. Brunner WM, Schreiner PJ, Sood A, Jacobs DR Jr. Depression and risk of incident asthma in adults. the CARDIA study. *Am J Respir Crit Care Med.* 2014;189(9):1044-1051.

91. Overman CL, Bossema ER, van Middendorp H, et al. The prospective association between psychological distress and disease activity in rheumatoid arthritis: a multilevel regression analysis. *Ann Rheum Dis.* 2012;71(2):192-197.

92. Okely J, Cooper C, Gale C. Wellbeing and arthritis incidence: the Survey of Health, Ageing and Retirement in Europe. *Ann Behav Med.* 2016;50(3):419-426.

93. Okely JA, Weiss A, Gale CR. Well-being and arthritis incidence: the role of inflammatory mechanisms. Findings from the English Longitudinal Study of Ageing. *Psychosom Med.* 2017;79(7):742-748.

94. Afari N, Ahumada SM, Wright LJ, et al. Psychological trauma and functional somatic syndromes: a systematic review and meta-analysis. *Psychosom Med.* 2014;76(1):2-11.

95. Hauser G, Pletikosic S, Tkalcic M. Cognitive behavioral approach to understanding irritable bowel syndrome. *World J Gastroenterol.* 2014;20(22):6744-6758.

96. Sibelli A, Chalder T, Everitt H, Workman P, Windgassen S, Moss-Morris R. A systematic review with meta-analysis of the role of anxiety and depression in irritable bowel syndrome onset. *Psychol Med.* 2016;46(15):3065-3080.

97. Koloski NA, Jones M, Kalantar J, Weltman M, Zaguirre J, Talley NJ. The brain–gut pathway in functional gastrointestinal disorders is bidirectional: a 12-year prospective population-based study. *Gut.* 2012;61(9):1284-1290.

98. Consoli G, Marazziti D, Ciapparelli A, et al. The impact of mood, anxiety, and sleep disorders on fibromyalgia. *Compr Psychiatry.* 2012;53(7):962-967.

99. Pearl SBP, Norton PJP. Transdiagnostic versus diagnosis specific cognitive behavioural therapies for anxiety: a meta-analysis. *J Anx Disord.* 2016;46:11-24.

100. Salters-Pedneault K, Steenkamp M, Litz B, Kring A, Sloan D. Suppression. In: Kring AM, Sloan DM, eds. *Emotion Regulation and Psychopathology: A Transdiagnostic Approach to Etiology and Treatment.* New York, NY: Guilford Press; 2010:137-156.

101. Appleton AA, Kubzansky LD. Emotion regulation and cardiovascular disease risk. In: *Handbook of Emotion Regulation.* 2nd ed. New York, NY: Guilford Press; 2014:596-612.

102. Chapman BP, Fiscella K, Kawachi I, Duberstein P, Muennig P. Emotion suppression and mortality risk over a 12-year follow-up. *J Psychosom Res.* 2013;75(4):381-385.

103. Spitzer RL, Kroenke K, Williams JB. Validation and utility of a self-report version of PRIME-MD: the PHQ primary care study. *JAMA.* 1999;282(18):1737-1744.

104. Matthews KA, Gallo LC. Psychological perspectives on pathways linking socioeconomic status and physical health. *Annu Rev Psychol.* 2011;62(1):501-530.

105. Arnett DK, Blumenthal RS, Albert MA, et al. 2019 ACC/AHA guideline on the primary prevention of cardiovascular disease: a report of the American College of Cardiology/American Heart Association Task Force on Clinical Practice Guidelines. *J Am Coll Cardiol.* 2019;74(10):e177-e232.

106. Lichtman JH, Froelicher ES, Blumenthal JA, et al. Depression as a risk factor for poor prognosis among patients with acute coronary syndrome: systematic review and recommendations: a scientific statement from the American Heart Association. *Circulation.* 2014;129(12):1350-1369.

107. World Health Organization. What is the WHO definition of health? Available at https://www.who.int/about/who-we-are/frequently-asked-questions. Accessed May 14, 2020.

108. VanderWeele TJ, Chen Y, Long K, Kim ES, Trudel-Fitzgerald C, Kubzansky LD. Positive epidemiology? *Epidemiology*. 2020;31(2):189-193.

109. Nahum-Shani I, Hekler EB, Spruijt-Metz D. Building health behavior models to guide the development of just-in-time adaptive interventions: a pragmatic framework. *Health Psychol*. 2015;34(S):1209-1219.

110. Kubzansky LD, Winning A. Emotion and health. In: Barrett LF, Lewis M, Haviland-Jones JM, eds. *Handbook of Emotions*. 4th ed. New York, NY: Guilford Press; 2016:613-633.

Emotion Dialogue in the Medical Encounter: When and How Often Does It Happen?

CHAPTER 4

Mollie A. Ruben, Morgan D. Stosic, and Debra L. Roter

There is evidence from nonverbal behavior research that a face can never be truly expressionless, emotionless, or neutral. Even if you ask someone to display a neutral face, they may still be feeling underlying emotion that leaks out in their expression through what is called a microexpression. Or, years of emotion-laden experiences may remain on the face through wrinkles or lines that make it appear expressive. Even when young adults' faces are in repose and deliberately "neutral," the features themselves connote emotion.[1] Similar to there being no truly neutral facial expressions, *medical interactions can never be truly emotionless.* Even if a doctor has a purely biomedical agenda or a patient only wants to know about the technical aspects of their diagnosis or treatment, they may still be feeling underlying emotion that leaks out in their verbal or nonverbal behavior. And even if on the surface what is being said does not appear to be emotional in nature, patients and doctors bring with them past experiences in medical interactions and in their personal lives that may impact how they feel, what they say, and how they behave.

Often, emotions in the medical dialogue are expressed in subtle ways and are not the focus of the interaction.[2] Some medical visits, on the other hand, are filled with intense emotion and are frequently one-sided, in that patients are the only ones expressing emotions. Stereotypes about which providers are good at dealing with emotions also likely influence the expression of emotion in the medical visit. For example, nurses are stereotyped as being able to handle and deal with patient emotions, and psychotherapists and palliative care physicians often have entire courses and supervision specific to managing, exploring, and coping with patient emotion. Because these providers are assumed to welcome emotion and be good at handling them, patients are likely to express their emotions more in these contexts and with these types of providers than with providers who are more biomedically focused and technical (e.g., surgeons).

While clinicians cannot ask about, recognize, or respond to every emotion that a patient has during the interaction (for the sake of time and energy), the current state of patient care lacks a crucial focus on emotion dialogue in the medical interaction. Emotions, not just of patients but also of physicians, must become a topic of learning in medical education and continuing education. This will benefit not only patients and their ability to cope, connect, and heal but also physicians in terms of their longevity in their career by potentially reducing the already high rates of burnout, depression, and suicide.

In this chapter, we discuss where emotions fit into conceptualizations of patient-centered care and patient-centered communication, why emotion dialogue matters in the medical interaction, how frequently emotion dialogue occurs and what facilitates or creates barriers in emotion dialogue, and finally make recommendations for educators and medical professionals to consider when training students and treating patients. In describing emotion-related talk, we draw extensively on studies that have used the most widely applied system for describing verbal and nonverbal emotion dialogue in medical interactions, the Roter Interaction Analysis System (RIAS).[3]

■ PATIENT-CENTERED CARE

Reports issued by the Institute of Medicine[4,5] and publication of the Charter on Medical Professionalism[6] have focused attention on the centrality of patient-centered communication as an essential element of patient care and the practice of ethical medicine. A growing body of research has also emerged linking "good" communication, often described in patient-centered terms, to a host of valued outcomes.[7,8] Within this context, patient-centeredness has become synonymous with care quality and an antonym of a narrow biocentric view of the patient. Indeed, the Institute of Medicine report "Crossing the Quality Chasm" listed patient-centeredness as one of six key indicators shaping the nation's future agenda for healthcare quality along with safety, effectiveness, efficiency, timeliness, and equity.[5] The popular embrace of patient-centeredness by policy makers, medical educators, researchers, and the general public reflects broad regard but little specificity. To this point, patient-centeredness has been used to describe a philosophy of medicine,[9] a clinical method,[10,11] a type of therapeutic relationship,[11] a quality-of-care indicator,[5] a professional and moral imperative,[6] and a communication style.[12]

Patient-centered ideas are not just evident in modern medical writings, but were foreshadowed by Plato some 2,000 years ago. In "The Dialogues"

Plato conveys a conversation between himself and his friend and philosopher, Cleinias, in which they discuss the difference between doctors treating slaves versus doctors treating freemen with striking resonance to modern concepts of patient-centeredness (see http://zackarysholemberger.com for further discussion).[13]

> [T]he slave doctors run about and cure the slaves or wait for them in the clinic. They never talk to their patients individually nor do they allow them to talk about their own individual complaints. The slave doctor diagnoses and prescribes a remedy on an empirical basis, [but does so] as if he had exact knowledge; He gives his orders [to the patient], like a tyrant, and then rushes off, to see some other slave who is ill, all the while projecting an air of confidence and assurance;...But the other doctor attends and practices upon freemen; and he carries his enquiries [with his patient] far back, and goes into the nature of the disorder in a scientific way; he enters into discourse with the patient and with his family, and is at once getting useful information from the sick person, and also instructing him as far as he is able. [The physician] will not prescribe for the patient until he has first convinced him; at last, when he has brought the patient more and more under his persuasive influences and set him on the road to health, he attempts to effect a cure.

This surely presages modern conceptualizations of patient-centeredness in a number of ways, including the value of forming an open and trusting bond by fully establishing the context and nature of the problem from the patient and family perspective, acknowledging the importance of sharing information—both giving and receiving—and finally, holding back on prescribing until the patient is willing to accept treatment. In line with these components, conceptual and empirical reviews of the modern concept of patient-centered care applicable to a narrower focus on patient-centered communication reflect a general consensus on four core domains: (1) biopsychosocial perspective to care, (2) recognition of the patient-as-person, (3) sharing of power and responsibility particularly in regard to treatment decisions, and (4) the establishment of a therapeutic alliance.[14,15]

The devil, it seems, is in the details; despite conceptual consensus, patient-centered care is characterized by vague language subject to wide interpretation.[15–17] Key concepts are often referred to in general descriptions but these have not led to anything near consensus, workable operational definitions or a distinguishable single model. To this point, Langbeg and colleagues[15] note that a third of the 80 study authors included in their systematic conceptual review of the topic commented that the language used to describe patient-centeredness is marked by ambiguity. Definitional vagueness is similarly noted by Epstein and colleagues[16] as characterizing the theoretical and practical weaknesses evident in assessment of patient-centered communication.

■ WHY EMOTION DIALOGUE MATTERS IN MEDICAL INTERACTIONS

While emotion is not explicitly stated in conceptualizations of patient-centered care, good medical visit communication, often described as "patient-centered" communication, *is characterized by patients and providers who are fully emotionally engaged with both positive and negative aspects of the patient's health and illness.* Epstein and Street[18] give examples of behaviors that clinicians and patients must engage in for effective communication. Clinicians must not only listen but also elicit and validate patients' emotions while patients must disclose needs that are often fraught with emotion; share information about concerns; share information about family, culture, and context; discuss expectations; and discuss options. Among all of these example behaviors of effective patient-centered communication, emotion is likely present.

There are also important outcomes related to this effective patient–clinician communication that come from the expression of emotion in the medical visit. In general, emotions have a powerful effect on well-being, health, and disease progression. Sharing emotions and feelings during medical interactions often leads to therapeutic benefits for patients.[19] In a similar vein, when patients hold back in sharing the emotions, particularly negative emotions, this may lead to more deleterious outcomes such as anxiety, depression, and confusion.[20] Not only is the disclosure and sharing of emotions mentally therapeutic, but it also contributes to physical symptom improvement.[21]

While most of the focus thus far in this chapter has been on outcomes related to emotion dialogue, there are contexts in which more or less emotion dialogue is to be expected in a medical interaction. While gender and culture are two large constructs that have been well-studied in basic research examining the expression of emotions, they are not usually considered in preparing providers for the healthcare force (see Chapter 11, Emotion and Gender, and Chapter 12, Culture and Emotions in the Medical Encounter). However, we know that culture (the beliefs, values, behavior, and material objects that constitute a people's way of life) has a profound impact on the way in which people express, perceive, and experience emotions.[22] In addition, gender and gender roles play a large part in who expresses emotions, what people's expectations are of how interactions will go, and the value placed on emotion in the interaction.[23] For example, women express verbally and nonverbally how they are feeling more than men and are expected to be more emotionally expressive and receptive to emotions because of gender roles that are instilled from an early age about women being nurturing and caring. Because of these gender roles, physicians and patients have expectations about what is appropriate behavior by men and women. These expectations can drive how an interaction goes and what space is left, if any, for emotional dialogue. For gender nonconforming individuals, gender roles likely play a part in expectations developed based on one's gender expression. However, in medical care, emotional dialogue among gender nonconforming individuals has yet to be systematically investigated.

Finally, larger expectations about the purpose of healthcare, the role of physicians, and a patient's wants/needs in terms of a patient-centered provider versus a more clinician-centered or biomedically based provider, can influence whether emotional talk occurs and how patients perceive emotions when their providers initiate conversations around these topics. For example, because a male military veteran is so used to a hierarchical system in which they receive and follow orders, they may want their provider to tell them exactly what choice to make when they have an important treatment decision to make, rather than embark on a shared decision-making journey. In order to understand what type of style a patient values in their healthcare, providers can simply ask the patient (if they can communicate verbally). Because there is no script for this in healthcare interactions, it is important that providers frame and contextualize why they are asking this of their patients.[24] There are also self-report measures such as the Patient Provider Orientation Scale (PPOS[25]) that assess a patient's degree of valuing a patient-centered versus clinician-centered provider. Example items on the PPOS include:

- "The doctor is the one who should decide what gets talked about during a visit."
- "When doctors ask a lot of questions about a patient's background, they are prying too much into personal matters."
- "It is not that important to know a patient's culture and background in order to treat the person's illness."

Those taking the PPOS indicate how much they agree or disagree with each item on a scale from 1 (strongly disagree) to 6 (strongly agree). For the example items listed above, higher scores indicate a more clinician-centered or biomedical value. Clinicians could give this to their patients during an initial appointment and once every year to ensure that those values have not changed. Then providers can tailor their communication style to patient preferences.

■ ASSESSING EMOTION DIALOGUE

Emotion dialogue often occurs as an exchange of verbal and nonverbal behaviors. For example, after hearing bad news, a patient may begin to cry, at which point a provider could provide comfort and support the patient by leaning in, making eye contact, and allowing space for silence and the processing of information. A family member could become distraught and angry at the care their older parent has received and start yelling at the healthcare team. A provider could ask the caregiver to sit with them, which acknowledges that the provider is going to really listen and take the time to hear them. Then the provider could verbally acknowledge that there has been a breakdown in communication and validate the caregiver's feelings by saying, "I can see that this breakdown has been very frustrating and upsetting." By using a combination of verbal and nonverbal behaviors to express and recognize emotions, there is a place for emotion in the interaction, and providers can form trusting relationships with their patients and families which ultimately will lead to higher quality patient care and better outcomes.

Context can also impact emotional dialogue as emotion does not happen in vacuum. In a medical interaction there could be family members, friends, healthcare teams consisting of attendings, fellows, residents, interns, medical students, and other healthcare professionals such as social workers or specialists. Emotions can impact any one of these people at any moment in the interaction.

While emotions and emotional dialogue appear to be easy to recognize in examples about a crying patient or angry family member, in the moment of the interaction there are subtle cues that are often expressed during a busy clinical day with many others' agendas present (e.g., the physician may be thinking about their next patient, the resident may be trying to gather the family or health history, the patient may be worried about their diagnosis, the caregiver may be worried about getting out of the appointment on time for their son's hockey game, and so on). Thus, assessing emotional dialogue in the medical interaction is not a task that can usually be remembered or even self-reported right after the interaction. Therefore, coding systems have been created to assess when, how often, and who initiates emotional dialogue during medical interactions (patients or providers). There are several validated and reliable systems in the literature that focus on coding emotional talk in these interactions (e.g., VR-Codes,[26] see Chapter 6, Emotion Cues as Clinical Opportunities, that describes the Empathic Communication Coding System[27]), as well as interaction analysis systems that are comprehensive and inclusive of all elements of medical interaction.

For the remainder of this chapter we focus on emotion talk as documented through the lens of the Roter Interaction Analysis System (RIAS),[25] the most commonly used and comprehensive medical interaction coding system.

■ ROTER INTERACTION ANALYSIS SYSTEM (RIAS) FOR CODING VERBAL AND NONVERBAL EMOTIONAL DIALOGUE

The many RIAS studies conducted since its development have established its utility to characterize medical visits and establish links between verbal dialogue and patient health outcomes. For example, the RIAS codes have been linked to patient satisfaction, adherence to treatment, level of control, and patient knowledge about their pathologies.[28-31] Specifically, the emotion categories are most often related to patient satisfaction.[32,33]

The goal of the present chapter is to take advantage of the many studies that have used the RIAS, in order to provide systematic empirical data about emotion expression in clinical visits. Although many studies using different measuring approaches have addressed emotional communication (see Chapter 6, Emotion Cues as Clinical Opportunities), research done with the RIAS affords the most extensive database available, with numerous studies that allow for a comprehensive summary and comparisons across research settings.

In order to establish clarity for readers, it is necessary first to set the stage by describing the RIAS. In doing so, we believe that clinicians will be able to not only grasp relevant methods, but also expand their understanding of what it means to discuss "emotion," and have a larger vocabulary and a broader set of concepts (both theoretically and practically) to help themselves and their patients cope with many emotions in practice. Our purpose is not to suggest that clinicians learn to use the RIAS (though some have used it in this way)[34-40]—it requires trained coders—but rather to help clinicians think in a more granular way about the various categories of emotional interaction that occur in clinical interactions. Also, understanding the emotion-related categories of the RIAS sets the stage for the findings we present.

The RIAS was developed by Debra Roter in the 1970s in the course of her doctoral research at the Johns Hopkins School of Public Health. The system was inspired by the seminal work of sociologist Robert Bales in assessing patterns of small group interaction during group problem-solving and decision-making[41] and an application of the Bales' Framework to pediatric visits.[42]

RIAS's features include:

- Interaction is coded directly from video or audio recordings without the need for transcription.
- Interaction is unitized into statements that represent complete thoughts.

- Each statement is assigned to a set of mutually exclusive categories (codes).
- All speakers present in the interaction can be coded.
- The overall affective nature of the interaction is captured through coders' global impressions of each speaker's positive and negative affect, for instance, irritation, anxiety, dominance, interest, and friendliness.
- RIAS-specific software logs each code entry by speaker, speaker turn characteristics such as density, duration and floor shift, and sequence.

The 37 categories of the RIAS relate to two broad interaction functions:

1. Affective codes include the expression of concerns, approval/disapproval, agreement, criticism, empathy, and legitimation, among others.
   o For example, a patient may express concern by saying, "I am really worried about the results of my upcoming test" while a provider may respond with legitimation such as, "Anyone who has gone through what you've gone through these past few years would be concerned."

2. Instrumental codes include exchange of clinical and therapeutically relevant information, questions, and facilitators of understanding and engagement through active and passive listening strategies.
   o For example, a provider may ask an *open-ended question* about *medical information*, in this case about family history, "tell me about your grandparents' and parents' health history." The patient may respond with *medical information*, "I actually don't know much about their health but I do know that my grandfather died of heart disease."

In what follows, we explain each of the nine primary RIAS codes that communicate emotionally focused dialogue. Table 4-1 lists individual codes within each affective domain and provides more code examples than what are described in text. These nine primary RIAS codes that communicate emotionally focused dialogue are often combined to form composites that reflect a common affective domain (see RIAS composites section). The affective domains reflect positive statements, negative statements, and explicitly emotional statements. In addition, a number of studies aggregate all emotionally focused talk as rapport statements (a combination of positive, negative, emotional, and social statements [i.e., personal remarks during greetings or chit chat that are not discussed below]).

Positive Statements

Approval

Approvals included compliments, expressions of approval, gratitude, praise, reward, respect, or admiration *directed to the other person present*. Examples of approvals include a patient expressing gratitude for a provider's diligence

■ **TABLE 4-1. RIAS Composites and Affect Ratings Related to Emotional Dialogue**

Code composites	Individual codes	Patient examples	Provider examples (Note: provider examples are independent of patient examples)
Positive talk	Approvals Compliments Agreements	You've been so helpful. Your nurse was so kind. Alright, Ok, I'll do that.	You look great. The lab tech was gentle. Ok, right. Yes.
Negative talk	Disagreements Criticisms	No. I didn't say that. Those people were rude.	Two pounds is not good enough. I don't like to rely on that lab.

Emotional talk	Concern
	Reassurance
	Empathy
	Legitimation
		I'm so upset.
		It is getting better.
		You must be worried to tell me
		   something.
		I know a lot of people feel this way.
			Your weight is a problem.
			You will be successful.
			You sound angry.
			Anyone coping with all that
			   would feel the same.

Rapport Statements		Positive talk (see above for examples) Negative talk (see above for examples) Emotional talk (see above for examples) Social talk (e.g., "Nice to meet you")	
GLOBAL AFFECT RATINGS			
Positive Patient Global Affect		Engagement/responsiveness Interest/attentiveness Friendliness/warmth Respectfulness Sympathetic/empathetic Interactive	
Negative Patient Global Affect		Irritation/anger Nervousness/anxiety Dominance/assertiveness Distress/upset Sad/depressed	
Positive Provider Global Affect		Engagement/responsiveness Interest/attentiveness Friendliness/warmth Respectfulness Sympathetic/empathetic Interactive	
Negative Provider Global Affect		Irritation/anger Nervousness/anxiety Dominance/assertiveness Hurried/rushed	

and time, "I really appreciate how much work it took to get me in with that specialist." A provider may use approvals to signal to the patient approval or compliment their hard work in maintaining their nutrition or physical activity such as by saying, "You're looking great today."

Compliment

Compliments vary from approvals, in that they include expressions of approval, gratitude, praise, reward, respect, or admiration *directed to another not present* during the exchange. A patient or provider may use a compliment toward another provider such as, "Dr. Smith is very thoughtful and competent, I really respect them."

Laughter

Laughter includes friendly jokes, trying to amuse or entertain, kidding around, good-natured teasing, morbid jokes (e.g., "I might blow away in a strong wind"), and all forms of laughter as well as laughter in response to jokes.

Agreement

Agreement includes any sign of agreement or understanding made by a patient or provider such as "I see" or "You were right."

Negative Statements

Disagreement

Disagreements include any indication of disapproval, criticism, complaint, rejection, coolness, or disbelief directed expressly *to the other person present.* This includes statements that contradict or refute something said by the other, or imply disagreement with or rejection of the others' hypotheses, ideas, or opinions. For example, a patient may disagree by saying, "I don't agree with our plan for me to stop smoking any longer" while a provider may disagree with a patient's statement by saying, "But you promised you would work on quitting by our next appointment which is now."

Criticism

Criticisms differ from disagreements, in that they include any indication of disapproval, complaint, rejection, coolness, or disbelief directed *toward another not involved* in the exchange. Criticisms include statements that contradict or refute something said by such a person, or imply disagreement with or rejection of such a person's hypotheses, ideas, or opinions. For example, a patient may be frustrated with a different clinic and push back when a provider suggests they go see a specialist there, "I just don't like the way they run things up there," while a provider may use criticism to signal disagreement with what another provider said to the patient in the past about their health, "I can't believe they told you that."

Emotional Statements

Empathy

Empathy statements include statements that paraphrase, interpret, name, or recognize the emotional state of the other person present during the visit. Most empathy statements are initiated by the provider toward the patient, such as "I understand that this continued pain must be distressing and frustrating for you." While likely rarer, a patient could also express empathy toward the provider by recognizing their busy day and the emotional toll it takes on them.

Legitimation

Legitimation statements are statements that indicate that the other's emotional situation, actions, or thoughts are understandable and normal. These statements indicate that it is understandable *why* the other feels or thinks a certain way, and not merely that they feel or think this way. A provider could use a legitimation statement in response to worry expressed, for example, by saying, "Who wouldn't be afraid of cancer?" Similar to empathy, the rate of patients using legitimation statements is likely lower than that of providers, given the context of the medical interaction, but it is possible that patients legitimize providers' actions or thoughts as normal or understandable.

Partnership

Partnership statements convey the physician's alliance with the patient in terms of help and support, decision-making, or the development of the therapeutic plan. These are only coded for providers' use of partnership statements. A provider could use a partnership statement with the use of "we" to show that they are in this with their patient or statements that show support and a joint plan such as "Let's figure out when would be the best time to meet again given what we just discussed."

Concern or Worry

Concern or worry statements, unlike the previous emotional statements described, are more likely to be initiated by a patient but again, providers could also express worry or concern about a patients' behaviors, actions, or emotional response among other things. Concern or worry statements are statements or nonverbal expressions indicating that a condition or event is serious, worrisome, distressing or deserving special attention (such as comforting or other special consideration), and is of particular concern at this point in time. These statements have a strong and immediate emotional or psychosocial component, and do not refer to a more general frame of mind or past issues. Voice tone, intonation, and/or verbal content may disclose worries, concerns, stress, nervousness, personal preferences, or uncertainties that are of *immediate* concern. A patient may express concern or worry about a procedure hurting, for example, "I'm afraid this will hurt." Likewise, a provider may express concern or worry about a patients' expectations about a terminal disease such as "I'm worried that you may not have as much time as you think and I'd like to talk about what happens if your disease progresses faster than we expect."

Reassurance/Optimism

These statements indicate optimism, encouragement, relief of worry, or reassurance. Unlike approvals or compliments, *reassurance* statements are more intensely personal, intimate or immediate (in other words, reflecting how the patient or physician feels at this point in time). These statements also include prognostic statements that are related to physical or emotional consequences. For example, a provider could use reassurance statements to comfort a patient, as in "I wouldn't worry about your past tests. These newer tests look a lot better." A patient may use reassurance or optimism statements to describe positive feelings in the moment, such as "I feel really good today."

RIAS Global Affect Ratings

In addition to explicit verbal statements, RIAS coders assign global ratings to both providers and patients across several positive and negative global affect dimensions (see Table 4-1). Coders assign ratings based on their overall impressions of the speakers after the entire interaction or after a given section (e.g., greeting vs. closing). In most studies, only the patients are rated on depression/sadness and emotional distress/upset while both patient and provider are rated separately on anxiety/nervousness, dominance/assertiveness, interest/attentiveness, friendliness/warmth, responsiveness/engagement, sympathetic/empathetic, respectfulness, hurried/rushed, and interactivity.

■ HOW OFTEN DOES EMOTION DIALOGUE OCCUR IN MEDICAL INTERACTIONS?

Using the common lens of RIAS-coded communication, we conducted a meta-analysis of this large body of empirical communication studies, addressing such fundamental questions such as *how much* emotion is conveyed, *what emotions* are conveyed, and *who conveys* more or less emotion during medical visits—doctors or patients, males or females, the young or the old, experienced or newly trained clinicians. Our review was limited to actual patients and healthcare providers (as opposed to simulated patients or avatars).

The summary below captures results from 77 research articles reflecting the experience of over 2,000 healthcare providers and over 7,000 patients (see Appendix A for list of all studies). Most studies were conducted in the United States, Europe, and Scandinavia, published from 1994 to 2020, with an average interaction length of 23.17 minutes ($SD = 16.17$) during mostly audio- or video-recorded routine visits. Providers were predominantly general practitioners, white, had a mean age of 40, and there were an equal number of males and females represented in the studies. Patients on average were 56 years old, predominantly white, and there were also an equal number of males and females represented in the studies.

We compared the amount of emotional talk to other types of dialogue (i.e., instrumental codes or codes that reflected more task-focused dialogue) across all studies. Instrumental utterances related to clinical and therapeutic information in the form of questions, paraphrases, and affirmations. As can be seen in Figs. 4-1 and 4-2, the percentage of emotional dialogue was

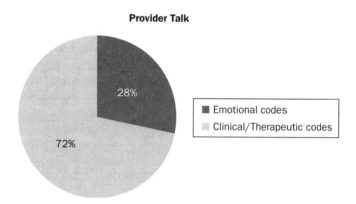

FIGURE 4-1. Percent of emotional and clinical/therapeutic provider talk across 77 research articles using the RIAS.

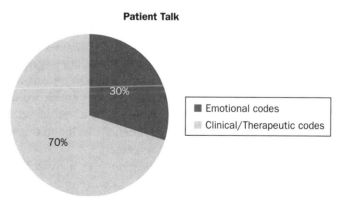

FIGURE 4-2. Percent of emotional and clinical/therapeutic patient talk across 77 research articles using the RIAS.

dramatically lower compared to the more clinical/therapeutic statements for both patients and providers. Only 28% of providers and 30% of patient statements were considered socioemotional or social and affective.

How Often Do Positive Statements Occur?

Among the nine emotional categories, positive statements, including approvals (e.g., "You've been so helpful"), compliments (e.g., "Your nurse was so kind"), laughter/jokes, and agreement (e.g., "Okay, I'll do that") were used most frequently by both patients and providers at about two positive statements per minute by patients and two positive statements per minute by providers, totaling four positive statements per minute on average. This means that every 15 seconds or so, a patient or provider would make a statement that showed approval, a compliment, a joke or laugh, or agreement. Said in another way, in an average 23.5-minute visit, there are some 94 positive statements made by patient or provider. While this category includes truly positive expressions such as compliments and approvals, the majority of exchanges in this category are usually agreements. While agreements are positive in nature, their function is largely passive acquiescence (e.g., "ok," "right," "aha"), cueing that a statement has been heard and understood rather than affirmatively endorsed.

Provider type was related to patient positive talk; patients' positive statements were significantly higher with physicians than with nurses. The effect of provider type on positive talk likely reflects power differentials: patients are more likely to acquiesce to physicians compared to nurses as reflected in patients' use of positive statements. Notably, this effect may be magnified by the gender disparity between physicians and nurses in our studies: the proportion of physicians in the studies was highly correlated with the number of male providers. Patients' greater positivity could reflect a pattern of socialization and verbal dominance which elicits high levels of patient passive assent, a pattern more characteristic of physicians than nurses. Passive assent likely means that patients are not engaged in their care or health decisions and instead simply defer. Based on this finding, providers should be aware of how their clinical role may influence the interaction when they ask for patient understanding and attempt shared decision making, as clinician type may play a role in patients' likelihood to use positive statements, particularly those that reflect agreement.

Finally, as publication year increased from 1994 to 2020, patients used fewer positive statements per minute. This finding could reflect that patients are becoming more activated and engaged in their care and health and are therefore less likely to passively agree with instructions delivered by clinicians in educational monologues. This may mark more clinician attention to inviting patient engagement in problem solving and counseling than didactic instruction. The former pattern of interaction was found to be predominant in 1997 but may have diminished over the subsequent 20 years with added emphasis in the literature on patient-centered communication.[43]

How Often Do Negative Statements Occur?

Negative statements, on the other hand, including criticisms (e.g., "I don't like the way they run that clinic") and disagreements (e.g., "No, that's not what I said") were rarely used by either patients or providers. On average, patients used negative statements at a rate of .11 per minute, which totals an average of two to three negative statements in an average 23.5-minute visit. Providers used negative statements at an even lower frequency, .04 per minute, totaling an average of one negative statement per 23.5-minute visit. While negative statements on the surface appear to harm the relationship between patients and providers, when used appropriately, they are essential to building rapport because they signal that the patient or the provider is comfortable enough to express disagreement or criticisms. It would be unusual for patients and providers to agree with every statement that someone has made; therefore, by holding back or not exchanging genuine feelings and thoughts that may be categorized as criticisms or disagreements, patients and providers may be consigning their relationship to one of superficiality. For instance, a patient statement "No, I don't think that medication is worth trying, it won't work for me" allows for a deeper discussion of why the patient feels this way and what they think would work for them rather than the patient simply not filling or taking the medication. Providers must be trained to become comfortable with patients disagreeing with a treatment recommendation and work on their own emotion regulation in order to respond to these statements effectively (see Chapter 7, Emotion Regulation in Patients, Providers, and the Clinical Relationship). Criticisms and disagreements initiated by providers must be done in a thoughtful and contextualized way so that patients do not withdraw or, worse, stop treatment or coming back for appointments.

Providers in general tend to use more negative statements with their male patients compared to their female patients. This could reflect assumptions about gender and gender roles such that providers think that males are more comfortable with disagreement and criticism than their female patients. It could also reflect a general difference in health and the content of appointments, in that males tend to be sicker than females when they seek healthcare, so more negative statements could be more likely in these interactions with males compared to females.[44]

How Often Do Emotional Statements Occur?

Emotional statements include statements of empathy, legitimation, partnership, concern/worry, and reassurance/optimism. On average, patients use .52 emotional statements per minute while providers use an average of .74 emotional statements per minute of the interaction. This translates to patients using approximately 12 emotional statements in a 23.5-minute visit while providers use slightly more at 17 emotional statements during the average 23.5-minute visit. Combined, patients and providers exchange approximately 29 emotional statements per 23.5-minute visit, approximately one emotional statement per minute of the interaction.

Older providers used more emotional talk than their younger counterparts. While age is not always tied to clinical experience, there was no consistent reporting of clinical experience across studies, so we took provider age as a reasonable proxy for clinical experience. Thus, this finding can be interpreted to mean that more experienced providers are more emotionally responsive than less experienced or younger providers. Perhaps older and more experienced providers have had the opportunity for higher continuity of relationships with their patients making emotional responsiveness more commonplace and natural. This is particularly true of the many resident studies with young providers who have limited opportunity to build long-term relationships with their patients. Medical educators should be particularly attuned to this when tailoring educational materials either in medical school programs or in continuing education curriculum and address the possible influence of continuity of care on emotional responsiveness.

We also found that patients used more emotional statements with physicians compared to nurses. Given stereotypes about nurses being better communicators and warmer than physicians, this finding was surprising.[45] This finding may be a function of the type of visit with a physician compared to a nurse by way of having more serious health conversations or concerns being addressed in medical rather than nursing sessions.

What Is the Average Global Affect of Interactions?

On average, patients were judged as conveying higher levels of positive affect and lower levels of negative affect than providers. Patients were rated on emotional distress and scored midscale on average while providers were on average rated as moderately to very responsive and engaged. Patients may be expressing more global positive affect than global negative affect compared to providers due to the power dynamics of interactions and the likely impression management that patients participate in. Providers are likely serious and rushed and this may be perceived as more negative than patients who are likely very engaged and want to appear positively to their providers.

As publication year increased from 1994 to 2020, providers expressed more positive affect, which could reflect initiatives such as emphasizing patient-centered care or the introduction of new ACGME clinical competencies relating to communication.

Both patient age and race were related to global coder affect ratings of emotional distress/upset. Studies with younger patients were rated by coders as displaying lower levels of patient emotional distress/upset than studies with older patients, and similarly, studies with more minority patients showed lower coder ratings of patient emotional distress/upset affect than studies with more white patients. We believe the effect of age likely has to do with younger patients having fewer health concerns, therefore appearing less emotionally distressed/upset than studies with older patients. In addition, minority patients may regulate their emotions more because the likelihood that they are paired with a provider of the same race is low. Race incongruent patient–provider dyads are characterized as being shorter, having patients with lower trust, satisfaction, and participation in their care compared to race congruent dyads (see Chapter 12, Culture and Emotions in the Medical Encounter).[46] Therefore, minority patients may feel as though they cannot truly express themselves or negative affect. This will be an important avenue of future educational interventions for medical educators and trainees—ensuring all patients, regardless of race or ethnicity, feel comfortable enough to express their emotions. In addition, medical schools should continue their work to reach, admit, and support diverse student bodies.

■ RECOMMENDATIONS FOR MEDICAL EDUCATORS AND MEDICAL PROFESSIONALS IN FACILITATING EMOTION DIALOGUE WITH THEIR PATIENTS

As mentioned prior, the RIAS is a useful tool for characterizing medical visits and establishing links between verbal dialogue and patient health outcomes. For example, the RIAS codes have been linked to patient satisfaction, adherence to treatment, level of control, and patient knowledge about their pathologies.[28-31] Specifically, the emotion categories are most often related to patient satisfaction.[32,33]

In this chapter, we highlight the rather limited expression of emotionally focused dialogue in the medical visit. When talk of this kind does occur, it tends to be positive rather than explicitly emotional. This positive talk, as discussed, may reflect passive assent or agreement rather than true positive emotion. The studies presented here have enabled the identification of shortcomings in emotional communication by providers, such as the predominance of instrumental (i.e., biomedical/therapeutic) communication.

The RIAS allows one to understand in a purely objective way (unlike many other assessment tools) the affective, instrumental, and nonverbal (as captured in the global ratings) components of communication that allow for more humanized, patient-centered, and effective care. While time intensive, using the RIAS as an assessment tool has greatly added the understanding of what providers and patients are doing, and how engaged their patients are in emotional and other types of dialogue. This type of assessment has allowed for the monitoring and continuous improvement of care by promoting satisfaction, reducing errors, and emotional difficulties by pointing out areas for improvement in the communication process and allowing for information about areas in which providers may need personalized communication skills training. Furthermore, for readers at all stages of clinical training and experience, familiarity not only with the research but also with the various categories of affective and emotional statements captured in the RIAS may help provide a more enriched and differentiated mental catalogue of relevant concepts to be drawn on in the process of clinical care.

While there are clearly a variety of positive aspects regarding the use of the RIAS, it is not without limitations. For instance, it is primarily a quantitative method of interaction analysis and while it does include some qualitative elements that allow for limited content analysis, it does not provide the kind of insight that qualitative methods of conversational and discourse analysis can provide. Therefore, while the RIAS can be a notably helpful tool for quantifying emotion in the medical dialogue, it should not be taken as a comprehensive assessment for all possible verbal and nonverbal exchanges.

■ CONCLUSION

The emotional world of routine medical practice is complex and varied. While these meta-analytic results show promise that the field of medicine may be moving toward a more emotion-focused approach to medical care, we must emphasize that the work here is not done. Patient-centeredness and the importance of emotions in the medical visit must continue to be incorporated into medical education through teaching the importance of outcomes related to emotional talk, how to engage in emotional talk, and practice and feedback about trainees' and providers' ability to participate in emotional talk with their patients. Providers must be given opportunities to practice emotional, patient-centered exchanges with opportunities for feedback, which ultimately may allow for patients to express their emotions more freely. Continuing to give attention to the role of emotional dialogue in medical information exchanges will not only benefit patient outcomes but will allow for this type of practice to become the criterion by which quality healthcare is judged.

REFERENCES

1. Montepare JM, Dobish H. The contribution of emotion perceptions and their overgeneralizations to trait impressions. *J Nonverbal Behav.* 2003;27(4):237-254.

2. Bensing JM, Verheul W, Van Dulmen AM. Patient anxiety in the medical encounter: a study of verbal and nonverbal communication in general practice. *Health Educ.* 2008;108(5):373-383.

3. Roter D, Larson S. The Roter Interaction Analysis System (RIAS): utility and flexibility for analysis of medical interactions. *Patient Educ Couns.* 2002;46(4):243-251.

4. Institute of Medicine. *Crossing the Quality Chasm: A New Health System for the 21st Century.* 2001.

5. Institute of Medicine (US) Committee on Quality of Health Care in America. In: Kohn LT, Corrigan JM, Donaldson MS, eds. *To Err Is Human: Building a Safer Health System.* Washington, D.C.: National Academies Press; 2000.

6. ABIM Foundation. Medical professionalism in the new millennium: a physician charter. *Ann Intern Med.* 2002;136(3):243-246.

7. Rathert C, Wyrwich MD, Boren SA. Patient-centered care and outcomes: a systematic review of the literature. *Med Care Res Rev.* 2013;70(4):351-379.

8. Zolnierek KBH, DiMatteo MR. Physician communication and patient adherence to treatment: a meta-analysis. *Med Care.* 2009;47(8):826-834.

9. Engel GL. The need for a new medical model: a challenge for biomedicine. *Science.* 1977;196(4286):129-136.

10. Lipkin M, Putnam S, Lazare A, eds. *The Medical Interview: Clinical Care, Education and Research.* New York, NY: Springer-Verlag; 1995.

11. McWhinney I. The need for a transformed clinical method. In: Stewart M, Roter DL, eds. *Communicating with Medical Patients.* Newbury Park, CA: Sage; 1989: 25-40.

12. Byrne PS, Long BEL. *Doctors Talking to Patients: A Study of the Verbal Behaviour of General Practitioners Consulting in Their Surgeries.* London: HMSO; 1976.

13. Plato, Jowett B, Kaplan JD, et al. *Dialogues of Plato.* New York, NY: Washington Square Press; 2001.

14. Mead N, Bower P. Patient-centredness: a conceptual framework and review of the empirical literature. *Soc Sci Med.* 2000;51(7):1087-1110.

15. Langberg EM, Dyhr L, Davidsen AS. Development of the concept of patient-centredness: a systematic review. *Patient Educ Couns.* 2019;102(7):1228-1236.

16. Epstein RM, Franks P, Fiscella K, et al. Measuring patient-centered communication in patient-physician consultations: theoretical and practical issues. *Soc Sci Med.* 2005;61(7):1516-1528.

17. Epstein RM, Street RLJ. The values and value of patient-centered care. *Ann Fam Med.* 2011;9(2):100-103.

18. Epstein RM, Street RL Jr. *Patient-Centered Communication in Cancer Care: Promoting Healing and Reducing Suffering;* 2007. NIH Publication No. 07-6225.

19. Carlick A, Biley FC. Thoughts on the therapeutic use of narrative in the promotion of coping in cancer care. *Eur J Cancer Care (Engl).* 2004;13(4):308-317.

20. Iwamitsu Y, Shimoda K, Abe H, Tani T, Kodama M, Okawa M. Differences in emotional distress between breast tumor patients with emotional inhibition and those with emotional expression. *Psychiatry Clin Neurosci.* 2003;57(3):289-294.

21. Rosenberg HJ, Rosenberg SD, Ernstoff MS, et al. Expressive disclosure and health outcomes in a prostate cancer population. *Int J Psychiatry Med.* 2002;32(1):37-53.

22. Kitayama SE, Markus HRE. *Emotion and Culture: Empirical Studies of Mutual Influence.* Washington, D.C.: American Psychological Association; 1994.

23. Manstead A, Oatley K. *Gender and Emotion: Social Psychological Perspectives.* Cambridge, UK: Cambridge University Press; 2000.

24. Wolfe HL, Fix GM, Bolton RE, Ruben MA, Bokhour BG. Development of observational rating scales for evaluating patient-centered communication within a whole health approach to care. *Explore.* 2020.

25. Krupat E, Yeager CM, Putnam S. Patient role orientations, doctor-patient fit, and visit satisfaction. *Psychol Health.* 2000;15(5):707-719.

26. Del Piccolo L, de Haes H, Heaven C, et al. Development of the Verona coding definitions of emotional sequences to code health providers' responses (VR-CoDES-P) to patient cues and concerns. *Patient Educ Couns.* 2011;82(2):149-155.

27. Bylund CL, Makoul G. Empathic communication and gender in the physician-patient encounter. *Patient Educ Couns.* 2002;48(3):207-216.

28. Sheldon LK, Ellington L, Barrett R, Dudley WN, Clayton MF, Rinaldi K. Nurse responsiveness to cancer patient expressions of emotion. *Patient Educ Couns.* 2009;76(1):63-70.

29. Gilbert DA, Hayes E. Communication and outcomes of visits between older patients and nurse practitioners. *Nurs Res.* 2009;58(4):283-293.

30. Kumar R, Korthuis PT, Saha S, et al. Decision-making role preferences among patients with HIV: associations with patient and provider characteristics and communication behaviors. *J Gen Intern Med.* 2010;25(6):517-523.

31. Siminoff LA, Graham GC, Gordon NH. Cancer communication patterns and the influence of patient characteristics: disparities in information-giving and affective behaviors. *Patient Educ Couns.* 2006;62(3):355-360.

32. Beach MC, Roter DL, Wang N-Y, Duggan PS, Cooper LA. Are physicians' attitudes of respect accurately perceived by patients and associated with more positive communication behaviors? *Patient Educ Couns.* 2006;62(3):347-354.

33. Haskard KB, Williams SL, DiMatteo MR, Rosenthal R, White MK, Goldstein MG. Physician and patient communication training in primary care: effects on participation and satisfaction. *Health Psychol.* 2008;27(5):513-522.

34. Roh H, Park KH, Park SY. Verbal communication of students with high patient-physician interaction scores in a clinical performance examination assessed by standardized patients. *Korean J Med Educ.* 2017;29(4):241-251.

35. Kubota Y, Yano Y, Seki S, et al. Assessment of pharmacy students' communication competence using the Roter Interaction Analysis System during objective structured clinical examinations. *Am J Pharm Educ.* 2011;75(3):43.

36. Kalet A, Earp JA, Kowlowitz V. How well do faculty evaluate the interviewing skills of medical students? *J Gen Intern Med.* 1992;7(5):499-505.

37. Stiefel F, Bourquin C, Layat C, Vadot S, Bonvin R, Berney A. Medical students' skills and needs for training in breaking bad news. *J Cancer Educ.* 2013;28(1):187-191.

38. Blanch DC, Hall JA, Roter DL, Frankel RM. Is it good to express uncertainty to a patient? Correlates and consequences for medical students in a standardized patient visit. *Patient Educ Couns.* 2009;76(3):300-306.

39. Price EG, Windish DM, Magaziner J, Cooper LA. Assessing validity of standardized patient ratings of medical students' communication behavior using the Roter Interaction Analysis System. *Patient Educ Couns.* 2008;70(1):3-9.

40. van Dulmen S, Tromp F, Grosfeld F, ten Cate O, Bensing J. The impact of assessing simulated bad news consultations on medical students' stress response and communication performance. *Psychoneuroendocrinology.* 2007;32(8-10):943-950.

41. Bales R. *Interaction Process Analysis.* Cambridge, MA: Addison-Wesley; 1950.

42. Korsch BM, Negrete VF. Doctor-patient communication. *Sci Am.* 1972;227(2):66-74.

43. Roter DL, Stewart M, Putnam SM, Lipkin MJ, Stiles W, Inui TS. Communication patterns of primary care physicians. *JAMA.* 1997;277(4):350-356.

44. Courtenay WH. Constructions of masculinity and their influence on men's well-being: a theory of gender and health. *Soc Sci Med.* 2000;50(10):1385-1401.

45. Sollami A, Caricati L, Mancini T. Ambivalent stereotypes of nurses and physicians: impact on students' attitude toward interprofessional education. *Acta Biomed.* 2015;86(Suppl 1):19-28.

46. Cooper LA, Roter DL, Johnson RL, Ford DE, Steinwachs DM, Powe NR. Patient-centered communication, ratings of care, and concordance of patient and physician race. *Ann Intern Med.* 2003;139(11):907-915.

■ APPENDIX A

RIAS-Coded Study References Included in Meta-Analysis

1. Aggarwal NK, Cedeno K, Lewis-Fernandez R. Patient and clinician communication practices during the DSM-5 cultural formulation interview field trial. *Anthropol Med.* 2020;27(2):192-211.

2. Agha Z, Roter DL, Schapira RM. An evaluation of patient-physician communication style during telemedicine consultations. *J Med Internet Res.* 2009;11(3):e36.

3. Badaczewski A, Bauman LJ, Blank AE, et al. Relationship between teach-back and patient-centered communication in primary care pediatric encounters. *Patient Educ Couns.* 2017;100(7):1345-1352.

4. Beach MC, Roter DL, Saha S, et al. Impact of a brief patient and provider intervention to improve the quality of communication about medication adherence among HIV patients. *Patient Educ Couns.* 2015;98(9):1078-1083.

5. Beach MC, Roter DL, Wang NY, Duggan PS, Cooper LA. Are physicians' attitudes of respect accurately perceived by patients and associated

with more positive communication behaviors? *Patient Educ Couns.* 2006;62(3):347-354.

6. Beach MC, Roter D, Korthuis PT, et al. A multicenter study of physician mindfulness and health care quality. *Ann Fam Med.* 2013;11(5):421-428.

7. Roter DL, Stewart M, Putnam SM, Lipkin M Jr, Stiles W, Inui TS. Communication patterns of primary care physicians. *JAMA.* 1997;277(4): 350-356.

8. Bensing JM, Tromp F, van Dulmen S, van den Brink-Muinen A, Verheul W, Schellevis FG. Shifts in doctor-patient communication between 1986 and 2002: a study of videotaped general practice consultations with hypertension patients. *BMC Fam Pract.* 2006;7:62.

9. Boss RD, Donohue PK, Larson SM, Arnold RM, Roter DL. Family conferences in the neonatal ICU: observation of communication dynamics and contributions. *Pediatr Crit Care Med.* 2016;17(3):223-230.

10. Cené CW, Haymore B, Laux JP, et al. Family presence and participation during medical visits of heart failure patients: an analysis of survey and audio-taped communication data. *Patient Educ Couns.* 2017;100(2):250-258.

11. Claramita M, Dalen JV, Van Der Vleuten CP. Doctors in a Southeast Asian country communicate sub-optimally regardless of patients' educational background. *Patient Educ Couns.* 2011;85(3):e169-e174.

12. Cox ED, Smith MA, Brown RL, Fitzpatrick MA. Assessment of the physician-caregiver relationship scales (PCRS). *Patient Educ Couns.* 2008;70(1):69-78.

13. Cruz M, Roter DL, Cruz RF, et al. Appointment length, psychiatrists' communication behaviors, and medication management appointment adherence. *Psychiatr Serv.* 2013;64(9):886-892.

14. Detmar SB, Muller MJ, Wever LD, Schornagel JH, Aaronson NK. The patient-physician relationship. Patient-physician communication during outpatient palliative treatment visits: an observational study. *JAMA.* 2001;285(10):1351-1357.

15. Eide H, Quera V, Finset A. Exploring rare patient behaviour with sequential analysis: an illustration. *Epidemiol Psichiatr Soc.* 2003;12(2):109-114.

16. Ellington L, Baty BJ, McDonald J, et al. Exploring genetic counseling communication patterns: the role of teaching and counseling approaches. *J Genet Couns.* 2006;15(3):179-189.

17. Ellington L, Clayton MF, Reblin M, Donaldson G, Latimer S. Communication among cancer patients, caregivers, and hospice nurses: content, process and change over time. *Patient Educ Couns.* 2018;101(3): 414-421.

18. Ellington L, Reblin M, Clayton MF, Berry P, Mooney K. Hospice nurse communication with patients with cancer and their family caregivers. *J Palliat Med.* 2012;15(3):262-268.

19. Ellington L, Roter D, Dudley WN, et al. Communication analysis of BRCA1 genetic counseling. *J Genet Couns.* 2005;14(5):377-386.

20. Ernesäter A, Winblad U, Engström M, Holmström IK. Malpractice claims regarding calls to Swedish telephone advice nursing: what went wrong and why? *J Telemed Telecare.* 2012;18(7):379-383.

21. Farquharson L, Noble LM, Barker C, Behrens RH. Health beliefs and communication in the travel clinic consultation as predictors of adherence to malaria chemoprophylaxis. *Br J Health Psychol.* 2004;9(Pt 2):201-217.

22. Ford S, Fallowfield L, Lewis S. Doctor-patient interactions in oncology. *Soc Sci Med.* 1996;42(11):1511-1519.

23. Forner D, Ungar G, Chorney J, Meier J, Hong P. Turn analysis and patient-centredness in paediatric otolaryngology surgical consultations. *Clin Otolaryngol.* 2020.

24. Gadomski AM, Fothergill KE, Larson S, et al. Integrating mental health into adolescent annual visits: impact of previsit comprehensive screening on within-visit processes. *J Adolesc Health.* 2015;56(3):267-273.

25. Guan Y, Roter DL, Erby LH, et al. Disclosing genetic risk of Alzheimer's disease to cognitively impaired patients and visit companions: findings from the REVEAL Study. *Patient Educ Couns.* 2017;100(5):927-935.

26. Hart CN, Drotar D, Gori A, Lewin L. Enhancing parent-provider communication in ambulatory pediatric practice. *Patient Educ Couns.* 2006;63(1-2):38-46.

27. Hausmann LR, Hanusa BH, Kresevic DM, et al. Orthopedic communication about osteoarthritis treatment: does patient race matter? *Arthritis Care Res.* 2011;63(5):635-642.

28. Havranek EP, Hanratty R, Tate C, et al. The effect of values affirmation on race-discordant patient-provider communication. *Arch Intern Med.* 2012;172(21):1662-1667.

29. Heyn L, Finset A, Eide H, Ruland CM. Effects of an interactive tailored patient assessment on patient-clinician communication in cancer care. *Psychooncology.* 2013;22(1):89-96.

30. Isenberg SR, Aslakson RA, Dionne-Odom JN, et al. Family companions' involvement during pre-surgical consent visits for major cancer surgery and its relationship to visit communication and satisfaction. *Patient Educ Couns.* 2018;101(6):1066-1074.

31. Ishikawa H, Roter DL, Yamazaki Y, Takayama T. Physician-elderly patient-companion communication and roles of companions in Japanese geriatric encounters. *Soc Sci Med.* 2005;60(10):2307-2320.

32. Ishikawa H, Takayama T, Yamazaki Y, Seki Y, Katsumata N, Aoki Y. The interaction between physician and patient communication behaviors in Japanese cancer consultations and the influence of personal and consultation characteristics. *Patient Educ Couns.* 2002;46(4):277-285.

33. Ishikawa H, Roter DL, Yamazaki Y, Takayama T. Physician-elderly patient-companion communication and roles of companions in Japanese geriatric encounters. *Soc Sci Med.* 2005;60(10):2307-2320.

34. Johnson KB, Serwint JR, Fagan LA, Thompson RE, Wilson ME, Roter D. Computer-based documentation: effects on parent-provider communication during pediatric health maintenance encounters. *Pediatrics.* 2008;122(3):590-598.

35. Katz MG, Jacobson TA, Veledar E, Kripalani S. Patient literacy and question-asking behavior during the medical encounter: a mixed-methods analysis. *J Gen Intern Med.* 2007;22(6):782-786.

36. Kim YM, Kols A, Bonnin C, Richardson P, Roter D. Client communication behaviors with health care providers in Indonesia. *Patient Educ Couns.* 2001;45(1):59-68.

37. Kindler CH, Szirt L, Sommer D, Häusler R, Langewitz W. A quantitative analysis of anaesthetist-patient communication during the pre-operative visit. *Anaesthesia.* 2005;60(1):53-59.

38. Koerber A, Gajendra S, Fulford RL, BeGole E, Evans CA. An exploratory study of orthodontic resident communication by patient race and ethnicity. *J Dental Educ.* 2004;68(5):553-62.

39. Lambert K, Lau TK, Davison S, Mitchell H, Harman A, Carrie M. Does a renal diet question prompt sheet increase the patient centeredness of renal dietitian outpatient consultations? *Patient Educ Couns.* 2020;103(8):1645-1649.

40. Langewitz WA, Loeb Y, Nübling M, Hunziker S. From patient talk to physician notes: comparing the content of medical interviews with medical records in a sample of outpatients in internal medicine. *Patient Educ Couns.* 2009;76(3):336-340.

41. Leone D, Borghi L, Del Negro S, et al. Doctor-couple communication during assisted reproductive technology visits. *Hum Reprod.* 2018;33(5):877-886.

42. Lerner B, Roberts JS, Shwartz M, Roter DL, Green RC, Clark JA. Distinct communication patterns during genetic counseling for late-onset Alzheimer's risk assessment. *Patient Educ Couns.* 2014;94(2):170-179.

43. Levinson W, Roter DL, Mullooly JP, Dull VT, Frankel RM. Physician-patient communication: the relationship with malpractice claims among primary care physicians and surgeons. *JAMA.* 1997;277(7):553-559.

44. Levinson W, Roter D. Physicians' psychosocial beliefs correlate with their patient communication skills. *J Gen Intern Med.* 1995;10(7):375-379.

45. Maatouk-Bürmann B, Ringel N, Spang J, et al. Improving patient-centered communication: results of a randomized controlled trial. *Patient Educ Couns.* 2016;99(1):117-124.

46. Maclachlan EW, Shepard-Perry MG, Ingo P, et al. Evaluating the effectiveness of patient education and empowerment to improve patient-provider interactions in antiretroviral therapy clinics in Namibia. *AIDS Care*. 2016;28(5):620-627.

47. Martin KD, Roter DL, Beach MC, Carson KA, Cooper LA. Physician communication behaviors and trust among black and white patients with hypertension. *Med Care*. 2013;51(2):151-157.

48. Martin L, Gitsels-van der Wal JT, Pereboom MT, Spelten ER, Hutton EK, van Dulmen S. Clients' psychosocial communication and midwives' verbal and nonverbal communication during prenatal counseling for anomaly screening. *Patient Educ Couns*. 2016;99(1):85-91.

49. Menendez ME, van Hoorn BT, Mackert M, Donovan EE, Chen NC, Ring D. Patients with limited health literacy ask fewer questions during office visits with hand surgeons. *Clin Orthop Relat Res*. 2017;475(5):1291-1297.

50. Mjaaland TA, Finset A. Frequency of GP communication addressing the patient's resources and coping strategies in medical interviews: a video-based observational study. *BMC Fam Pract*. 2009;10:49.

51. Muller I, Kirby S, Yardley L. The therapeutic relationship in telephone-delivered support for people undertaking rehabilitation: a mixed-methods interaction analysis. *Disabil Rehabil*. 2015;37(12):1060-1065.

52. Ong LM, Visser MR, Lammes FB, de Haes JC. Doctor-patient communication and cancer patients' quality of life and satisfaction. *Patient Educ Couns*. 2000;41(2):145-156.

53. Paasche-Orlow M, Roter D. The communication patterns of internal medicine and family practice physicians. *J Am Board Fam Pract*. 2003;16(6):485-493.

54. Pelicano-Romano J, Neves MR, Amado A, Cavaco AM. Do community pharmacists actively engage elderly patients in the dialogue? Results from pharmaceutical care consultations. *Health Expect*. 2015;18(5):1721-1734.

55. Pourhabib S, Chessex C, Murray J, Grace SL. Elements of patient-health-care provider communication related to cardiovascular rehabilitation referral. *J Health Psychol*. 2016;21(4):468-482.

56. Reblin M, Baucom BRW, Clayton MF, et al. Communication of emotion in home hospice cancer care: implications for spouse caregiver depression into bereavement. *Psychooncology*. 2019;28(5):1102-1109.

57. Reblin M, Clayton MF, Xu J, et al. Caregiver, patient, and nurse visit communication patterns in cancer home hospice. *Psychooncology*. 2017;26(12):2285-2293.

58. Reich CM, Hack SM, Klingaman EA, et al. Consumer satisfaction with antipsychotic medication-monitoring appointments: the role of

consumer-prescriber communication patterns. *Int J Psychiatry Clin Pract.* 2018;22(2):89-94.

59. Roter DL, Larson S. The relationship between residents' and attending physicians' communication during primary care visits: an illustrative use of the Roter Interaction Analysis System. *Health Commun.* 2001;13(1):33-48.

60. Roter DL, Geller G, Bernhardt BA, Larson SM, Doksum T. Effects of obstetrician gender on communication and patient satisfaction. *Obstet Gynecol.* 1999;93(5 Pt 1):635-641.

61. Roter DL, Larson S, Fischer GS, Arnold RM, Tulsky JA. Experts practice what they preach: A descriptive study of best and normative practices in end-of-life discussions. *Arch Intern Med.* 2000;160(22):3477-3485.

62. Roter DL, Stewart M, Putnam SM, Lipkin M Jr, Stiles W, Inui TS. Communication patterns of primary care physicians. *JAMA.* 1997;277(4):350-356.

63. Roter DL, Larson S, Fischer GS, Arnold RM, Tulsky JA. Experts practice what they preach: a descriptive study of best and normative practices in end-of-life discussions. *Arch Intern Med.* 2000;160(22):3477-3485.

64. Schouten BC, Meeuwesen L, Tromp F, Harmsen HA. Cultural diversity in patient participation: the influence of patients' characteristics and doctors' communicative behaviour. *Patient Educ Couns.* 2007;67(1-2):214-223.

65. Shaw WS, Chin EH, Nelson CC, Reme SE, Woiszwillo MJ, Verma SK. What circumstances prompt a workplace discussion in medical evaluations for back pain? *J Occup Rehabil.* 2013;23(1):125-134.

66. Sondell K, Söderfeldt B, Palmqvist S. Underlying dimensions of verbal communication between dentists and patients in prosthetic dentistry. *Patient Educ Couns.* 2003;50(2):157-165.

67. Street RL Jr, Marengo MF, Barbo A, et al. Affective tone in medical encounters and its relationship with treatment adherence in a multi-ethnic cohort of patients with rheumatoid arthritis. *J Clin Rheumatol.* 2015;21(4):181-188.

68. Tilburt J, Yost KJ, Lenz HJ, et al. A multicenter comparison of complementary and alternative medicine (CAM) discussions in oncology care: the role of time, patient-centeredness, and practice context. *Oncologist.* 2019;24(11):e1180-e1189.

69. van den Brink-Muinen A, Caris-Verhallen W. Doctors' responses to patients' concerns: testing the use of sequential analysis. *Epidemiol Psichiatr Soc.* 2003;12(2):92-97.

70. Wakefield BJ, Bylund CL, Holman JE, et al. Nurse and patient communication profiles in a home-based telehealth intervention for heart failure management. *Patient Educ Couns.* 2008;71(2):285-292.

71. Washington Cole KO, Roter DL. Starting the conversation: patient initiation of weight-related behavioral counseling during pregnancy. *Patient Educ Couns.* 2016;99(10):1603-1610.

72. Watanabe S, Yoshida T, Kono T, et al. Relationship of trainee dentists' self-reported empathy and communication behaviors with simulated patients' assessment in medical interviews. *PLoS One.* 2018;13(12):e0203970.

73. Wissow LS, Roter DL, Wilson ME. Pediatrician interview style and mothers' disclosure of psychosocial issues. *Pediatrics.* 1994;93(2):289-295.

74. Wittenberg-Lyles E, Oliver DP, Kruse RL, Demiris G, Gage LA, Wagner K. Family caregiver participation in hospice interdisciplinary team meetings: how does it affect the nature and content of communication? *Health Commun.* 2013;28(2):110-118.

75. Wolff JL, Roter DL. Older adults' mental health function and patient-centered care: does the presence of a family companion help or hinder communication? *J Gen Intern Med.* 2012;27(6):661-668.

76. Wolff JL, Roter DL, Barron J, et al. A tool to strengthen the older patient-companion partnership in primary care: results from a pilot study. *J Am Geriatr Soc.* 2014;62(2):312-319.

77. Zaleta AK, Carpenter BD. Patient-centered communication during the disclosure of a dementia diagnosis. *Am J Alzheimer's Dis Other Demen.* 2010;25(6):513-520.

Clinical Emotional Intelligence

II

Perception of Emotion in the Medical Visit

Morgan D. Stosic, Mollie A. Ruben, and Danielle Blanch-Hartigan

The process of interpersonal accuracy can be defined as an accurate judgment about any verifiable characteristic of a person such as their affective states, personality traits, values, and intentions.[1] One of the more relevant dimensions of interpersonal accuracy to the medical encounter is that of *emotion perception*. Clinicians who notice and accurately interpret their patient's emotional reactions will be better equipped to foster rapport and trust with their patients, as well as better able to tailor treatment plans and goals during the medical visit.[2] This chapter introduces the concept of interpersonal accuracy as it refers to emotion perception, discusses the outcomes associated with this skill, reviews psychometrically validated tests of emotion perception, and recommends ways to train and improve emotion recognition as a clinical skill.

■ EMOTION PERCEPTION ACCURACY

In order for clinicians to accurately assess their patient's emotional state, they must first be able to detect and correctly utilize emotion cues expressed by their patients.[3-5] Emotional content is expressed by patients in a majority of consultations.[6-8] Moments within the exchange when a patient presents emotional content to a clinician have been operationalized and labeled in a variety of ways, as "windows of opportunity,"[9] "clues,"[10,11] or "empathic opportunities."[6,12-15] A group of researchers in this area agreed to call these moments "cues,"[16,17] which is the terminology we will use in this chapter. Chapter 4 (Emotion Dialogue in the Medical Encounter : When and How Often Does It Happen?) and Chapter 6 (Emotion Cues as Clinical Opportunities) in the present volume specifically address the use of verbal emotion cues in the clinical interaction.

Emotion cues can be both verbal (e.g., "I am scared that my treatment won't work") and nonverbal. These nonverbal cues can manifest as visual cues from the face or body (e.g., smiling or body posture) as well as vocal and speech-related cues (e.g., tone and intensity; see Table 5-1 for a list of possible nonverbal cues). Nonverbal cues are equally, if not more, fundamental to the process of emotion detection than are verbal cues. Indeed, nonverbal cues occur more often than verbal cues, and healthcare providers are more likely to use information from nonverbal cues than verbal cues when judging patient emotions.[18,19] Furthermore, patient anxiety is more easily diagnosed when providers have access to full video information in comparison to a simple transcript of the interaction, again suggesting the importance of nonverbal emotion cues.[20] However, patients' nonverbal cues tend to be conveyed more subtly and can be more difficult to detect (e.g., they may tap their foot repeatedly or fidget while talking about what to expect during an upcoming test), in comparison to verbal cues (e.g., a patient may explain verbally, "I'm nervous about my upcoming test"). It is important to note, however, that verbal cues can still sometimes be ambiguous (as when a patient says, "I'm sorry I was late, there is a lot going on at home," which could be referencing the family babysitter getting the wrong time, or could be referencing to a far more emotionally consequential event). With both verbal and nonverbal cues that are subtler in nature, it is important that clinicians explore these cues with patients by asking follow-up questions.

Emotion cues can also differ in terms of their valence. Positively valenced cues result from an individual's subjective feeling of pleasantness or intention to convey positive information while negatively valenced cues result from an individual's subjective feeling of unpleasantness or intention to convey negative information.[21] Some researchers have added a second dimension of *arousal* to the categorization of emotion cues. Arousal refers to a subjective state of feeling activated or deactivated. In this way, emotion cues can be positive-high arousal, positive-low arousal, negative-high arousal, and negative-low arousal (see Fig. 5-1 for a list of some emotions in the medical visit). Interestingly, most emotion perception work within clinical settings has focused on the perception of negatively valenced cues. In fact, one widely used coding system for capturing these moments in medical interactions, the Verona Coding Definitions of Cues and Concerns (VR-CoDES), defines emotion cues as "verbal or nonverbal hints which suggest an underlying *unpleasant* [emphasis added] emotion and would need clarification from the health provider."[16,17] (See Chapter 6, Emotion Cues as Clinical Opportunities, in the present volume.) While it is often the case that high arousal and negative cues are the most salient during a medical interaction, physicians must learn to accurately perceive and respond to the entirety of emotion cues being

■ TABLE 5-1. Examples of Nonverbal Cues to Notice in Medical Visits	
Cue channel	**Nonverbal behavior**
Cues in the face	
	Facial expressions
	Facial muscle movement
	Eye movement
	Eye contact
	Gaze directions
	Mutual gaze
	Smiling
Vocal and speech-related cues	
	Tone
	Pitch
	Speaking rate
	Speaking time
	Pausing
	Silence
	Volume
	Expressivity
	Interruptions
	Back-channeling
Cues in the body	
	Nodding
	Head shaking
	Gesturing
	Fidgeting
	Self-touching
	Body position
	Posture
	Body orientation
	Touch

expressed by the patient (verbal and nonverbal, negative and positive, high arousal and low arousal) in order to achieve optimal medical interaction outcomes such as accurate diagnoses, appropriate treatment plans, patient satisfaction, and a quality patient–provider relationship.

While some emotion cues may be inherently easier to decode than others, patients also differ markedly in their ability to validly *encode* (i.e., reveal or express) the emotion they are experiencing. In order to assess emotion

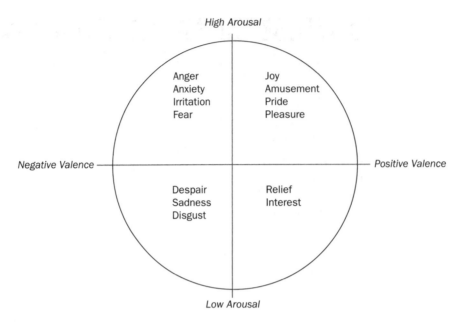

FIGURE 5-1. Examples of emotions in medical visits.

perception accuracy, researchers must disambiguate the clinician's ability or skill in accurately assessing their patient's emotions from their patient's tendency to express their emotions validly.[22] For example, a provider who is able to detect that their patient is irritated may only be accurate at detecting such a state because their patient is expressing clear and intense irritation cues. On the other hand, a provider may not be able to detect that their patient is irritated if that patient is not effectively expressing emotion cues associated with this internal state, or is expressing this irritation so subtly that only a very attuned provider would be able to perceive it.

While it may be that some individuals are naturally better or worse at expressing their internal emotional states, or are more or less willing to do so, others may purposely adapt their behaviors in order to control the impression they believe they are making—a term often referred to as impression management.[23] This process is a precursor for *metaperception* (i.e., how an individual perceives others' perceptions of themselves),[24] by which individuals evaluate whether the impression they were trying to create was successful. In the context of patient—provider interactions, patients may think that their provider will not believe how much pain they are in and thus control expressions and complaints about pain or exaggerate their claims in order to get the provider's attention. Additionally, patients may try to control their negative emotions (e.g., distress, anxiety, fear, or anger) because they have acquired the belief over time that a provider's office is not the place to deal with emotions.

One's tendency to regulate their emotion cues during a clinical interaction may vary according to a patient's gender, race, or cultural upbringing (see Chapter 11, Emotion and Gender, and Chapter 12, Culture and Emotions in the Medical Encounter). For instance, males, to a greater degree than females, become socialized at a very young age to withhold their internal affective state in order to create a more socially acceptable external representation of their emotions (or lack thereof).[25] This male-specific social norm has been referred to as "restrictive emotionality."[26] It is therefore likely that the emotion cues expressed by male patients may be much more subtle than those expressed by female patients, and require particular attention from providers. Display rules (i.e., informal norms regarding how one should express their emotions) also differ according to one's culture. For example, more individualistic cultures tend to normalize emotional expressivity to a greater degree than more collectivist cultures.[27] However, individuals of *all* cultures endorse expressing emotions to a greater degree with in-group members in comparison to out-group members.[27] This is likely due to greater feelings of vulnerability and mistrust that stem from intergroup interactions. In this way, providers must take into consideration the gender, race, and cultural upbringings of their patients in order to better understand how a patient may be engaging in impression management of emotions.

Beyond these considerations, providers must also work to establish an understanding of their patients' baseline behavioral cues. That is, providers need to take into consideration whether the emotional expressivity of their patient is different from how that same patient normally expresses emotion, instead of comparing a patient's emotional expression to the average expression of other patients. It may be that certain patients always express their emotions with low intensity, making it important to recognize that even the subtlest changes in emotion may carry significant meaning, whereas they may not for highly expressive patients. While we understand that not all medical visits allow for this type of baseline to be assessed (e.g., emergency department interactions or any type of initial consultation), when possible, this allows for a more individualized approach to assessing emotion during medical visits that accounts for a patient's general levels of emotional expressivity.

While it is essential that providers be accurate in their judgments of their patient's emotional states, there are often additional parties present within the medical visit whose emotions are crucial to address as well. Family members regularly accompany loved ones to medical visits, and in some cases, may be the ones responsible for advocating on behalf of the patient if they cannot communicate their wants or needs themselves (e.g., parents for children or informal caregivers for patients with dementia). In cases such as this, providers must learn to be sensitive to the emotion cues of the family or friends who are present within the medical visit and respond appropriately to those cues. Additionally, it is common for nurses, trainees, or additional providers to be present during a patient's medical visit. As with the patient's family members and friends, the affective states of these colleagues cannot be ignored. Doctors must learn to integrate and understand the emotions of the entire care team in order to better understand the environment the patient is experiencing. Chapter 8, Managing Emotion in Medical Encounters with Children, speaks in detail to this issue in the context of pediatric medicine.

■ WHAT EMOTION PERCEPTION IS NOT

Given the significance of emotion perception as a skill within clinical settings, it is important to distinguish this concept from the other interpersonal skills with which it overlaps. One of these constructs, which has received a great deal of attention within the medical literature, is empathy. As a result of a growth in empathy research across multiple psychological and medical fields, the collection of definitions and measurement techniques regarding this construct has grown exponentially as well. Converging evidence from multiple reviews of the empathy literature seems to identify four facets of the construct: the ability to *perceive* the affective state of another, an *understanding* of another's cognitive experience or perspective, an emotional *reaction* to another's state, and an interpersonally effective *behavioral response* to another.[28,29] Although some researchers strictly limit the definition of empathy to emotion perception abilities,[30] it is more common within the medical literature for empathy to be considered an effective behavioral or communication style.[31] Thus, perceiving and responding to patients' emotion cues are components of providing empathic healthcare.

Another construct which encompasses the processes of emotional perception is emotional intelligence. In a similar manner to the theoretical components of empathy, emotional intelligence comprises one's ability to perceive emotions accurately, use emotions to facilitate thinking, understand emotions and emotional language, and manage emotions.[32] Within the healthcare setting, personal accomplishment, less burnout, greater job satisfaction, and a series of other positive outcomes have been associated with physicians who are more emotionally intelligent.[33,34]

Given that emotion perception is often incorporated as a necessary skill within larger interpersonal processes, it is important for researchers and providers to designate exactly what it is they are interested in, instead of using catch-all terms such as emotional intelligence or empathy. This will allow for a more individualized approach for educating and training providers on the specific facets of interpersonal skills which comprise a patient-centered approach to healthcare.

■ PATIENT-CENTERED CARE AND EMOTION PERCEPTION ABILITY

Perceiving patient emotions is implicit in almost every definition of patient-centered care. Patient-centered care is defined by the Institute of Medicine as "providing care that is respectful of, and responsive to, individual patient preferences, needs and values, and ensuring that patient values guide all clinical decisions."[36] Differing from the biomedical model of healthcare that stresses the importance of physical processes, patient-centered care is about fostering provider–patient relationships with effective communication that allows patients to express their emotions and feelings openly and providers to respond to these cues in empathic and validating ways.[37]

Many models have been developed to outline the characteristics of patient-centered communication. While there is not an accepted definition or model of patient-centered communication, Epstein and Street created a framework for patient-centered communication in the context of cancer care in their 2007 monograph for the National Cancer Institute describing six core functions (Fig. 5-2).[14] These six core functions share many of the characteristics described in other models of patient-centered care, and perceiving patients' emotions is crucial to all six functions. These six functions

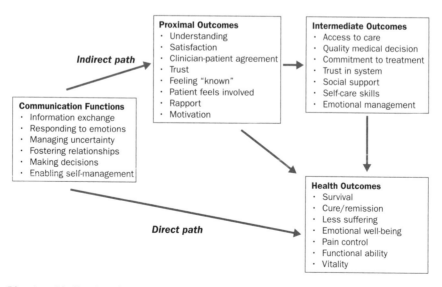

FIGURE 5-2. **Direct and indirect pathways from communication to health outcomes.**

include: Fostering the patient–clinician relationship, exchanging information, responding to emotions, managing uncertainty, making decisions, and enabling self-management. While it is possible to connect the ability to perceive emotions with all six core functions, we will focus on the first three as they are most relevant to perceiving emotions.

The first relevant function is fostering the patient–clinician relationship. Patient-centered care requires patient–clinician relationships that are high in mutual trust and rapport. Patient-centered relationships are more than sources or exchanges of biomedical information. These relations are characterized by the provision of emotional support, guidance, and understanding by providers. *Providers cannot give effective support, guidance, or show understanding if they do not first accurately perceive their patients' emotions, thoughts, feelings, or physical sensations.* The first step in fostering the patient–clinician relationship is for clinicians to perceive their patients' cues accurately. Emotion perception ability is an important component of rapport building because providers must accurately sense their patients' intentions, needs, wants, values, and so on in order to respond in a way that avoids miscommunication or disappointment.

The second relevant function is exchanging information. *Patient-centered care involves the exchange of not only biomedical information but also psychosocial information.* Providers should be aware that not all patients want a complete exchange of information so the ability to perceive emotions is exceptionally important in order to understand patients' comfort level and desire to exchange information. Patients' information needs may differ not only from patient to patient but also from session to session or even from minute to minute. It is important that providers monitor patients' information needs both in what they say they want to know and how their nonverbal behaviors change as they are given more information (see Table 5-1). For instance, if a patient is shifting their eyes away, fidgeting, or orienting their body away during difficult conversations, a provider may want to verbally check in with the patient in order to re-assess their comfort level with the current informational exchange. Additionally, if a patient is failing to nod their head, furrowing their brows, pursing their lips, or frowning, the patient may be experiencing confusion and again, providers may want to verbally check in with the patient and check for understanding. Often information is given as medical jargon and patients can become overwhelmed or tune out. Checking for understanding with both verbal and nonverbal cues is very important. In addition, as information becomes more negative, patients may detach or become distressed. The absence of providers' ability to perceive this distress and effectively address it may explain why many patients and family members remain dissatisfied with the timing and amount of information they are given by providers.[38]

Finally, the third, and potentially most important relevant function to perceiving patients' emotions is responding to emotions. This function is also part of one of Zulman et al.'s [39] five practices that have the potential to enhance physician presence and meaningful connection with patients in the clinical encounter, labeled exploring emotional cues (notice, name, and validate the patient's emotions). Throughout the course of a clinical encounter and depending on the type and context, a patient may experience a range of emotions, feelings, and thoughts from fear, to sadness, anger, anxiety, depression, pain, happiness, hope, or relief, to name a few. These cues may be expressed in verbal behavior, nonverbal behavior, or through both verbal and nonverbal channels. In addition, cues from different modalities may even contradict one another (e.g., a patient verbally expresses that they are feeling good about a treatment procedure but expresses nonverbal cues of doubt or despair). They are rarely static and may change over the course of the interaction. It is particularly important that providers recognize and respond to these patient cues as some of them may impact patient quality of life and satisfaction of patients,[40] change their tolerance of a painful procedure,[41] reflect symptoms of larger issues (e.g., anxiety or depression), help to build rapport and trust, and signal adherence to a treatment regimen or a patient's willingness to come back for follow-up appointments.

Providers, however, are not always good at perceiving their patients' emotional cues, nor are they necessarily effective at uncovering patients' fears and concerns.[42,43] In order to respond to patient emotions, providers must be able to read a patient's verbal and nonverbal emotional cues (e.g., changes in the patient's tone of voice, facial expressions, and body language), elicit patient emotions through questions (e.g., "How are you feeling about this?"), and reflect and validate patient's emotions (e.g., "That sounds very difficult" or "I can see that this is affecting you deeply"). However, providers rarely initiate conversations about emotions (see Chapter 4, Emotion Dialogue in the Medical Encounter: When and How Often Does it Happen?).

It is important to acknowledge here that part of the patient-centered approach not only takes into account the patient's emotions but also acknowledges that providers have emotions too. When providers show their own appropriate emotions during clinical interactions, it can humanize providers for their patients and further the development and trust in the relationship. Providers should learn how to both acknowledge and manage their emotions effectively (see Chapter 7, Emotion Regulation in Patients, Providers, and the Clinical Relationship) so that they can balance empathy for their patients with potentially distressing effects on their own mind and body (see Chapter 16, Striving and Thriving: Challenges and Opportunities for Clinician Emotional Wellness).

■ ADAPTABILITY

Although most research and clinical recommendations suggest a patient-centered communication style, recent research suggests that providers should adapt their communication style to fit that which their patients prefer in order to have the most satisfied patients.[44] The Behavioral Adaptability Model was developed to describe how adapting one's behavior can lead to better outcomes, in this case for patients.[45] The model posits that the *ability to perceive patients' emotions* leads to better social interaction outcomes because it enables providers to understand their patients' expectations and to adapt their behavior accordingly. Providers should utilize both verbal and nonverbal emotion cues in order to determine what a patient's expectations of the interaction may be in order to feel confident in shaping their interaction style to meet these needs. When patients' expectations are met, they tend to be more satisfied (Expectation Confirmation Theory).[46] Thus, in order to have effective and quality interactions with patients, and subsequently better outcomes, providers should consider adapting their behavior to match their patients' expectations, as long as these expectations are within the bounds of professional judgment.

To measure providers' adaptability, Carrard, Schmid Mast, and Cousin[47] objectively measured the nonverbal dominance behaviors (i.e., loudness of voice, speaking time, gazing, nodding, and visual dominance) of 32 physicians interacting with two of their patients and compared it with each patient's preference for a more paternalistic physician (i.e., one who is dominant, treats the medical problem as the central concern, and expects the patient to defer to their judgment) versus a more patient-centered physician (i.e., one who is caring and values emotions, treats the patient as a person, and makes decisions together with the patient) as measured by the Patient Provider Orientation Scale (PPOS).[48] Carrard, Schmid Mast, and Cousin[47] also measured patient-reported outcomes including patient satisfaction, trust in the physician, and evaluation of physician competence. When the physicians' nonverbal dominance behavior was adapted to the patient's preferred level of paternalism or patient-centeredness, patients reported higher satisfaction, more trust, and increased perceptions of competence. This study suggests that, instead of exhibiting the same patient-centered behaviors to all patients, it may be advantageous for a provider to adapt their behavior depending on their patient's wants and values. This can be done with a simple question specific to their treatment, diagnosis, or health (i.e., "What are your hopes for this treatment?") or by giving a validated and reliable measure that assesses general values and expectations of providers in medical care such as the Patient-Practitioner Orientation Scale (PPOS).[48] Scores on the PPOS could then be used by providers to understand how they should behave and what types of questions or responses they use with patients based on individual patient preferences.

■ BURNOUT

Communication, and in particular, the ability to perceive patients' emotions, is not always easy and does take its toll on the individual; it can be considered cognitive work. On the other hand, decoding clinical and health cues generally becomes second nature to physicians as they practice more and more. The same, we believe, should be true of communication cues if trained and practiced enough. While rarely ever directly measured, there does appear to be a link between quality of communication and burnout. Providers who tend to show more care and concern (as rated by their patients) tend to have one of two outcomes related to burnout—they either become tired, observe and internalize too much distress and become burnt out, or they find joy and purpose in their work which buffers the negative impact of this cognitive work.[49] In the first research of its kind,[50] medical students completed a test of emotion perception ability specific to the clinical context, the Test of Accurate Perception of Patient Affect,[51] and completed self-reported validated and reliable measures of positive and negative empathy (the ability to share in patients' positive vs. negative emotions) and burnout. The ability to accurately perceive patients' emotions had no relationship to burnout. However, providers' negative empathy (the ability to share in negative emotions with patients) predicted higher levels of burnout while positive empathy (the ability to share in positive emotions with patients) predicted lower levels of burnout. It appears that a combination of positive empathy, while still responding to negative emotions (but not sharing in those negative emotions), may be the most important combination for providers' well-being and longevity in their respective field and patient outcomes, though more research is needed on this topic.

■ CORRELATES OF PERSON PERCEPTION

As with many different skills, researchers have identified specific groups of individuals who tend to excel in emotion perception accuracy in comparison to others. Perhaps the most prominent and well-documented correlate of this skill is gender. Multiple reviews of the literature have concluded that females reliably excel in perceiving the emotions of others in comparison to males.[52-54] Females are more accurate regardless of the gender of the person they are judging, the cue channel (e.g., vocal or visual), and the type of emotion being expressed by the person being judged. The one exception to this rule, which is especially relevant within the medical context, is in reference to perceptions of pain, in which there is evidence of a male superiority in accuracy.[55] No differences have been observed in male and female's accuracy in detecting lies however, which can also be a relevant skill within the clinical context.[56] These differences in emotion perception skill, combined with females' greater use of patient-centered communication, have been linked to a host of positive clinical implications for patients of female providers. For instance, patients treated by female doctors in comparison to male doctors have significantly lower mortality and readmission rates.[57] While the causes of this general female advantage in accuracy are unknown, researchers have speculated that they may be the result of evolution, motivation, differences in knowledge bases, the result of gender socialization, or a combination of any of these factors.[54] Whatever the case may be, this female advantage needs to be recognized and appreciated in healthcare settings as it may have practical implications for patients' treatment and welfare.

Other correlates of person perception accuracy in clinicians include clinical specialty. However, it is unclear whether these advantages or disadvantages are due to differences in clinical training, more focus on recognizing and responding to emotions in clinical practice, or a self-selection bias into these specialties. Interestingly, medical students may be particularly poor at accurately perceiving others or at least have not emerged as especially skilled compared to nonclinical samples or compared to their peers who are not in scientific fields.[58,59] Medical students considering specialties less characterized by patient interaction, such as radiology and surgery, demonstrate even lower person perception abilities than medical students interested in primary care.[58] However, personal experience and education also play a role. In nonclinical contexts, there is evidence that those who have acquired knowledge of nonverbal cues, perhaps through taking a class on nonverbal behavior in college or participating in a nonverbal training, are more accurate perceivers of emotion cues.[60]

■ OUTCOMES OF PERSON PERCEPTION

A large body of research suggests that providers' ability to perceive patient emotions accurately benefits not only patients, but also providers, the interaction in general, and the healthcare system at large. Although we have touched upon some of these positive clinical outcomes thus far, in this section we will directly highlight the existing research on emotion perception outcomes in each of these domains.

Outcomes for Patients

According to Street and colleagues,[61] communication functions including recognizing and responding to patient emotions, indirectly and directly impact health outcomes. As shown in Fig. 5-2, communication can impact health through a direct path by which recognizing and responding to patient emotions can be therapeutic by reducing fear or anxiety and improving psychological well-being. In terms of direct effects of provider communication on patient health outcomes, a meta-analysis by Kelley et al.[62] showed that among 13 randomized controlled trials which systematically manipulated the communication of providers (e.g., via improved communication skills, increased empathy, better attention to nonverbal signals, not interrupting, sitting down, or making appropriate eye contact), patients had significantly improved objective (e.g., blood pressure) and validated subjective (e.g., pain score) health outcomes. In other empirical work, higher quality provider communication including perceiving and responding to patient emotions is related to higher patient satisfaction, more appointment adherence, and better patient health outcomes.[2,35,63–66]

Clinicians' accuracy in perceiving patient emotion cues may also influence patients' learning of medical information and cognitive response. In a study of genetic counselors, increased sensitivity to patient cues was associated with more knowledge gained by role-playing patients as a result of the visit.[67] Not responding appropriately to emotion cues is also associated with decreased patient recall of educational information in the visit.[68]

In most cases, however, accurately perceiving patients' emotions can impact health through a more indirect or mediated route. These mediated processes can affect health at the proximal outcome level (e.g., understanding, satisfaction, trust, rapport) or through intermediate outcomes that are affected by proximal outcomes (e.g., trust in system, social support, enhanced patient empowerment, improved self-care skills, better emotion management). For example, research suggests that analogue patients appreciate provider attempts to elicit and recognize their emotional cues, even when the provider is incorrect in their assessment of the felt emotion (see Fig. 5-3).[3] This likely shows the patient that the provider is attentive to them and is putting in effort to understand the psychosocial dimensions of the healthcare interaction.

Outcomes for Providers

Not only does emotion perception ability benefit the patient, but there are also impacts on providers themselves when they are more accurate perceivers of their patients. First, providers who are more accurate perceivers of

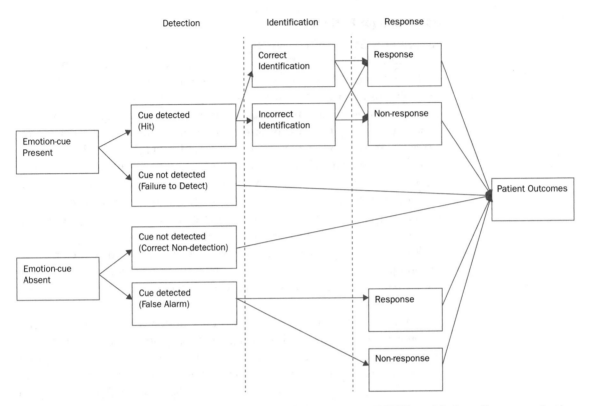

FIGURE 5-3. The detection, identification, and response to emotion cue (DIREC) model of emotion processing in the physician–patient interaction.

emotion tend to perform better in the clinical domain than those who are less accurate. For example, occupational therapy students who scored higher on tests of emotion perception accuracy performed better in clinical fieldwork examinations than those who scored lower.[69] In addition, psychotherapists who perceived emotions more accurately were evaluated by their supervisors as having better clinical skills.[60] Similarly, medical students who were more accurate at perceiving emotions received higher interpersonal skill ratings from simulated patients.[51]

In addition, colleagues and subordinates of providers who are more accurate at perceiving emotions may also benefit from this ability. For example, in one study outside of the healthcare domain, leaders who scored higher on a test of perceiving emotions had more satisfied subordinates after a role-play.[70] It is likely that by contributing to the satisfaction of others around them, those who are more accurate at perceiving emotions also feel more satisfied in their work, which may buffer symptoms of burnout as discussed earlier.

Another study based upon real reports from workplace employees revealed that not only did supervisors who more accurately perceived emotional expression receive greater performance and satisfaction ratings from their subordinates, but that also *how managers used this emotional information* (e.g., to support employees) mattered.[71] This finding highlights the notion that a positive workplace environment, as well as a positive clinical interaction, does not begin and end with an accurate perception of emotion, but that the *encoding* of understanding and support for various emotional expressions is also a critical component.

Outcomes for the Healthcare System

While there is a dearth of research on how emotion perception ability impacts the overall healthcare system, including factors like cost and medical errors, there is certainly reason to believe that this ability is beneficial. For example, when providers were more responsive to a simulated patient's emergency pain, the visit length was shorter, which allowed the patient to access effective pain-reducing care faster.[72] It is likely that effective engagement with patient emotion does in fact decrease visit length, all the while increasing patient satisfaction[11] because providers are getting the information that they need to engage with and treat the patient the first time. *It is likely that providers who miss or inaccurately perceive their patients' emotions are also missing other signs and symptoms that the patient is displaying which may be crucial in understanding what types of tests to run or treatments to prescribe.* This would not only create a burden on the healthcare system, but also elicit frustration and distrust from the patient. It is also possible, as discussed above, that those who are more accurate in perceiving emotions have lower symptoms of burnout. Past literature suggests that burnout is intimately tied to medical errors where those higher in burnout tend to make more medical errors.[73] It is assumed then that if burnout is reduced through increased emotion perception ability, medical errors would also be reduced.

Outcomes in Life

While most of the research discussed so far has taken place in the context of clinical interactions (i.e., with clinicians and patients), there is a host of social psychology research that examines correlates of emotion perception ability in a nonclinical context. While this research is often not done in the context of the clinical interaction, many of the factors related to emotion perception ability are highly relevant to providers and are discussed briefly in this section. As mentioned previously, those who are more accurate in perceiving others' emotions have more successful interactions and higher quality relationships.[74] In a meta-analysis, those higher in the ability to perceive others accurately (including emotion perception ability) were more empathic, affiliative, extraverted, conscientious, open, tolerant, had higher internal locus of control, and more positive adjustment. In addition, those higher on interpersonal accuracy were less neurotic, shy, and depressed.[74] In other fields outside of healthcare, those with higher perception ability are more likely to have better sale rates, better negotiation outcomes, salary increases, and higher customer ratings.[75–77] Finally, those better at perceiving others tend to be less guided by their stereotypes when evaluating others,[78] which may be especially relevant when treating patients of various backgrounds, races, ethnicities, and genders.

Limitations

Nearly all studies discussed above are correlational in nature and do not manipulate emotion perception ability. Therefore, it is unknown whether there is a causal relationship between emotion perception accuracy and outcomes. If the relationship is causal, it is also unclear what mechanisms are responsible for explaining the relationship between higher emotion perception ability and better outcomes. For example, what are the behavioral expressions or verbalizations that make someone who is a better perceiver have patients that are more satisfied or more likely to come back for their next appointment? It is possible that there are many contributing factors. Some research has begun to understand these mechanisms. For example, among medical students, those who score higher on emotion perception accuracy behave in a more engaged way with their patients.[79] This engagement may directly relate to patient satisfaction and appointment adherence.

■ MEASUREMENT OF EMOTION RECOGNITION ABILITY

In order to quantify the accurate assessment of another's emotion both inside and outside of medical visits, researchers have developed numerous assessments of emotion recognition ability. While the overarching aim of these measurements is to assess emotion recognition ability, they often differ in their response format, the type of stimuli used, and even the criteria by which accuracy is defined. Each of these different methods of measurement has specific benefits; however, each method also has its own set of limitations which researchers as well as providers must acknowledge and understand.

One of the most commonly employed methods of assessing emotion recognition accuracy is to ask individuals to self-report on their own emotion recognition ability. Several self-report measures of emotion recognition exist and have been utilized within the clinical setting as a way of assessing providers' understanding of their own emotion recognition skills. The Empathy Quotient (EQ),[80] for example, asks participants about the extent to which they agree with a series of statements regarding their general reactions to the observed experiences of another. While this measure is generally considered a measure of trait empathy, it taps into one's general disposition to perceive, as well as understand and react to another's emotional state. Likewise, the Social Skills Inventory (SSI)[81] is another self-report measure of skill in both encoding and decoding of nonverbal and verbal information (sample item: "I always seem to know what people's true feelings are, no matter how hard they try to conceal them").

While self-report measures have the benefit of being easily distributed, they are often not accurate assessments of one's true emotion perception ability as people rarely know how good they are at this skill.[74,82] Indeed, self-reports of abilities are only valid to the extent that a person has the metacognitive ability to know how good or accurate they truly are and are immune to any self-presentation motives while reporting this information, which is often not the case.[83] Physicians often report that they recognize and respond appropriately to patient emotions.[84,85] However, numerous studies have shown that patient emotions are often missed or not responded to appropriately by providers.[8,11,14,15,42,68,86–91] Further, results from three separate meta-analyses regarding medical students' self-assessment of their own technical and interpersonal skills find that medical students are more likely to overestimate their own interpersonal skills, such as emotion recognition, than they are their technical skills.[92] This may be due to the fact that feedback regarding one's own interpersonal accuracy is not frequently received, leaving room for individuals to over or underestimate their own skills.

A more objective assessment of emotion perception ability comes in the form of standardized tests. These empirically validated tests assess an individual's emotion recognition skill by asking them to identify emotions from nonverbal cues apparent in static pictures (e.g., Reading the Mind in the Eyes; RME),[93] audio clips (e.g., Diagnostic Analysis of Nonverbal Accuracy—Voice; DANVA),[94] or audiovisual clips (e.g., Test of Accurate Perception of Patients' Affect; TAPPA).[52] Unlike self-report measures of emotion recognition ability, these standardized tests consist of items which each have an objectively correct response. What is considered to be a "correct response" differs from test to test, however. For example, the accuracy criterion (i.e., correct response) may be an answer agreed upon via a panel of experts and researchers. Sometimes it is the self-reported emotion of the person displaying the emotion in the photograph or video (e.g., "When this picture was taken, I was feeling X"). In some cases, where stimuli were formed via actors trying to display different emotions, the correct answer is the emotion which the actor was trying to display or pose. In the TAPPA test alluded to above, the correct answer is what actual patients said they were feeling or thinking at specific moments during real medical visits, which was determined via videotape review and commentary by the patient after their medical visit.

In addition to having different assessments of criteria by which accuracy is assessed, standardized tests of emotion perception can differ in their response format. Some measures require that individuals categorize emotion displays into a series of predetermined categories by determining which category is the best fit. Other measures require that individuals determine the extent to which any type of emotion is present within a stimulus. This type of response format requires that individuals go above and beyond categorizing the correct emotion by asking individuals to identify the *intensity* of the emotions expressed. Finally, some tests do not explicitly ask individuals about emotions, but instead ask individuals to infer the emotional states of the target person by discriminating between different emotionally laden contexts. For instance, the Profile of Nonverbal Sensitivity (PONS)[60] shows a series of short clips of an individual acting out specific scenes, and asks participants to identify whether the individual is, for example, talking about the death of a friend (i.e., implying sadness) or threatening someone (i.e., implying anger).

While these tests are generally far better assessments of an individual's objective emotion recognition skill in comparison to self-report measures, most are not specifically designed for clinical contexts. Nonclinically relevant tests are still able to assess an individual's emotion recognition ability for a majority of emotions but may fail to capture key clinical elements such as expressions of pain. Those which are clinically relevant, however, can be particularly important tools within the medical field (e.g., the Test of Accurate Perception of Patients' Affect [TAPPA][52]; the Patient Emotion Cue Test [PECT][95]). For example, employing these types of tests for medical students or trainees either for a medical school intake or during an initial communication course allows individuals to receive direct feedback regarding their aptitude in perceiving emotions. Receiving feedback in this manner is important as it allows the participant to adjust their perceptions of their own accuracy (i.e., were they over- or underestimating their own skill). Given that patients do not often provide this kind of direct feedback regarding their provider's assessments of emotions, employing standardized tests can be helpful for providing these evaluations. Additionally, emotion perception accuracy aligns well with the American Medical Colleges (AAMC)'s "Interpersonal" domain of the core competencies for entering medical students. Therefore, incorporating these types of tests into medical school curricula is important to facilitate conversations and understanding regarding the importance of interpersonal skills for a successful clinical encounter.

■ TRAINING EMOTION RECOGNITION

As we have discussed, accurate perceptions of patients, particularly accurate recognition of patient emotions, is an ability associated with better patient care, and more satisfied and more adherent patients. Given that emotion cue recognition is an important skill for clinicians, the next step is to develop ways to foster and improve this ability. One potential approach is to develop training interventions. While many researchers have examined the correlates of accuracy,[74] literature on approaches to improving emotion perception accuracy is less well developed.[96,97] In fact, there was some debate as to whether this was a skill that was amenable to training in adults or whether it was something innate or learned through development; however, meta-analysis has revealed that even short trainings can be effective to increase emotion perception accuracy.[97] Simply providing someone instruction, in a textbook or a classroom, may not be enough on its own to increase accuracy. *What appears to matter most is not the length of the training, but the ability for trainees to practice and receive feedback on the accuracy of their judgments.*[98,99]

In clinical interactions, clinicians have a lot of exposure to patient emotion cues. This might lead to the assumption that clinicians are constantly practicing and receiving feedback and that formal training is less important than experience. However, clinicians rarely receive explicit feedback about their *accuracy* in perceiving their patient's emotion cues. For example, patients rarely stop and say, "Hey, I just sighed and you failed to realize that I was nervous about the side effects that you were describing" or "Hey, I just looked away and you failed to notice that I was frustrated." Without immediate feedback about accuracy, clinicians may not realize when they have missed or misinterpreted an emotion cue. Training that focuses specifically on accurately perceiving emotion cues may fill this gap.

Training can improve accuracy even for those who are already skilled. In a small study, 24 first-year medical students took the Micro Expression Training Tool (METT), designed to improve their ability to recognize fear, sadness, happiness, contempt, disgust, anger, and surprise in facial expressions.[100] As part of the training, students practiced labeling example facial expressions, got feedback on their overall score, received narrated instructions on the nonverbal signals of the various emotions, and received more practice and feedback on individual items before taking a posttest. Students who were predefined as good communicators in previous patient interactions actually improved more than students who were predefined as poor communicators. The authors posited that this could have occurred for several reasons including differences in attention, motivation, interest, anxiety, or learning.

Although accurately perceiving patients' nonverbal emotion cues is associated with positive patient outcomes,[2] medical education in most cases does not specifically train healthcare providers to recognize patient emotion cues as part of the communication curricula.[11] Communication courses are only a small part of the medical school curriculum and these courses typically include training in a wide range of behaviors including gathering medical information and being an ethical provider.[101] When they do address patient cues, communication training programs often focus on eliciting emotion cues and responding appropriately to them.[102] Communication training that focuses on providing space for patients to share emotions and practice appropriate responses to patients expressing emotions is vital. However, if a provider is unable to accurately recognize an emotion cue when it is present, then getting a patient to convey more cues or being able to respond appropriately to a cue when it is noticed are of secondary importance.[4,5]

■ CONCLUSION

During a given patient–provider interaction, it is likely that a patient will express any number of emotions varying both in how they are expressed (i.e., verbally and/or nonverbally) and in their intensity. A patient may begin a medical visit by verbally stating how *proud* they feel of their process during treatment (e.g., "I am feeling much better and have started going back to work"). This same patient may then, upon being told that new complications have arisen due to their treatment, furrow their eyebrows and cast their eyes away (i.e., indicating a state of *annoyance or frustration*). As the consultation progresses, the patient may then bring their hand to their face, lower their tone of voice, and let out a sigh (i.e., indicating a state of *grief or sadness*). While this example scenario illustrates three different common emotions that a patient may experience in a short consultation, it is likely that, within any given medical consultation, a patient will express numerous emotion cues varying in both arousal and valence. Given this, accurate perception of these cues by providers, along with the communication of these perceptions, is critical to the success of the interaction.

The studies reviewed above discuss what exactly emotion perception accuracy *is* along with how to measure it, its fundamental relationship to patient-centered care, who generally excels at this skill and the outcomes associated with being accurate, and the ways in which this ability can be trained. The literature overwhelming suggests that this skill is a necessary component of the medical visit. Educating medical professions about the importance of emotion recognition along with providing practice and feedback regarding the implementation of this skill is imminently important in both medical education and continuing education programs. Following these recommendations will not only likely improve the satisfaction of patients with their medical visit, but may also buffer against physician burnout and lead to more accurate diagnoses and treatments of patients.

REFERENCES

1. Hall JA, Schmid Mast M, West TV. Accurate interpersonal perception: many traditions, one topic. In: Hall JA, Schmid Mast M, West TV, eds. *The Social Psychology of Perceiving Others Accurately*. Cambridge, UK: Cambridge University Press; 2018:2-33.

2. Hall JA. Clinicians' accuracy in perceiving patients: its relevance for clinical practice and a narrative review of methods and correlates. *Patient Educ Couns.* 2011;84(3):319-324.

3. Blanch-Hartigan D. Patient satisfaction with physician errors in detecting and identifying patient emotion cues. *Patient Educ Couns.* 2013;93(1):56-62.

4. Funder DC. On the accuracy of personality judgment: a realistic approach. *Psychol Rev.* 1995;102(4):652-670.

5. Funder DC. *Personality Judgment: a Realistic Approach to Person Perception.* Amsterdam: Elsevier; 2007.

6. Bylund CL, Makoul G. Empathic communication and gender in the physician-patient encounter. *Patient Educ Couns.* 2002;48(3):207-216.

7. Duric V, Butow P, Sharpe L, et al. Reducing psychological distress in a genetic counseling consultation for breast cancer. *J Genet Couns.* 2003;12(3):243-264.

8. Zimmermann C, Del Piccolo L, Finset A. Cues and concerns by patients in medical consultations: a literature review. *Psychol Bull.* 2007;133(3):438-463.

9. Branch WT, Malik TK. Using 'windows of opportunities' in brief interviews to understand patients' concerns. *JAMA.* 1993;269(13):1667-1668.

10. Floyd MR, Lang F, McCord RS, Keener M. Patients with worry: presentation of concerns and expectations for response. *Patient Educ Couns.* 2005;57(2):211-216.

11. Levinson W, Gorawara-Bhat R, Lamb J. A study of patient clues and physician responses in primary care and surgical settings. *JAMA.* 2000;284(8):1021-1027.

12. Bylund CL, Makoul G. Empathic communication and gender in the physician–patient encounter. *Patient Educ Couns.* 2002;48(3):207-216.

13. Bylund CL, Makoul G. Examining empathy in medical encounters: an observational study using the empathic communication coding system. *Health Commun.* 2005;18(2):123-140.

14. Eide H, Frankel R, Haaversen AC, Vaupel KA, Graugaard PK, Finset A. Listening for feelings: identifying and coding empathic and potential empathic opportunities in medical dialogues. *Patient Educ Couns.* 2004;54(3):291-297.

15. Street RL, Epstein RM. *Patient-Centered Communication in Cancer Care: Promoting Healing and Reducing Suffering.* Bethesda, MD: U.S. Department of Health and Human Services, National Institutes of Health, National Cancer Institute; 2007.

16. Morse DS, Edwardsen EA, Gordon HS. Missed opportunities for interval empathy in lung cancer communication. *Arch Intern Med.* 2008;168(17):1853-1858.

17. Piccolo LD, Goss C, Zimmermann C. The Third Meeting of the Verona Network on Sequence Analysis. Finding common grounds in defining patient cues and concerns and the appropriateness of provider responses [published correction appears in Patient Educ Couns. 2005;59(1):111]. *Patient Educ Couns.* 2005;57(2):241-244.

18. Davenport S, Goldberg D, Millar T. How psychiatric disorders are missed during medical consultations. *Lancet.* 1987;2(8556):439-441.

19. Yogo Y, Ando M, Hashi A, Tsutsui S, Yamada N. Judgments of emotion by nurses and students given double-bind information on a patient's tone of voice and message content. *Percept Mot Skills.* 2000;90(3 Pt 1):855-863.

20. Waxer PH. Channel contribution in anxiety displays. *J Res Pers.* 1981;15(1):44-56.

21. Barrett LF. Discrete emotions or dimensions? the role of valence focus and arousal focus. *Cogn Emot.* 1998;12(4):579-599.

22. Snodgrass SE, Hecht MA, Ploutz-Snyder R. Interpersonal sensitivity: expressivity or perceptivity? *J Pers Soc Psychol.* 1998;74(1):238-249.

23. Schlenker BR. *Impression Management: the Self-Concept, Social Identity, and Interpersonal Relations.* Monterey, CA: Brooks/Cole Pub. Co.; 1980.

24. Carlson EN, Barranti M. Metaperceptions: do people know how others perceive them? In: Hall JA, Schmid Mast M, West TV, eds. *The Social Psychology of Perceiving Others Accurately.* Cambridge, UK: Cambridge University Press; 2018:165-182.

25. Zeman J, Garber J. Display rules for anger, sadness, and pain: it depends on who is watching. *Child Dev.* 1996;67(3):957-973.

26. Levant RF. Toward the reconstruction of masculinity. In: Pollack WS, Levant RF, eds. *A New Psychology of Men.* New York: Basic Books; 2007:229-252.

27. Matsumoto D, Yoo SH, Fontaine J. Mapping expressive differences around the world. *J Cross Cult Psychol.* 2008;39(1):55-74.

28. Hall JA, Schwartz R. Empathy present and future. *J Soc Psychol.* 2019;159(3):225-243.

29. Stosic MD, Fultz AA, Brown J, Bernieri FJ. Are you choosing the wrong empathy measure? Poster presented at: The Society for Personality and Social Psychology Annual Meeting; February, 8, 2020; Portland, OR.

30. Ekman P, Friesen W. *Unmasking the Face: A Guide to Recognizing Emotions from Facial Cues.* Englewood Cliffs, NJ: Prentice-Hall; 1975.

31. Dow AW, Leong D, Anderson A, Wenzel RP; VCU Theater-Medicine Team. Using theater to teach clinical empathy: a pilot study. *J Gen Intern Med.* 2007;22(8):1114-1118.

32. Mayer JD, Salovey P. What is emotional intelligence? In: Salovey P, Sluyter DJ, eds. *Emotional Development and Emotional Intelligence: Educational Implications.* New York, NY: Basic Books; 2001:3-31.

33. Năstasă L-E, Fărcaş AD. The effect of emotional intelligence on burnout in healthcare professionals. *Procedia Soc Behav Sci.* 2015;187:78-82.

34. Weng HC, Hung CM, Liu YT, et al. Associations between emotional intelligence and doctor burnout, job satisfaction and patient satisfaction. *Med Educ.* 2011;45(8):835-842.

35. Weng HC, Steed JF, Yu SW, et al. The effect of surgeon empathy and emotional intelligence on patient satisfaction. *Adv Health Sci Educ Theory Pract.* 2011;16(5):591-600.

36. Institute of Medicine. *Crossing the Quality Chasm*. Washington, D.C.: National Academy Press; 2003.

37. Stein T, Frankel RM, Krupat E. Enhancing clinician communication skills in a large healthcare organization: a longitudinal case study. *Patient Educ Couns*. 2005;58(1):4-12.

38. Leydon GM, Boulton M, Moynihan C, et al. Cancer patients' information needs and information seeking behaviour: in depth interview study. *BMJ*. 2000;320(7239):909-913.

39. Zulman DM, Haverfield MC, Shaw JG, et al. Practices to foster physician presence and connection with patients in the clinical encounter [published correction appears in *JAMA*. 2020 Mar 17;323(11):1098]. *JAMA*. 2020;323(1):70-81.

40. Clark PA, Drain M, Malone MP. Addressing patients' emotional and spiritual needs. *J Comm J Qual Saf*. 2003;29(12):659-670.

41. Ruben MA, Blanch-Hartigan D, Hall JA. Nonverbal communication as a pain reliever: the impact of physician supportive nonverbal behavior on experimentally induced pain. *Health Commun*. 2017;32(8):970-976.

42. Beach WA, Easter DW, Good JS, Pigeron E. Disclosing and responding to cancer "fears" during oncology interviews. *Soc Sci Med*. 2005;60(4):893-910.

43. Osse BH, Vernooij-Dassen MJ, Schadé E, de Vree B, van den Muijsenbergh ME, Grol RP. Problems to discuss with cancer patients in palliative care: a comprehensive approach. *Patient Educ Couns*. 2002;47(3):195-204.

44. Carrard V, Schmid Mast M, Jaunin-Stalder N, Junod Perron N, Sommer J. Patient-centeredness as physician behavioral adaptability to patient preferences. *Health Commun*. 2018;33(5):593-600.

45. Palese T, Schmid Mast M. Interpersonal accuracy and interaction outcomes: why and how reading others correctly has adaptive advantages in social interactions. In: Sternberg RJ, Kostić Aleksandra, eds. *Social Intelligence and Nonverbal Communication*. Cham, Switzerland: Palgrave Macmillan; 2020.

46. Jiang JJ, Klein G. Expectation-confirmation theory: capitalizing on descriptive power. In: Dwivedi YK, ed. *Handbook of Research on Contemporary Theoretical Models in Information Systems*. Hershey, PA: Information Science Reference; 2009:384-401.

47. Carrard V, Schmid Mast M, Cousin G. Beyond "one size fits all": physician nonverbal adaptability to patients' need for paternalism and its positive consultation outcomes. *Health Commun*. 2016;31(11):1327-1333.

48. Krupat E, Yeager CM, Putnam S. Patient role orientations, doctor-patient fit, and visit satisfaction. *Psychol Health*. 2000;15(5):707-719.

49. Wilkinson H, Whittington R, Perry L, Eames C. Examining the relationship between burnout and empathy in healthcare professionals: a systematic review. *Burn Res*. 2017;6:18-29.

50. Ruben MA, Stosic MD, Aleksanyan T, Blanch-Hartigan D. Where's the discussion on positive empathy in medical education? the relationship between positive and negative empathy and burnout among medical students. Manuscript in prepration.

51. Hall JA, Ship AN, Ruben MA, et al. The test of accurate perception of patients' affect (TAPPA): an ecologically valid tool for assessing interpersonal perception accuracy in clinicians. *Patient Educ Couns*. 2014;94(2):218-223.

52. Hall JA. Gender effects in decoding nonverbal cues. *Psychol Bull.* 1978;85(4):845-857.

53. Hall JA. *Nonverbal Sex Differences: Communication Accuracy and Expressive Style.* Baltimore, MD: Johns Hopkins University Press; 1984.

54. Hall JA, Gunnery SD, Horgan TG. Gender differences in interpersonal accuracy. In: Hall JA, Schmid Mast M, West TV, eds. *The Social Psychology of Perceiving Others Accurately.* Cambridge, UK: Cambridge University Press; 2018:309-327.

55. Ruben MA, Hall JA. "I know your pain": proximal and distal predictors of pain detection accuracy. *Pers Soc Psychol Bull.* 2013;39(10):1346-1358.

56. Aamodt MG, Custer H. Who can best catch a liar?: A meta-analysis of individual differences in detecting deception. *The Forensic Examiner.* 2006;15(1):6-11.

57. Tsugawa Y, Jena A, Figueroa J, Orav E, Blumenthal D, Jha A. Comparison of hospital mortality and readmission rates for medicare patients treated by male vs female physicians. *JAMA Intern Med.* 2017;177(2):206.

58. Giannini AJ, Giannini JD, Bowman RK. Measurement of nonverbal receptive abilities in medical students. *Percept Mot Skills.* 2000;90(3 Pt 2):1145-1150.

59. Evans BJ, Stanley RO, Burrows GD. Measuring medical students' empathy skills. *Br J Med Psychol.* 1993;66 (Pt 2):121-133.

60. Rosenthal R, Hall JA, DiMatteo MR, Rogers PL, Archer D. *Sensitivity to Nonverbal Communication: the PONS Test.* Baltimore, MD: Johns Hopkins University Press; 1979.

61. Street RL Jr, Makoul G, Arora NK, Epstein RM. How does communication heal? Pathways linking clinician-patient communication to health outcomes. *Patient Educ Couns.* 2009;74(3):295-301.

62. Kelley JM, Kraft-Todd G, Schapira L, Kossowsky J, Riess H. The influence of the patient-clinician relationship on healthcare outcomes: a systematic review and meta-analysis of randomized controlled trials [published correction appears in PLoS One. 2014;9(6):e101191]. *PLoS One.* 2014;9(4):e94207. Published 2014 April 9.

63. DiMatteo MR, Taranta A, Friedman HS, Prince LM. Predicting patient satisfaction from physicians' nonverbal communication skills. *Med Care.* 1980;18(4):376-387.

64. DiMatteo MR, Hays RD, Prince LM. Relationship of physicians' nonverbal communication skill to patient satisfaction, appointment noncompliance, and physician workload. *Health Psychol.* 1986;5(6):581-594.

65. Stewart MA. Effective physician-patient communication and health outcomes: a review. *CMAJ.* 1995;152(9):1423-1433.

66. Zolnierek KB, DiMatteo MR. Physician communication and patient adherence to treatment: a meta-analysis. *Med Care.* 2009;47(8):826-834.

67. Roter D, Erby L, Hall J, Larson S, Ellington L, Dudley W. Nonverbal sensitivity: consequences for learning and satisfaction in genetic counseling. *Health Educ.* 2008;108(5):397-410.

68. Jansen J, van Weert JC, de Groot J, van Dulmen S, Heeren TJ, Bensing JM. Emotional and informational patient cues: the impact of nurses' responses on recall. *Patient Educ Couns.* 2010;79(2):218-224.

69. Tickle-Degnen L. Working well with others: the prediction of students' clinical performance. *Am J Occup Ther.* 1998;52(2):133-142.

70. Schmid Mast M, Jonas K, Cronauer CK, Darioly A. On the importance of the superior's interpersonal sensitivity for good leadership. *J Appl Soc Psychol.* 2011;42(5):1043-1068.

71. Byron K. Male and female managers' ability to read emotions: relationships with supervisor's performance ratings and subordinates' satisfaction ratings. *J Occup Organ Psychol.* 2007;80(4):713-733.

72. Ruben MA, Blanch-Hartigan D, Blum R, Waisel D, Meyer EC, Laquidara JR, Hall JA. Anesthesiology residents' verbal and nonverbal responses to pain. Manuscript under review.

73. Tawfik DS, Profit J, Morgenthaler TI, et al. Physician burnout, well-being, and work unit safety grades in relationship to reported medical errors. *Mayo Clin Proc.* 2018;93(11):1571-1580.

74. Hall JA, Andrzejewski SA, Yopchick JE. Psychosocial correlates of interpersonal sensitivity: a meta-analysis. *J Nonverbal Behav.* 2009;33(3):149-180.

75. Byron K, Terranova S, Nowicki S. Nonverbal emotion recognition and salespersons: linking ability to perceived and actual success. *J Appl Soc Psychol.* 2007;37(11):2600-2619.

76. Puccinelli NM, Andrzejewski SA, Markos E, Noga T, Motyka S. The value of knowing what customers really want: the impact of salesperson ability to read non-verbal cues of affect on service quality. *J Mark Manag.* 2013;29(3-4):356-373.

77. Elfenbein HA, Foo MD, White J, Tan HH, Aik VC. Reading your counterpart: the benefit of emotion recognition accuracy for effectiveness in negotiation. *J Nonverbal Behav.* 2007;31(4):205-223.

78. Frauendorfer D, Schmid Mast M. Hiring gender-occupation incongruent applicants. *Pers Psychol.* 2013;12(4):182-188.

79. Hall JA, Ship AN, Ruben MA, et al. Clinically relevant correlates of accurate perception of patients' thoughts and feelings. *Health Commun.* 2015;30(5):423-429.

80. Baron-Cohen S, Wheelwright S. The empathy quotient: an investigation of adults with Asperger syndrome or high functioning autism, and normal sex differences. *J Autism Dev Disord.* 2004;34(2):163-175.

81. Riggio RE, Tucker J, Coffaro D. Social skills and empathy. *Pers Indiv Diff.* 1989;10(1):93-99.

82. Murphy BA, Lilienfeld SO. Are self-report cognitive empathy ratings valid proxies for cognitive empathy ability? Negligible meta-analytic relations with behavioral task performance. *Psychol Assess.* 2019;31(8):1062-1072.

83. Nisbett RE, Wilson TD. Telling more than we can know: verbal reports on mental processes. *Psychol Rev.* 1977;84(3):231-259.

84. DeCoster VA, Egan M. Physicians' perceptions and responses to patient emotion: implications for social work practice in health care. *Soc Work Health Care.* 2001;32(3):21-40.

85. Smith RC, Zimny GH. Physicians' emotional reactions to patients. *Psychosomatics.* 1988;29(4):392-397.

86. Doblin BH, Klamen DL. The ability of first-year medical students to correctly identify and directly respond to patients' observed behaviors. *Acad Med.* 1997;72(7):631-634.

87. Easter DW, Beach W. Competent patient care is dependent upon attending to empathic opportunities presented during interview sessions. *Curr Surg.* 2004;61(3):313-318.

88. Kim YM, Kols A, Prammawat S, Rinehart W. Sequence analysis: responsiveness of doctors to patient cues during family planning consultations in Mexico. *Patient Educ Couns.* 2005;58(1):114-117.

89. Oguchi M, Jansen J, Butow P, Colagiuri B, Divine R, Dhillon H. Measuring the impact of nurse cue-response behaviour on cancer patients' emotional cues. *Patient Educ Couns*. 2011;82(2):163-168.

90. Ryan H, Schofield P, Cockburn J, et al. How to recognize and manage psychological distress in cancer patients. *Eur J Cancer Care (Engl)*. 2005;14(1):7-15.

91. Uitterhoeve R, De Leeuw J, Bensing J, et al. Cue-responding behaviours of oncology nurses in video-simulated interviews. *J Adv Nurs*. 2008;61(1):71-80.

92. Blanch-Hartigan D. Medical students' self-assessment of performance: results from three meta-analyses. *Patient Educ Couns*. 2011;84(1):3-9.

93. Baron-Cohen S, Wheelwright S, Hill J, Raste Y, Plumb I. The "Reading the Mind in the Eyes" Test revised version: a study with normal adults, and adults with Asperger syndrome or high-functioning autism. *J Child Psychol Psychiatry*. 2001;42(2):241-251.

94. Nowicki S, Duke MP. Individual differences in the nonverbal communication of affect: the Diagnostic Analysis of Nonverbal Accuracy scale. *J Nonverbal Behav*. 1994;18(1):9-35.

95. Blanch-Hartigan D. Measuring providers' verbal and nonverbal emotion recognition ability: reliability and validity of the Patient Emotion Cue Test (PECT). *Patient Educ Couns*. 2011;82(3):370-376.

96. Costanzo M. Training students to decode verbal and nonverbal cues: effects on confidence and performance. *J Educ Psychol*. 1992;84(3):308-313.

97. Blanch-Hartigan D, Andrzejewski D, Hill KM. Training people to be interpersonally accurate. In: Hall JA, Schmid Mast M, West TV, eds. *The Social Psychology of Perceiving Others Accurately*. Cambridge, UK: Cambridge University Press; 2018:253-269.

98. Blanch-Hartigan D. An effective training to increase accurate recognition of patient emotion cues. *Patient Educ Couns*. 2012;89(2):274-280.

99. Schlegel K, Vicaria IM, Isaacowitz DM, Hall JA. Effectiveness of a short audiovisual emotion recognition training program in adults. *Motiv Emot*. 2017;41(5):646-660.

100. Endres J, Laidlaw A. Micro-expression recognition training in medical students: a pilot study. *BMC Med Educ*. 2009;9(47).

101. Hargie O, Dickson D, Boohan M, Hughes K. A survey of communication skills training in UK schools of medicine: present practices and prospective proposals. *Med Educ*. 1998;32(1):25-34.

102. Butow P, Cockburn J, Girgis A, et al. Increasing oncologists' skills in eliciting and responding to emotional cues: evaluation of a communication skills training program. *Psychooncology*. 2008;17(3):209-218.

Emotion Cues as Clinical Opportunities

Lidia Del Piccolo and Arnstein Finset

■ INTRODUCTION

How Do We Define a Cue and Why is it Important to Attend to Emotion Cues in the Clinical Setting?

In medical consultations, patients often feel vulnerable or emotionally tense due to their illness and the circumstances related to it. However, there is evidence that they seldom verbalize their concerns and emotions directly and spontaneously to their health providers.[1,2] Research has indicated that they rather tend to offer indirect cues and hints which suggest potential underlying concerns ("and then the pain really stabs me"; "I am starting to snap, I am starting to a little bit snap now…").[3–5] These hints need to be further explored in order to be correctly understood. The danger of missing their significance is twofold: to overlook important issues brought by the patient or to make erroneous assumptions about the core message they want to bring into the consultation.[6]

As defined in Oxford Advanced Learner's Dictionary a *cue* is "an action (also a few words) or event that is a signal for somebody to do something."[7] Similarly, a *hint* is defined as "something that you say or do in an indirect way in order to show somebody what you are thinking." In the latter definition, the implicit aspect of the signal is underlined, suggesting how such verbal or nonverbal signals are ambiguous and vague by nature, making them difficult to detect. There is a nuance in the meaning of cue and hint: the term cue points to communication process rather than content, in that a cue is a signal from the patient to the clinician, directing the clinician's attention to something. In some definitions of cue, it is specified that a cue from the patient requires a clarification by the provider.[8] A hint, on the other hand, is more a reference to the content rather than the process.

Why are emotional issues introduced in an allusive and nonexplicit way rather than being explicitly expressed? Piccinelli et al. have suggested that patients most often prefer to express the organic components related to the reason for the consultation rather than emotional concerns.[9] Moreover, physical symptoms and emotional distress frequently coexist, which can further muddle consultation priorities. The difficulty of making emotional issues explicit is also associated with several other aspects, both health provider and patient related: such as the clinician's attitudes toward psychosocial themes,[10,11] gender,[12,13] the patient's personality and life experiences,[14] cultural expectations,[15–17] severity and type of medical illness,[18] health beliefs of the patient,[19] and a general tendency by patients to consider emotional aspects as a private and reserved aspect of personal life.

Therefore, very often patients seem to test the ground during medical consultations. At the outset, they cautiously introduce a vague or ambiguous expression to check how the health provider reacts. Then, on the basis of the interest and the attention they receive, they may make the emotional aspect more explicit. However, emotions are not always made explicit. The expression of emotion will depend on the capacity by both participants to name emotions and correctly recognize them (a topic explored further in Chapter 5, Perception of Emotion in the Medical Visit). The same difficulty in recognizing the presence of emotional talk in medical consultations emerged when researchers tried to study emotional communication in healthcare scientifically. This gave rise to several methodological questions on how to grasp the complexities of verbal expressions and nonverbal behaviors which could be related to an emotion. To respond to this issue, researchers have attempted to develop various coding schemes with specified criteria to help raters grasp and then classify, in an operationalized and reliable way, all expressions containing references to some kind of emotion. The difficulty in operationalizing emotional expressions is related to the fact that emotional talk is strongly context dependent[20] and it may contain several verbal and paraverbal (tone of voice, fluency, prosody) nuances which give room to alternative possible reactions by a listener, contributing to the difficulty in finding consensus in coding emotional expressions. These same ambiguities can also partially explain why health providers find it difficult to recognize, acknowledge, and then respond appropriately to patients' expressions of emotion.

Suchman et al. suggested the term "empathic opportunities" to denote patients' expression of emotion either explicitly or by a statement from which a clinician might infer an underlying emotion not explicitly expressed (potential empathic opportunities). "Empathic opportunities" are very close conceptually to the terms "cue," "clue," or "hint." Stone et al. reported a study where a group of experts tried to understand more deeply what contributes to the complexity of emotion identification in medical consultations and found this endeavor to be complex and multifaceted.[5] They identified three types of ambiguity which made the task particularly challenging: (1) presentations of emotion cues can be "fuzzy" and varied; (2) expressions of illness can be emotionally loaded in the absence of explicit "emotion words"; and (3) empathic opportunities vary in length and intensity. All these aspects made the study of emotional expressions far subtler than these authors had thought. Nevertheless, they concluded that "the gap between theory and practice in recognizing and responding to patients' emotions, in all their forms, offers a great opportunity for improvement and skills development for physicians, and an equally exciting opportunity for researchers to develop more nuanced methodologies in studying clinical empathy" (p. 67).[5] Indeed, an active attention to cues, either referring to emotional issues or to other aspects of the patient's life, including illness, will usually be the quickest way for health providers to discover important areas that require attention. Cues are often introduced spontaneously, refer to intimate issues, and might help the health provider open a window to the patient's inner world.

Brief Outline of the Chapter

Given the difficulty in operationalizing the recognition and the coding of emotional expressions, we decided to present an overview of the main attempts in the literature to define and distinguish, among the different utterances given by a patient during a consultation, those which refer to emotional issues and are variously reported as *cues, clues, hints, prompts, "empathic and potential empathic opportunities," concerns, or similar expressions with a reference to the patient's affect.* For the clinician, some of the passages may seem technical, but some knowledge of coding routines may be helpful to get a more detailed understanding of how emotions are expressed and therefore may have practical relevance in clinical situations.

A chronological overview of quantitative studies on emotion *cues* will be followed by a brief section on qualitative approaches in the tradition of conversation analysis. Then psychophysiological and nonverbal correlates of emotion cues will be reported, as well as empirical studies reporting actual evidence for the relation between cues and health provider responses or other clinical outcomes, whenever possible. Finally, the role of emotion cues in communication skills training will be outlined, delineating how attending to cues may help students to become more active listeners and potentially more empathic clinicians, with positive implications for their clinical work.

■ QUANTITATIVE APPROACHES TO STUDYING EMOTION CUES

In this section we chronologically report quantitative approaches that have introduced new definitions of patient utterances related to emotion issues. Only the main systems described in the literature will be mentioned here. A more detailed description of the early literature on this topic has been provided by Zimmermann et al.[4]

First Studies on "Emotion Cues" in General Practice

The first studies that introduced the idea of paying attention to *emotion cues* (defined as "any verbalization of emotion, whether hinted or fully expressed") were published in the 1970s and 1980s by a group of British psychiatrists,[21-25] who were interested in exploring how doctors could improve their ability to detect emotional distress during their consultations with patients. Epidemiological research in general practice demonstrated that not only anxiety and depressive states, but also less well-defined subthreshold conditions of emotional distress, were common among patients with physical disease, with prevalence rates of 20–40%,[26,27] but that the detection rate of emotional distress in this population was low.[28] Therefore, these researchers proposed a more comprehensive approach to patient care that was more sensitive to the nuances characterizing emotional talk, either by the patient or the health provider, during a consultation. More recently, Mitchell et al. have confirmed low detection rates in general practice.[29]

Based on the classification of all utterances expressed during the consultation, Goldberg and his group identified *"emotion cues"* (see Table 6-1 for the definition), and demonstrated that (1) training could increase sensitivity to these cues[21-25]; (2) there was a relationship between the general practitioner's ability to detect distress (by using the General Health Questionnaire, GHQ-12, as screening tool for emotional distress) and the number of cues given by patients; (3) good detectors of emotional distress (able identifiers who were able to correctly identify a higher percentage of patients with emotional distress) elicited more verbal and vocal cues than poor detectors (poor identifiers), who instead tended to suppress patients' verbal and vocal cues.[30,31] Goldberg et al. also showed that patient-led interviews were associated with greater cue emission; doctor-led interviews were associated with lower rates of cue emission, but when using patient-centered behaviors, able identifiers had an increase in cue emission, whereas poor identifiers had an unaltered or lower cue emission.[30]

■ TABLE 6-1. Summary of the Different Definitions for Emotional Expressions and Health Provider Response

Coding system	Definition of patient's emotional expression	Classification of health provider responses to patient's emotional expression
Goldberg et al.,[22,23] Davenport et al.[31]	*Emotional cue*: *movement* (agitated, restless, demonstrative, gesticulating, immobile), *vocal* (monotonous, sighing, tense, strained, distressed, weeping, plaintive, whining, angry), and *postural* (dejected, tense, on edge, gaze avoidance). Emotional cues are all rated on a three-point scale of severity.	Cue detected/nondetected
"Patient-Centred Score Sheet" (PCSS)[33]	**Offer:** any verbal expression through which patients indicate their *symptoms* (verbal descriptions of experiences or sensations representing the subjective evidence of disease or physical disorder), *expectations, thoughts* (ideas, opinions, beliefs related or not to the disease, its causes and implications), *sensations* (the state or emotional reactions that accompany the symptoms, expressed directly by the patient or in response to a specific question from the doctor), *prompts* (signals that aim to solicit the doctor's attention on a given topic, spontaneously expressed by the patient and not consequent to particular facilitations the doctor), and *nonspecific cues* (signals that cannot be classified until after further clarification).	Evaluated according to four possible values: 0: Completely ignores 1: Use a closed answer 2: Use an open answer 3: It explicitly facilitates the expression of expectations, thoughts, and sensations experienced by the patient. The total score is divided by the number of offers and corresponds to the patient centeredness index of the scale (range from 0 to 3).
Booth and Maguire Rating System to assess interactions between cancer patients and health professionals[34]	*Verbal cue:* an utterance with some level of psychological depth. Level 0 = facts only. Level 1 = a hint of feelings. Level 2 = feeling can be identified. Level 3 = feelings clearly expressed.	Percentage of all health professionals' utterances with some level of psychological depth about diagnosis, prognosis, or adverse physical, psychological, and social sequelae of patient's disease and treatment within each interview.

(Continued)

■ **TABLE 6-1. Summary of the Different Definitions for Emotional Expressions and Health Provider Response (Continued)**

Coding system	Definition of patient's emotional expression	Classification of health provider responses to patient's emotional expression
Roter Interaction Analysis System (RIAS)[37]	**Shows concern or worry**: a statement or nonverbal expression indicating that a condition or event is serious, worrisome, distressing or deserving special attention, and of particular concern right now during the medical interview. Voice, tone, intonation, or verbal content may disclose worries, concerns, stress, nervousness, personal preferences, or uncertainties which are of immediate concern. Includes negative emotional description of the medical situation, statements that ask for pardon, self-criticism. **Asks for reassurance**: questions that convey the need or desire to be reassured or encouraged. Voice tone, intonation, and emotional content may be of significance. **Gives psychosocial information**: statements related to psychosocial concerns or problems (e.g., stress, feelings, and emotions, general state of mind, philosophical outlook, values, and beliefs).	All health provider utterances as classified according to their "socio-emotional" or "task-focused" function.
Medical Interview Aural Rating Scale (MIARS)[47]	**Cue**: whether the patient has said something, which contains a hint or clear expression that something (content) is or may be important or distressing or a cause of concern to the interviewee. Linguistic rules to identify cues are also given (i.e., any expression of wishing, wanting, desire, longing, hoping, uncertainty, the use of metaphors, expressions of should's, ought, guilt, relief from something distressing, swear words...). **Concerns** are the areas of concern as expressed by the patient, they are broad in content and may correspond to a number of different cues which relate to one concern area. All patient expressions are rated at different levels: Level 0 (neutral): straightforward information exchange. No element of feeling. Level 1: Hints of worry and concern.	Health provider responses to cues are distinguished in five categories: 1. Exploration (eliciting, clarification, or educated guess). 2. Acknowledgment (empathic statement, reflection, or checking). 3. Factual clarification about the content (not the emotion) of the cue. 4. Distancing strategy (blocking further disclosure, switching focus, giving premature reassurance or inappropriate advice). 5. Overt blocking when changing completely away from the all content of the interviewees speak.

■ TABLE 6-1. Summary of the Different Definitions for Emotional Expressions and Health Provider Response (*Continued*)

Coding system	Definition of patient's emotional expression	Classification of health provider responses to patient's emotional expression
	Level 2: Clear mention of feeling. Direct expressions of worry and concern. Level 3: Clear expressions of intense emotions (e.g., crying).	
Empathic and potential empathic opportunities[1]	***Empathic opportunity***: a direct and explicit description of an emotion by a patient. ***Praise opportunity:*** an explicit statement about something praiseworthy (e.g., adopting a health promoting behavior). ***Potential empathic opportunity:*** patient statement from which a clinician might infer an underlying emotion that has not been explicitly expressed which needs further elaboration to move toward a more explicit expression of the emotion.	*Continuer*: a clinician's statement following a (potential) empathic opportunity that facilitates further exploration of the implied emotion. *Empathic* response: a clinician's explicitly expressed recognition of patient's expressed emotion. *(Potential) empathic opportunity terminator*: a clinician's statement that immediately follows a (potential) empathic opportunity directing the interview away from the (hinted) stated emotion.
Empathic Communication Coding System (ECCS)[62]	**Empathic opportunities:** patient statements that include an explicit (i.e., clear and direct) statement of emotion, progress, or challenge by the patient.	Responses are placed into one of seven distinct categories: 6. *Shared feeling or experience*: Physician self-discloses, making an explicit statement that he or she either shares the patient's emotion or has had a similar experience, challenge, or progress. 5. *Confirmation:* Physician conveys to the patient that the expressed emotion, progress, or challenge is legitimate. 4. Pursuit: Physician explicitly acknowledges the central issue in the empathic opportunity and pursues the topic with the patient by asking the patient a question, offering advice or support, or elaborating on a point the patient has raised. 3. *Acknowledgment*: Physician explicitly acknowledges the central issue in the empathic opportunity but does not pursue the topic.

(Continued)

■ **TABLE 6-1. Summary of the Different Definitions for Emotional Expressions and Health Provider Response (*Continued*)**

Coding system	Definition of patient's emotional expression	Classification of health provider responses to patient's emotional expression
		2. *Implicit recognition*: Physician does not explicitly recognize the central issue in the empathic opportunity but focuses on a peripheral aspect of the statement and changes the topic.
		1. *Perfunctory recognition*: Physician gives an automatic, scripted-type response, giving the empathic opportunity minimal recognition.
		0. *Denial/disconfirmation*: Physician either ignores the patient's empathic opportunity or makes a disconfirming statement.
Verona Medical Interview Classification System (VR-MICS)[72,75,77]	*Cue*: a spontaneous introduction of new elements: a. By directing the doctor's attention to an issue which is different from the one dealt with immediately before. b. By attempts to explain the situation spontaneously introduced using clarifications or switching to other contents and themes. c. By taking up a theme already emerged during the consultation, redirecting the doctor's attention to it. Variations in voice quality (crying, laughing, anger), in content or speech (i.e., unsolicited new information, topic changes, emphasis, metaphors, repetitions, profanities, unusual words), are also included to identify a cue. *Statement*: a. Expressions solicited by the doctor's questions or comments. b. Yes/no answers to the doctor's questions. c. Interventions developing themes or cues previously introduced.	All health provider utterances as classified according to their function and content: Questions to gather information or to involve the patient; expressions to facilitate or support the patient; negative talk; orienting expressions; orienting explanations.
Patient clues[79]	*Clue:* a "direct or indirect comment that provides information about any aspect of a patient's life circumstances or feelings."	*Positive response*: supports or encourages the patient to express personal, psychological, or family-related concerns.

■ TABLE 6-1. Summary of the Different Definitions for Emotional Expressions and Health Provider Response (*Continued*)

Coding system	Definition of patient's emotional expression	Classification of health provider responses to patient's emotional expression
	It "offers a glimpse into the inner world of patients and creates an opportunity for empathy and personal connection." Clues are distinguished as either *emotional* (they are associated with an emotion or implicitly request support from the physician) or *social* (an expression referring to patient's life but not associated to an emotion).	*Missed opportunity*: physician does not support or encourage the discussion about emotional concerns or avoided the subject.
Medical Interaction Process System (MIPS)[80]	*Concern*: a general issue raised by the patient. *Cue*: any expression by the patient which requires (and allows for) a response or some action to be taken by the clinician. Cues tend to be much subtler in nature than concerns and are seldom overt requests for a response from the clinician. Doctor- or patient-initiated verbal cues may be to *ask information* or "I wasn't told very much about what is wrong with me" or *reassurance/information* on side effects, e.g., "I fear the treatment will make me ill."	Fifteen content and eight affective independent modes are defined. Four global affective (paralinguistic) categories are coded for the health provider: *Friendliness, Sensitivity, Nervousness,* and "*patient centredness*" (which is rated according to how much the clinician attempts to understand and respond to the patient's cues and emotions). Seven nonverbal (kinesic) categories are used to code nonverbal behavior.
Oncologists' Reactions to Cancer Patients' Verbal Cues[88]	*Patient-initiated verbal clue*: a statement in a non-question-asking form that is given by the patient to signal a need for information or emotional support. No distinction is made on the degree of explicitness of the emotion the patient refers to, but on the intensity of the cue, which is defined on a three-point scale.	Responses to emotional cues are coded as appropriate if they demonstrate sufficient empathy by addressing patient's feelings and cover relevant content.
Verona Coding Definitions of Emotional Sequences (VR-CoDES)[8,93]	*Cue*: a verbal or nonverbal hint which suggests an underlying unpleasant emotion and would need a clarification from the health provider. Instances include: a. Words or phrases in which the patient uses vague or unspecified words to describe his/her emotions ("I feel so strange").	Responses to the patient cues and concerns are coded according to two dimensions: 1. Whether or not the response *explicitly or not explicitly* refers to the cue/concern. This dimension indicates whether the response of the health provider maintains the wording or the key elements of the cue/concern it refers to.

(Continued)

■ **TABLE 6-1. Summary of the Different Definitions for Emotional Expressions and Health Provider Response (*Continued*)**

Coding system	Definition of patient's emotional expression	Classification of health provider responses to patient's emotional expression
	b. Verbal hints to hidden concerns (emphasizing, "it is terrible!," unusual words, unusual description of symptoms, "My body is boiling," profanities, exclamations, metaphors, "I have a knot in the stomach," ambiguous words, double negations, expressions of doubt, uncertainty, and hope).	2. Whether or not the provider response *provides space or reduces space* for further disclosure of the cue or concern. This dimension represents the function of the response, as it allows or reduces space to talk about the cue/concern.
	c. Words or phrases which emphasize (verbally or nonverbally) physiological or cognitive correlates (regarding sleep, e.g., "my nights are sleepless," appetite, physical energy, excitement or motor slowing down, sexual desire, concentration) of unpleasant emotional states. Physiological correlates may be described by words such as weak, dizzy, tense, restless, low, or by reports of crying whereas cognitive correlates may be described by words such as poor concentration or poor memory.	A third element relates to the timing of health provider response, all immediate responses are coded default, but also delayed responses might be considered if present.
	d. Neutral expressions that mention issues of potential emotional importance which stand out from the narrative background and refer to stressful life events and conditions (e.g., "My wife is fed up with me!" "My work is very stressful").	Once defined the two main dimensions, the specific type of behavior being used by the health provider may be coded by using 17 categories.
	e. A patient-elicited repetition of a previous neutral expression (repetitions, reverberations, or echo of a neutral expression within a same turn are not included).	Provider responses which do not follow a patient cue or concern or do not explicitly relate to a cue/concern are not coded
	f. Nonverbal cue: clear expressions of negative or unpleasant emotions (crying), or hint to hidden emotions (sighing, silence after provider question, frowning, etc.).	
	g. A clear and unambiguous expression of an unpleasant emotion which is in the past (more than one month ago) or is referred to an unclear period of live ("I was worried about..."; "I was terrified...").	

▨ **TABLE 6-1. Summary of the Different Definitions for Emotional Expressions and Health Provider Response (Continued)**		
Coding system	**Definition of patient's emotional expression**	**Classification of health provider responses to patient's emotional expression**
	Concern (explicit negative emotion/affect): a clear and unambiguous expression of an unpleasant current or recent emotion where the emotion is explicitly verbalized ("I worry about ..."; "I am upset"), with a stated issue of importance for the patient ("I am so worried about my husband's illness"; "Since the illness of my husband I feel very helpless") or without ("I am so anxious"; "I am nervous"). Included are patient expressions confirming health provider's explicit assumption or question about an unpleasant current or recent emotion (Health Provider: "are you anxious? or "you must have been shocked!" Patient: "Yes"). The source, i.e., who (patient or health provider) solicited the emotional expression is also coded.	

"Offers" in the "Patient-Centred Score Sheet" (PCSS)

Inspired by Levenstein's model of patient-centered consultation,[32] Henbest and Stewart in 1989 introduced the "Patient-Centred Score Sheet."[33] The starting point for the analysis of patient-centered interaction is the patient's "*offers*" (see Table 6-1 for the definition).

The sheet is based on a coding form where the *offers* are briefly reported and the doctor's response to them is evaluated according to four possible values: (0) completely ignores; (1) uses a closed answer; (2) uses an open answer; (3) explicitly facilitates the expression of expectations, thoughts, and sensations experienced by the patient. The total score is then divided by the number of offers and corresponds to the patient-centeredness index of the scale (range from 0 to 3). Therefore, the Score Sheet provides an overall "outcome" of the consultation, which measures the patient-centeredness of the clinician's responses to all *offers* given by the patient. The aims of the system are broader than analyzing only emotional talk. What makes the coding system of interest here is the distinction made by the authors between the source of the offer (whether it is spontaneously expressed by the patient or elicited by the clinician) and the degree of explicitness (a prompt needs to be clarified by the clinician). Clinician responses are coded starting by the *offer* expressed by the patient, introducing the sequence of interaction as a target of the analysis.

Booth and Maguire's Rating System to Assess Interactions between Cancer Patients and Health Professionals

The rating system elaborated by Booth and Maguire aimed to assess the form, function, and content of each patient and interviewer utterance as well as the emotional level of patient utterances.[34]

A *verbal cue* was defined as an utterance with some level of psychological depth (level 0 = facts only; level 1 = a hint of feelings; 2 = feeling can be identified; 3 = feelings clearly expressed).

In 1996, they published two papers on the effect of communication skills training in cancer care, demonstrating that the rate of hinted feelings was more than double (37.6%) that of explicitly mentioned feelings (16%). They reported that patient disclosure of significant information (utterances including perceptions of disease or prognosis or adverse sequelae of cancer and treatment: severity of pain, worry about prognosis, or concerns about loneliness) was promoted by the use of open directive questions, focusing on and clarifying psychological aspects, empathic statements, summarizing, and making educated guesses. The use of leading questions, focusing on and clarifying physical aspects, and moving into advice and reassurance mode, inhibited patient disclosure.[35] In a following paper they partially confirmed these results, showing that significant gains in promoting patients' disclosure were still evident 6 months later, but that there had been some decline over time, indicating that the ability and the attention toward emotional issues needs additional practice by the health provider.[36]

Roter Interaction Analysis System (RIAS)

The Roter Interaction Analysis System (RIAS) is the most widely used classification system of doctor–patient interaction (also discussed in Chapter 4, Emotion Dialogue in the Medical Encounter: When and How Often Does it Happen?).[37] It is devoted to coding all consultation utterances by provider and patient. Among them, three categories are of interest for our purposes: *Shows concern or worry; Asks for reassurance; Gives psychosocial information* (see Table 6-1 for the definition).

No distinction is made between indirect and explicit expressions of emotion. Examples are reported in the manual and tend to focus mainly on fully verbalized emotions, even if verbal utterances accompanied by a nonverbal expression of emotion, for example, voice pitch, may be coded as an affective expression. The RIAS is based mainly on frequencies of coded utterances. Most of the research using this system reports the rate of occurrences of coded expressions based on frequency counts; nevertheless, some authors tried to consider the temporal aspects of interaction process related to affective discourse by analyzing how the sequence of coded utterances was related to specific outcomes.[38–44] These studies confirmed previous observations that the likelihood of a patient expressing a concern was higher after physicians' open questions than after closed ones[41] or after silence or minimal facilitations[40–45]; and that health provider affective responses after concerns were rare,[44–46] being more frequently facilitations[40–43] or expressions of agreement, understanding, or information.[44]

Medical Interview Aural Rating Scale (MIARS)

Heaven and Green developed the MIARS specifically for oncology settings.[47] The basic unit of observation is the "turn," which is "the complete segment of speech from one person, finished when another person speaks" (p. 2)[47] and it is coded for both the patient and the health provider. Any *patient cue* is counted when the patient has said something, which contains "a hint or clear expression that something (content) is or may be important or distressing or a cause of concern to the interviewee" (p. 12).[47]

Concerns denote the areas of concern as expressed by the patient. They are broad in content and may correspond to a number of different cues which relate to one area of concern. As in the Booth and Maguire Rating System,[34] all patient expressions are rated at different levels. Moreover, health provider responses to cues are distinguished in five categories (see Table 6-1 for more detail).

The MIARS accomplishes several goals: (1) it gives clear rules on how to recognize a cue (which can be a hint or an explicit expression of emotion); (2) even if based on an observer's evaluation, it requires reporting emotional intensity level; (3) healthcare provider responses are coded in terms of sequence, i.e., given a patient's utterance, healthcare provider responses are subsequently evaluated.

Eleven publications so far have reported the use of MIARS to code the type and number of cues and the level of health provider (mainly nurse) responses. In several studies, results showed that patients gave more informational than emotion cues,[48–51] that they were more often expressed in an implicit than explicit way,[52] and that distressed patients gave more verbal cues.[53] Moreover, all the studies applying the MIARS were focused on the effect of health provider responses to cues, suggesting that it is more difficult to respond to emotional than to informative cues[48,54]; that training on cue-responses needs subsequent clinical supervision in the workplace[55]; that responding to emotion cues increases patient satisfaction,[56] self-reported adherence,[51] and information recall[48,57]; and that, compared to physicians, nurses are generally more competent in responding appropriately to emotion cues,[52] although a recent study in Taiwan showed nurses to respond to patients' emotion cues with more inappropriate strategies.[58]

Finally, Uitterhoeve et al. demonstrated that the way nurses responded to cues influenced subsequent expressions of concern and emotion by the patient; specifically, disclosure of a concern was two times higher after exploration or acknowledging a preceding cue than after a distancing response.[59] This highlighted how attention to sequence analysis may help providers understand the process related to emotional disclosure.

Empathic and Potential Empathic Opportunities and the Empathic Communication Coding System (ECCS)

Suchman et al. built the term "*empathic opportunity*"[1] on the expression "window of opportunity" introduced by Branch and Malik[60] to describe cases wherein patients discussed emotional, personal, or family concerns. Eide et al. found significant overlap between empathic opportunities as defined by Suchman et al. and the code "showing concern" in RIAS.[61] Detailed definitions for patients' expressions and health provider responses are reported in Table 6-1.

The authors do not refer to their approach as a coding system but as a model based on the operationalization of observable behaviors, aimed at emphasizing both the early stages of recognition and facilitation and the dynamics of interactional sequences that attend to the emergence of patients' emotions.

Based on this model, Bylund and Makoul built the Empathic Communication Coding System (ECCS), which divides patient-initiated empathic opportunities (EOs) into statements of emotion (an affective state of consciousness in which joy, sorrow, fear, hate, or the like, is experienced), progress, or challenge.[62] Progress is defined as a positive development in physical condition that has improved quality of life, a positive development in the psychosocial aspect of the patient's life, or a recent, very positive, life-changing event. Challenge is defined as a negative effect that a physical or psychosocial problem is having on the patient's quality of life, or a recent, devastating, life-changing event. The ECCS is used to measure empathic communication in terms of behavior expressed by the use of emotionally focused talk, psychosocial discussion, positive talk, and positive nonverbal communication. After identifying EOs expressed by the patient, the doctor's responses to them are distinguished in seven levels (ranging from Level 0—the doctor's denial of the patient's perspective—right through to Level 6—the doctor and the patient share a feeling or experience, see also Table 6-1 for more detail) which account for the emotional responsiveness of the health provider in terms of a hierarchy of empathic behaviors.

The model by Suchman et al.[1] and the ECCS[62] have been widely applied in clinical and teaching contexts, showing that:

- Regardless of the clinical setting, healthcare providers were often not very attentive to empathic opportunities offered by patients and tended to "terminate" the empathic opportunity by changing the topic from the patient's concerns to a salient biomedical issue that was a more comfortable matter for health providers.[63–67]
- Female physicians tended to score higher on the ECCS in response to the empathic opportunities created by patients.[62,64]
- The higher the professionals' ECCS responses to emotional opportunities, the more satisfied patients were with their consultations.[68,69]
- Training might be useful in improving empathy competencies by helping health providers to become aware and then to learn which verbal behaviors are felt as empathic by patients, going beyond the mere sharing of the patient's feeling.[70,71]

The Verona Medical Interview Classification System (VR-MICS)

The Verona Medical Interview Classification System (VR-MICS) was originally built for studying interactions between general practitioners (GPs) and patients within a biopsychosocial perspective with the aim of helping doctors improve detection of emotionally distressed patients.[72–75]

The VR-MICS includes a separate coding system for patients (VR-MICS/P),[72] inspired by the systems proposed by Henbest and Stewart[33] and Stewart et al.,[76] and for physicians (VR-MICS/D[77] which is an adaptation of the RIAS[37]). The VR-MICS/P comprises 21 categories and distinguishes between *cues* and *statements* (see Table 6-1 for the definition).

All cues and statements are defined by seven different content categories: (1) Psychological (emotions, worries, feelings); (2) Social (events or situations referring to work, finance, family, and other interpersonal relationships); (3) Lifestyle (usual behaviors or changes in habits); (4) Life episodes (occasional/sporadic and isolated behaviors, circumscribed in time, and intended or adopted by patients in response to particular situations or events); (5) Illness management (content related to physical illness and its treatment); (6) Impact on function (the impact of illness on daily life); (7) Other (cue undefined by content). Six other verbal behaviors, undefined by content, complete the classification system (asking questions, a bid for repetition, social conversation, positive talk, negative talk, illness opinions/expectations).

The VR-MICS differentiated between distressed and nondistressed patients in terms of number and type of cues and also in GPs' approach to these two groups of patients, showing that distressed patients gave more cues regarding social problems, emotions, and feelings than nondistressed patients.[3] Other cues concerning life events, personal episodes, and occasional behaviors were also significantly more frequent in consultations with emotionally distressed patients, but these patients were not recognized by their GP as being distressed.

The VR-MICS was also applied for sequence analysis purposes, showing that emotional distress of the patient was related to an increased number of cues,[78] confirming the initial observations reported by Davenport et al.[31] and Goldberg et al.,[30] and that, in terms of sequence of talk, cues were preceded by the use of facilitations, by supportive expressions showing appraisal, reassurance, agreement (handling of emotion), and by asking open-ended questions on psychological issues. At the same time, the study showed that open-ended inquiry and active listening skills, as well as handling of emotion by the physician and active participation by the patient throughout the consultation, all contributed to reduce the overall number of cues in the consultation, as they developed as explicit expressions of psychosocial content, defined as statements by the VR-MICS.

Patient Clues

Very similar to that of "empathic opportunity" is the definition of *clue* indicated by Levinson et al. (see Table 6-1 for the definition).[79] Like earlier studies on cues which differentiated between doctor-led and patient-led cues,[22–25,30,31] Levinson et al. distinguished between patient-initiated and physician-initiated clues, where physician-initiated clues were "physician questions that encouraged the patient to discuss a personal topic" (p. 1022).[79] Health provider responses were distinguished as either positive or missed opportunities. They applied the coding system in routine primary care and surgical settings, reporting results very similar to those based on the model by Suchman et al.[1] with the additional indication that most of the clues were patient initiated.[79]

Medical Interaction Process System (MIPS)

The MIPS[80–83] draws upon a patient-centered approach, viewing "patients as providing cues to their feelings and fears which if responded to appropriately will lead to their disclosure" (p. 557).[80] The system classifies interactions in terms of modes of exchange (function of an utterance) and content (topics being addressed). The system provides seven global affective categories, among which the level of "*patient centeredness*" is rated according to "how much the clinician attempts to understand and respond to the patient's cues and emotions" (p. 559).[80] Regarding cues, the authors state that "if a patient expresses a concern which requires (and allows for) a response or some action to be taken by the clinician, then a cue is also coded. Thus, cues can exist separately or in conjunction with concerns. When coded separately, cues tend to be much subtler in nature than concerns and are seldom overt requests for a response from the clinician" (p. 558).[80] Cues may implicitly request information ("I wasn't told very much about what is wrong with me," p. 558) or reassurance/support ("I'm terrified the treatment will make me ill (anxious tone)," p. 558) and may relate to a series of concerns (similarly to the definition reported in the MIARS). Research applying the MIPS's concept of patient centeredness showed that enabling consultations were more patient-centered with doctors facilitating socioemotional interchange[84] and that the odds of poor medication adherence were greater when patient–provider interactions were low in patient centeredness and did not address patients' sociodemographic circumstances.[85]

Cancer Patients' Verbal Cues

Butow and her group started to publish papers on doctor–patient communication in the oncology setting during the 1990s,[86,87] but the first publication where the term cue was introduced dates to 2002,[88,89] focusing on patient provision of indirect cues of emotional and informational need. In these studies, a *cue* is defined as "a statement in a non-question asking form that is given by the patient to signal a need for information or emotional support" (p. 50).[88] Examples of cues are: Informational cue (Patient), "I really don't know much about the different treatments" (p. 50), and Emotion cue (Patient), "I get so upset sometimes that I can't stop crying" (p. 50). Cues are differentiated on the degree of their intensity without considering the explicitness of the emotion the patient refers to. In these papers the focus is on the fact that the patient is actually, but indirectly, asking for something (treatments or how to cope with difficult emotions). Such indirect requests may be expressed as an experience of uncertainty, for instance by saying "I wonder how this will work out" instead of asking explicitly for treatment options. Also, the content being discussed at the time the cue occurred is coded (history, diagnosis, prognosis, treatment, other medical, psychosocial, social support/counseling/stress management, social exchange, and other/nonspecific), together with the following response by the health provider. Responses to emotion cues are coded as appropriate if they demonstrate sufficient empathy (by addressing the patient's feelings) and cover relevant content. The main findings were that patients gave, and doctors responded to, more informational than emotion cues,[88] but the capacity to be flexible and to respond to emotion cues was relevant in successful consultations.[89] Other studies regarded the relation between emotional distress and cues during genetic counseling in oncology,[90] the influence of family in patients' cues/concerns,[91] and the evaluation of a communication skills training program on cue emission by comparing an intervention and a control group of oncologists.[92] Those in the intervention group displayed more creating environment and fewer blocking behaviors immediately and 6 months after the communication skills training; although these differences did not reach statistical significance.

The Verona Coding Definitions of Emotion Sequences (VR-CoDES)

The Verona Coding Definitions of Emotion Sequences (VR-CoDES)[8,93,94] is the result of a consensus process involving several experts in communication coming from different countries in Europe and the United States, forming the "Verona Network of Sequence Analysis," who began meeting in Verona in 2003. This consensus process involved several steps, alternating between group discussions, individual and group coding exercises, and pilot reliability tests between annual meetings, leading to progressive refinements of the coding definitions and the conceptual framework. During this time, some other new coding systems were published,[95,96] reconsidering previous models like the MIARS and the MIPS. The consensus process was focused on finding a common definition and an operationalized way to capture any expression of worry or distress by the patient, either explicit or implicit. The final system distinguishes between patient expressions in terms of *cues* and *concerns* (see Table 6-1 for the definition), focusing on the process related to their expression (the type of patient emotional expression, whether cue or concern, whether the patient or health provider solicited the emotional expression, and the nature of the health provider's immediate response). Detailed coding rules for cues and concerns are defined by Zimmermann et al.,[8] whereas those for health provider responses are described by Del Piccolo et al.[93]

The main conceptual framework for VR-CoDES is based on the idea of studying emotional communication in terms of a sequential process, where the elicit-express-response sequence represents a basic triadic structure of emotional communication. The principle leading to this choice, as expressed by Bensing, is that "doctor-patient communication is a reciprocal give-and-take, in which each statement bears a relationship to the preceding and subsequent statements" (p. 79).[97]

The responses to cues are described according to two main dimensions: whether or not the provider refers explicitly to the cue and the extent to which he or she provides room for further disclosure of the emotions. A constructed example may illustrate the different response categories. The patient says

"*I often ponder if my pain will ever cease.*" The provider may choose *not* to invite further talk about the topic, by ignoring both the pain and the pondering in the next turn, or by referring to the cue without opening up for further talk ("*Pain is common after such an injury*"). Alternatively, the provider may open up for further talk, either nonexplicitly with a minimal encourager ("*Mmmhmm*") or with an explicit reference either to the pain ("*On a scale from 0 to 10, how would you describe your pain?*") or to the pondering ("*How does that pondering over pain make you feel?*").

An important principle of the VR-CoDES is the descriptive nature of health provider response categorization. The idea is not to judge a response as good or bad, but to analyze its function in cue/concern evolution within the consultation. The main dimensions to be considered in health provider responses are described in Table 6-1.

The conceptual framework on which the system is built is described by Del Piccolo et al.[94]

Empirical Studies Using VR-CoDES

Over the course of the 10 years since the VR-CoDES was published, more than 80 papers have been published based on studies applying the method. These studies represent a large variety in terms of healthcare context, patient categories, age, type of disease, and the nature of the consultation. There is no significant pattern across studies regarding associations between the number of cues and variables such as patient age and gender. However, in a number of studies there is a significant positive association between psychological distress and the number of cues and concerns. Across patient category, age, and setting, patients with a higher degree of anxiety, as measured with standard anxiety questionnaires, most often expressed more cues in medical consultations.[98–101] Interestingly, in one study of cancer patients the number of cues was more strongly related to the oncologist's attribution of anxiety, rather than anxiety test screening, evidencing how relevant is the role of the doctor and the attribution of anxiety in eliciting cues in the patient.[102] On the other hand, patients who gave more cues were more easily considered anxious by oncologists, independently of screening results.

A special example of distress is the fear of cancer recurrence (FCR). In one study of head and neck cancer patients, the researchers found that expression of negative emotion in terms of cues and concerns was related to a lowering of FCR over the treatment period.[103] One explanation could be that patients with lower FCR were more actively using the medical visit to vent their emotions. Interestingly, a higher frequency of cues and concerns in consultations predicted lower FCR over time.[104] Such findings are in keeping with experimental evidence indicating that putting feelings into words (affect labeling) may attenuate emotional experience, due to downregulation of centers of negative emotion in the brain.[105] Similarly, in another study of cancer patients, the number of expressed cues and concerns was associated with the oncologist's ability to pick up on the patient's worries, indicating that consultation characteristics may influence the expression of cues.[102]

Physiological measures have been applied in a number of studies of cues and concerns, but few results have been published. An exception is a study using voice pitch as an indicator of arousal.[106] In that study, the voice pitch associated with cues and concerns was significantly higher than in neutral statements, confirming the physiological aspect of verbal expression of emotion. In a clinical setting high pitch may be an indicator of emotion, but should also be understood in relation to context.

Emotion Cues in Conversation Analysis

Emotional communication in medical interviews has also been investigated by researchers who have applied qualitative methodology. In the quantitative study referred to above, the emotion cues and other relevant utterances were coded and counted according to specific coding schemes. In qualitative analysis of interpersonal interaction, researchers observe and analyze verbal and nonverbal behavior, looking for patterns or principles of interaction. Within the qualitative tradition of conversation analysis (CA), a main principle is to study conversation in natural environments in terms of sequences, with less emphasis on counting events and more emphasis on the patterns of interaction embedded in the conversation.

As pointed out above, clinician–patient communication is a reciprocal give-and-take.[97] A basic concept in the sequential analysis of CA to describe this reciprocity is *turn design*. Turn design refers to the interplay between what one speaker is doing in a current turn and what the other speaker did in the previous turn and will do in the subsequent one.[107] A typical finding in CA studies of informal talk is that speakers consistently design their turns with a reference or connection to prior turns. A speaker will typically display that connection to the other speaker for instance by repeating a word from the other speaker, by referring to the prior turn with a pronoun ("it"), or simply with an omission (an unstated reference to a prior turn). A speaker's cue to an emotion, as defined and described above, may be the element of a turn which is picked up by the other speaker in designing the next turn. Not only do speakers refer back to the previous turn, there is evidence that during informal talk-in-interaction speakers actually may also adjust to one another's terminology, repeating expressions from turn to turn and even imitating each other's verbal as well as nonverbal behavior.[108]

In CA, emotional concerns are often referred to as trouble talk. The sequential nature of trouble talk has been investigated in depth by Gail Jefferson, in a large corpus of conversations from daily life.[109] Jefferson argued that trouble talk is a sequential phenomenon that moves from an engagement with business as usual to a focus on trouble talk and back to business as usual. A similar pattern may be seen in medical consultations. The main topic is the patient's health complaint, but the conversation may in certain sequences focus on the patient's worry and concern.

Jefferson proposed a number of stages of trouble talk.[109] For the study of cues, the first main phase, the buildup, is the most interesting. The buildup phase will often start when one of the speakers, not necessarily the trouble-teller, raises an issue of potential trouble. The trouble teller has a number of ways to attend to the troublesome and emotionally charged topic. One response type is to downplay the potential trouble, but often in an ambiguous way that subtly indicates an element of trouble. Such an implicit expression of trouble or emotion is referred to by Jefferson as an *Approach* step. Next, the trouble-teller may be slightly more explicit (the *Arrival* phase) before trouble is expressed more clearly (the *Delivery* phase).

A similar pattern may be seen in medical consultations. Mellblom et al. combined the VR-CoDES and CA in a study of follow-up consultations with young cancer survivors in tertiary cancer care.[110] From a corpus of 66 consultations, they studied seven consultations in which patients expressed emotions a number of times during the consultation. They identified 32 sequences or segments and analyzed to what extent the stages of buildup, provider response, workup, and topic shift occurred.

A passage from Mellblom et al.'s study can serve as an example (p. 79).[110] A young adolescent girl comes to a follow-up consultation. This is how the consultation starts:

1. *Dr. So, how are you?*
2. *Pt. Mmm it's going OK (feebly)*
3. *Dr. Fine yeah (doctor nods)*
4. *Pt. Am so weary and stuff ... so*
5. *Dr. Are you weary all the time?*
6. *Pt. Yes*
7. *Dr. Yeah*
8. *Pt. And I have so many problems*

In line 2, the patient downplays the potential emotion ("it's going OK"), but the tone of voice indicates an underlying emotion and may be understood as a cue, or an *Approach to emotion,* in Jefferson's sense. After a minimal response from the doctor, the patient presents another cue, the first explicit verbal indicator of trouble, the *Arrival stage* in Jefferson's terminology ("am so weary and stuff"). After a closed question by the doctor, the patient's discomfort is being more clearly expressed, but again without using explicit emotion words ("I have so many problems")—the *Delivery phase*. In about half the segments Mellblom and her collaborators identified a pattern of upgrading the initial cue to a more explicit cue or concern. Most typically, upgrading occurred when doctors clearly facilitated the patients' cues.

The buildup sequence from cue to an explicit concern has also been investigated with a quantitative approach by Del Piccolo et al.[98] The authors analyzed a corpus of 104 first psychiatric consultations, showing that in almost all of them at least one emotional explicit concern was present, but that almost half (48%) were not linked to previous cues, which means that several of the emotion cues reported by patients had no further elaboration. Cues which became concerns and concerns which were further elaborated by the patient were those that had been acknowledged and handled by the psychiatrist by actively providing space to their expression.

Below is an example taken from the paper (p. 157)[98]:

1. *P: in October, it was bad (abortion). Now I take a pill until the end of January. In February, we start with a second trial. . . They say they can't give a 100% guarantee, they just say I should try, as any normal person. They have statistics of other women, who succeeded in becoming pregnant, although in much more serious conditions than me. However, my fixed point is that I do not accept my illness, this situation which in the past has not been treated adequately. (cue elicited by the patient)*
2. *D: mmhmm (Back channel—space provision)*
3. *P: I do not accept that! If it comes to the worst, that I cannot have any. . .(starts crying) . . .Sorry, but. . . (verbal and nonverbal –crying - cue elicited by the psychiatrist)*
4. *D: don't mind, just let it out. . . with all what has happened to you... (Explicit empathy providing space)*
5. *P: I don't know, I changed a lot. I am always sad, depressed. I have attacks of anxiety, panic, things which never happened to me before (concern elicited by the psychiatrist).*

Based on these results, authors concluded that the psychiatrist's competence in providing space by using active listening skills was essential to uncover the patient's emotions.

In the extensive CA literature on doctor–patient communication there are few studies on cues to emotion, which is surprising, given the theoretical and empirical framework given by Jefferson. An exception is Ruusuvuori's studies on managing affect in consultations in general practice and homeopathy.[111,112]

In her analysis of sequences, Ruusuvuori follows Jefferson's framework, but is more concerned with how cues are responded to than on the buildup phase. She found that doctors' responses to cues often are oriented toward closing the sequence of trouble-telling, in an attempt to shift back to problem-solving activity. Pino et al. studied how patients in palliative consultations presented cues to explicit talk about end-of life themes.[113] The researchers found several examples of how doctors followed up on cues given by patients, but they did not find evidence that doctors actually considered patients' cues as intentions to express end-of-life concerns.

The Role of Emotion Cues in Communication Skills Training

Over the past 60 years there has been a shift in expectations of health provider behavior during the consultation, moving from "detached concern" toward "clinical empathy."[114] A similar shift took place regarding research on clinical communication. A number of researchers started to pay more attention to emotion cues, as this chapter has documented. After seminal works by Goldberg and his group where they demonstrated that training could increase sensitivity to emotion cues,[23-25] contributing to emotional distress recognition,[30] more recent papers devoted their attention either toward the effect of training on emotion cue-responding in health providers or students and also on the most effective approaches in using cues as teaching tools.

Following Vinson and Underman, the ability to respond to emotion cues is not only a form of reasoning that attends to the patient's expressed feeling, but it also implies a change in the attitude and the emotional awareness of the health provider, requiring the ability "to induce or suppress feeling in order to sustain the outward countenance that produces the proper state of mind in others" (p. 2)[114] (see Chapter 7, Emotion Regulation in Patients, Providers, and the Clinical Relationship, for further discussion of emotion regulation). As they suggested, "Proper emotional conduct in the clinical encounter includes eliciting patients' emotions, often through the use of emotion words, sensing patients' cues about emotions, such as being attentive to disengagement or fear; and addressing patients' emotions, both with emotion words and by inviting patients to speak about their emotions" (p. 3).[114] Similarly, Dean and Street suggested a three-stage model for addressing patients' emotional distress, based on recognition (by the use of strategies such as mindful practice, active listening, and facilitative communication skills), exploration (by providing space for patients to talk about their emotions through open-ended questions, eliciting concerns, clarifying emotional concerns, naming emotions, showing respect and be a partner), and therapeutic action (by actively acknowledging emotions and providing support or referral when needed).[115]

Most training programs for either practitioners or students are based on this model.

A recent systematic review of curricula for "empathy and compassion" training in medical education found that all 52 suitable study curricula included in the review incorporated "teaching some aspect of taking time to listen and/or having awareness of the patient's emotional state" (p. 16)[116] and that among the skills and behaviors that demonstrated an increase in real patients' perception of compassion were "detecting patients' facial expressions and nonverbal cues of emotion; recognizing and responding to opportunities for compassion; nonverbal communication of caring; incorporating statements of support, worry, acknowledgement, emotion naming, and validation" (e.g., "Most people would feel the way you do") (p. 16).[116] Moreover, the most effective training methods were based on actual patients' involvement as well as video recording of interviews. In line with this observation, Schmitz et al. demonstrated that the use of specific hints during video-based examples displayed for training purposes was the most effective method for students' performance, compared to purely text or video-based examples.[117] Nevertheless, teaching method did not affect the tendency to respond to unpleasant emotions by space-providing techniques, which in any case proved to be the most appropriate behavior across conditions, compared to space-reducing.

Three recent studies reported the use of the VR-CoDES for medical students' training. Ortwein et al. adopted the VR-CoDES to code medical students' written responses to written case scenarios, demonstrating its applicability for direct speech phrased answers and its usefulness for coding students' ways of responding to hinted (cues) or explicit (concerns) expressions of emotion by simulated patients.[118] Zhou et al. coded 40 Objective Structured Clinical Examinations (OSCEs) using the VR-CoDES, showing that medical students responded differently according to emotion cue types expressed by simulated patients (i.e., students provided space to emotion cues when expressed in vague and unspecific words and reduced space to cues emphasizing physiological or cognitive correlates).[119] (See Table 6-1 for definitions of providing and reducing space.) The authors also found that patients' emotional distress exploration depended on consultation timing (what point they were at in the visit), patient speech duration, and the number of cumulative emotion cues (a decrease in cue exploration was observed near the end of the consultation, with longer patient turns and higher cumulative frequency of cues).

Recently, Barbosa et al. adopted the VR-CoDES to assess the effectiveness of a brief training program in relational/communication skills for medical residents, showing that after the training program residents provided more space for further disclosure of cues and concerns according to VR-CoDES definitions.[120]

The main terms from the VR-CoDES may be useful keywords also when teaching more experienced providers. Teaching clinicians to listen for cues is an obvious starting point, which easily may be implemented in standard communication skills training programs, such as the Four Habits framework.[121,122] Moreover, training clinicians to provide room in the encounter for clarification of cues is a common strategy in relevant training programs.

The effects of different approaches for training clinicians how to respond to emotion cues, using real and simulated patients, were also analyzed by applying other coding systems (mainly the MIARS, MIPS, Empathic opportunities model) in the professional context. Both in oncological[55,81,82,92,123,124] and in other medical settings[70,125] interventions were usually effective, but mainly on enhancing clinicians' (who were mostly nurses) ability to respond to, rather than to elicit cues. Heaven et al. also demonstrated that 4 weeks of clinical supervision after training could enhance the clinical effectiveness of communication skills training programs, because of the immediate transfer of communication skills training from workshop to workplace.[55]

Recently, and in line with the need to extend training strategies by using virtual reality, Gibbon et al. proposed an original and effective online module using a gamebook format, which prompted internal medicine residents to engage in focused and repetitive practice of three well-defined skills for responding to emotion cues in a simulated family conference and analyzed their reactions in response to emotion cues.[126] The three skills for responding to emotion cues were: (1) Distinguish emotion cues hinting at some form of distress from information cues which request a medical explanation; (2) Respond to emotion cues with empathic NURSE (name, understand, respect, support, explore); (3) Explore emotion cues when the conversation is stuck, or when providers, patients, and families are in conflict.

■ IMPLICATIONS OF RESEARCH ON CUES FOR CLINICAL WORK

One of the challenges in the medical encounter is to relate to the emotional needs of patients in a way that is helpful to the patient. For the clinician, knowledge about how patients tend to signal underlying emotions by emitting cues or hints, rather than spontaneously expressing their emotions in an explicit form, may be useful either when collecting information or when dealing with the patient's reaction to a specific situation. Often patients do not convey emotions overtly, but have thoughts and feelings which might interfere with their attention and memory functions and consequently with their ability to cope with illness. Paying attention and exploring cues becomes helpful because they function as a shortcut to important areas requiring clinicians' attention and, as demonstrated by Levinson et al.,[79] might also contribute to shortened visits.

Cues are both common and rare in medical consultations. Cues are common in the sense that when patients express their emotions, they tend to do so by alluding to the emotion in an indirect way rather than expressing the feeling explicitly. Most research on cues and concerns has shown that cues are much more frequent than explicit expressions of emotion.[13,99,102,127–129] At the same time, cues are rare in the sense that in most clinical encounters they are erratic and sporadic, depending on consultation duration[18] and health provider sensitivity toward their appearance.[130] If the healthcare provider responds and acknowledges the cue, this reflects an attentive attitude and increases the probability of creating an atmosphere conducive to more disclosure.

A second aspect is that for the clinician, it is useful to recognize that the most common cues tend to be rather allusive in nature. In the VR-CoDES, the use of emphasis ("it is terrible!"), unusual words, unusual description of symptoms ("my body is boiling"), profanities, exclamations ("I feel that I'm stuck"; "This is terribly unbelievable!"), metaphors ("I have a knot in the stomach"), and ambiguous words are the most frequent cues in most of the studies that have applied the system.[99,127–129,131]

Third, as discussed above, there is some evidence that the expression of emotion in the clinical encounter may develop in a buildup from a vague hint to a somewhat clearer expression of emotion.[13,132] It is useful for the clinician to be attentive to this potentially gradual exposure of emotion. More research is needed to investigate the buildup phenomenon in order to provide clinicians with more knowledge on the process of developing cues into explicit expressions.

Fourth, knowledge on how cues are expressed may provide the clinician with more insight on the cultural and ethnic differences in how emotions are expressed. For instance, in a study of hospital consultations in Norway, Kale et al. found that ethnic minority patients with low second language proficiency tended to be particularly vague in their expression of emotion cues.[16,133] In a recent study on consultations with HIV-positive patients in general practice in the United States, Park et al. found that African American patients initiated expressions of emotion less frequently than White patients, and that they more often than Whites gave cues to an underlying emotion by spontaneously repeating a seemingly neutral utterance.[134] It might seem that instead of simply expressing their worries, some African American patients repeated the cause of worry, such as a symptom, hoping that the doctor would take the cue. One could speculate that this behavior indicates a reluctance to disclose emotions in the medical encounter. (Chapter 12, Culture and Emotions in the

Medical Encounter, further explores cultural and ethnic differences in emotion communication.)

These different aspects of cues are all relevant topics in communication skills training, where students are often explicitly encouraged to listen for verbal and nonverbal cues, to be attentive to how and when cues are expressed, and to consider ways to respond to these cues so that the emotional content is clarified and the emotions are being acknowledged. As mentioned above, these general approaches may successfully be implemented in regular programs of communication skills training. However, in the further development of the field, there is a need to be more specific. A general instruction to listen for cues and respond with "empathy" is not sufficient for the clinician to learn how to handle patients' emotion in practice. The challenge ahead for researchers, educators, and clinicians is therefore to move beyond the mere description of how emotions are expressed and responded to, to the investigation of which strategies are most effective in different situations. For instance, a recent study tested the use of VR-CoDES categories to judge the appropriateness of emotion handling communication behavior.[135] Future studies should translate more specific findings on cues, such as their rarity in most consultations, the vagueness of the expression, the sequential nature of emotional talk, and the subtle cultural differences in how cues are expressed, into more specific training modules, making students and clinicians better prepared to adequately attend to patients' emotions in medical encounters.

REFERENCES

1. Suchmann AL, Markakis K, Beckman HB, Frankel RM. A model of empathic communication in the medical interview. *JAMA*. 1997;277:678-682.

2. Eide H, Eide T, Rustøen T, Finset A. Patient validation of cues and concerns identified according to Verona coding definitions of emotional sequences (VR-CoDES): a video- and interview-based approach. *Patient Educ Couns*. 2011;82:156-162.

3. Del Piccolo L, Saltini A, Zimmermann C, Dunn G. Differences in verbal behaviors of patients with and without emotional distress during primary care consultations. *Psychol Med*. 2000;30:629-643.

4. Zimmermann C, Del Piccolo L, Finset A. Cues and concerns by patients in medical consultations: a literature review. *Psychol Bull*. 2007;133:438-463.

5. Stone AL, Tai-Seale M, Stults CD, Luiz JM, Frankel RM. Three types of ambiguity in coding empathic interactions in primary care visits: implications for research and practice. *Patient Educ Couns*. 2012;89:63-68.

6. Silverman J, Kurtz S, Draper J. *Skills for Communicating with Patients*. London: Radcliffe Publishing; 2013:85.

7. *Oxford Advanced Learner's Dictionary*.

8. Zimmermann C, Del Piccolo L, Bensing J, et al. Coding patient emotional cues and concerns in medical consultations: the Verona coding definitions of emotional sequences (VR-CoDES). *Patient Educ Couns*. 2011;82:141-148.

9. Piccinelli M, Pini S, Bonizzato P, et al. Results from the Verona Centre. In: Üstün TB, Sartorius N, eds. *Mental Illness in General Health Care: An International Study*. New York, NY: John Wiley & Sons; 1995:301-321.

10. Kaplan SH, Gandek B, Greenfield S, Rogers WH, Ware JE. Patient and visit characteristics related to physicians' participatory decision-making styles. *Med Care*. 1995; 12:1176-1187.

11. Kaplan SH, Greenfield S, Gandek B, Rogers WH, Ware JE. Characteristics of physicians with participatory decision-making styles. *Ann Intern Med*. 1996;124:497-504.

12. Hall JA, Irish JT, Roter DL, Ehrlich CM, Miller LH. Gender in medical encounters: an analysis of physician and patient communication in a primary care setting. *Health Psychol*. 1994;13:384-392.

13. Del Piccolo L, Mazzi MA, Goss C, Rimondini M, Zimmermann C. How emotions emerge and are dealt with in first diagnostic consultations in psychiatry. *Patient Educ Couns*. 2012; 88:29-35.

14. Purnamaningsih EH. Personality and emotion regulation strategies. *Int Psychol Res*. 2017;10(1):53-60.

15. De Maesschalck S, Deveugele M, Willems S. Language, culture and emotions: exploring ethnic minority patients' emotional expressions in primary healthcare consultations. *Patient Educ Couns*. 2011;84: 406-412.

16. Kale E, Finset A, Eikeland HL, Gulbrandsen P. Emotional cues and concerns in hospital encounters with non-western immigrants as compared with Norwegians: an exploratory study. *Patient Educ Couns*. 2011;84(3):325-331.

17. Schouten BC, Schinkel S. Emotions in primary care: are there cultural differences in the expression of cues and concerns? *Patient Educ Couns*. 2015;98:1346-1351.

18. Zhou Y, Lundy JM, Humphris G, Mercer SW. Do multimorbidity and deprivation influence patients' emotional expressions and doctors' responses in primary care consultations? an exploratory study using multilevel analysis. *Patient Educ Couns*. 2015; 98:1063-1070.

19. Mechanic D. The concept of illness behaviour: culture, situation and personal predisposition. *Psychol Med*. 1986;16:1-7.

20. Watzlawick P, Beavin JH, Jackson DD. *The Pragmatics of Human Communication: A Study of Interactional Patterns, Pathologies and Paradoxes*. New York, NY: WW Norton; 1967.

21. Maguire P, Rutter DR. History taking for medical students. *Lancet*. 1976;11:556-557.

22. Maguire P, Goldberg D, Hobson RF, Margison F, Moss S, O'Dowd T. Evaluating the teaching of a method of psychotherapy. *Br J Psychiatry*. 1984;144:575-580.

23. Goldberg D, Steele JJ, Smith C. Teaching psychiatric interview techniques to family doctors. *Acta Psychiatrica Scandinavica*. 1980;62:41–47.

24. Gask L, Goldberg D, Lesser A, Millar T. Improving the psychiatric skills of the general practice trainee: an evaluation of a group training course. *Med Educ*. 1988;22:132-138.

25. Gask L, McGrath G, Goldberg D, Millar T. Improving the psychiatric skills of established general practitioners: evaluation of group teaching. *Med Educ.* 1987;21:362-368.

26. Ford S, Lewis S, Fallowfield L. Psychological morbidity in newly referred patients with cancer. *J Psychosom Res.* 1995;39:193-202.

27. Ustun TB, Sartorius N. *Mental Illness in General Health Care: An International Study.* New York: Wiley. 1995.

28. Fallowfield L, Ratcliffe D, Jenkins V, Saul J. Psychiatric morbidity and its recognition by doctors in patients with cancer. *Br J Cancer.* 2001;84:1011-1015.

29. Mitchell AJ, Rao S, Vaze A. Can general practitioners identify people with distress and mild depression? a meta-analysis of clinical accuracy. *J Affect Disord.* 2011;130(1-2):26-36.

30. Goldberg D, Jenkins L, Miller T, Faragher EB. The ability of trainee general practitioners to identify psychological distress among their patients. *Psychol Med.* 1993;23:185-193.

31. Davenport S, Goldberg D, Millar T. How psychiatric disorders are missed during medical consultations. *Lancet.* 1987;22:439-441.

32. Levenstein JH, McCracken EC, McWhinney IR, Brown JB, Weston WW, Stewart MA. The patient-centred clinical method: a model for the doctor-patient interaction in family medicine. *Fam Pract.* 1986;3:24-30.

33. Henbest RJ, Stewart MA. Patient-centredness in the consultation. 1: a method for measurement. *Fam Pract.* 1989;4:249-253.

34. Booth C, Maguire P. *Development of a Rating System to Assess Interactions Between Cancer Patients and Health Professionals.* London: Report to Cancer Research Campaign; 1991.

35. Maguire P, Faulkner A, Booth K, Elliot C, Hillier V. Helping cancer patients disclose their concerns. *Eur J Cancer.* 1996a;32:78-81.

36. Maguire P, Booth K, Elliot C, Jones B. Helping health professionals involved in cancer care acquire interviewing skills: the impact of workshops. *Eur J Cancer.* 1996;32:1457-1459.

37. Roter DL. *The Roter Method of Interaction Process Analysis.* Baltimore, MD: Johns Hopkins University; 1993.

38. Bensing JM, Verheul W, Jansen J, Langewitz WA. Looking for trouble: the added value of sequence analysis in finding evidence for the role of physicians in patients' disclosure of cues and concerns. *Med Care.* 2010;48(7):583-588.

39. Butalid L, Verhaak PFM, Bensing JM. Changes in general practitioners' sensitivity to patients' distress in low back pain consultations. *Patient Educ Couns.* 2015;98(10): 1207-1213.

40. Eide H, Quera V, Graugaard P, Finset A. Physician-patient dialogue surrounding patients' expression of concern: applying sequence analysis to RIAS. *Soc Sci Med.* 2004;59(1):145-155.

41. Langewitz W, Nübling M, Weber H. A theory-based approach to analysing conversation sequences. *Epidemiologia e Psichiatria Sociale.* 2003;12(2):103-108.

42. Roter DL, Larson SM, Beach MC, Cooper LA. Interactive and evaluative correlates of dialogue sequence: a simulation study applying the RIAS to turn taking structures. *Patient Educ Couns.* 2008;71(1):26-33.

43. Van den Brink-Muinen A, Caris-Verhallen W. Doctors' responses to patients' concerns: testing the use of sequential analysis. *Epidemiologia e Psichiatria Sociale.* 2003;12(2):92-97.

44. Van Dulmen S, Nübling M, Langewitz W. Doctors' responses to patients' concerns; an exploration of communication sequences in gynaecology. *Epidemiologia e Psichiatria Sociale*. 2003;12(2):98-102.

45. Eide H, Quera V, Finset A. Exploring rare patient behaviour with sequential analysis: an illustration. *Epidemiologia e Psichiatria Sociale*. 2003;12(2):109-114.

46. Kim YM, Kols A, Prammawat S, Rinehart W. Sequence analysis: responsiveness of doctors to patient cues during family planning consultations in Mexico. *Patient Educ Couns*. 2005;58:114-117.

47. Heaven C, Green C. Medical Interview Aural Rating Scale. Unpublished report, Cancer Research UK Psychological Medicine. Group, University of Manchester, Manchester, the United Kingdom. 1999.

48. Jansen J, van Weert JCM, de Groot J, van Dulmen S, Heeren TJ, Bensing JM. Emotional and informational patient cues: the impact of nurses' responses on recall. *Patient Educ Couns*. 2010;79(2):218-224.

49. Noordman J, van Dulmen S. Shared medical appointments marginally enhance interaction between patients: an observational study on children and adolescents with type 1 diabetes. *Patient Educ Couns*. 2013;92(3):418-425.

50. Aarts JWM, Van Oers AM, Faber MJ, et al. Communication at an online infertility expert forum: provider responses to patients' emotional and informational cues. *J Psychosom Obstet Gynaecol*. 2015;36(2):66-74.

51. Driesenaar JA, De Smet PAGM, van Hulten R, Noordman J, van Dulmen S. Cue-responding behaviors during pharmacy counseling sessions with patients with asthma about inhaled corticosteroids: potential relations with medication beliefs and self-reported adherence. *Health Commun*. 2016;31(10):1266-1275.

52. Repping-Wuts H, Repping T, van Riel P, van Achterberg T. Fatigue communication at the out-patient clinic of rheumatology. *Patient Educ Couns*. 2009;76(1):57-62.

53. Sheldon LK, Blonquist TM, Hilaire DM, Hong F, Berry DL. Patient cues and symptoms of psychosocial distress: what predicts assessment and treatment of distress by oncology clinicians? *Psychooncology*. 2015;24(9):1020-1027.

54. Farrell C, Chan EA, Siouta E, Walshe C, Molassiotis A. Communication patterns in nurse-led chemotherapy clinics: a mixed-method study. *Patient Educ Couns*. 2020;103(8):1538-1545.

55. Heaven C, Clegg J, Maguire P. Transfer of communication skills training from workshop to workplace: the impact of clinical supervision. *Patient Educ Couns*. 2006;60(3):313-325.

56. Uitterhoeve R, Bensing J, Dilven E, Donders R, DeMulder P, Van Achterberg T. Nurse-patient communication in cancer care: does responding to patient's cues predict patient satisfaction with communication. *Psychooncology*. 2009;18(10):1060-1068.

57. Tol F, Jansen J, Bensing J, Weert JV. Older cancer patients' anxiety, information preference, coping style and participation during consultation: effects on recall of information. In: *Psychology of Cancer*. New York, NY: Nova Science Publishers; 2012:165-180.

58. Lin M, Lee A, Chou C, Liu T, Tang C. Factors predicting emotional cue-responding behaviors of nurses in Taiwan: an observational study. *Psychooncology*. 2017;26(10):1548-1554.

59. Uitterhoeve R, De Leeuw J, Bensing J, et al. Cue-responding behaviours of oncology nurses in video-simulated interviews. *J Adv Nurs*. 2008;61(1):71-80.

60. Branch WT, Malik TK. Using "Windows of opportunities" in brief interviews to understand patients' concerns. *JAMA.* 1993;269(3):1667-1668.

61. Eide H, Frankel R, Haaversen ACB, Vaupel KA, Graugaard PK, Finset A. Listening for feelings: identifying and coding empathic and potential empathic opportunities in medical dialogues. *Patient Educ Couns.* 2004;54(3):291-297.

62. Bylund CL, Makoul G. Empathic communication and gender in the physician-patient encounter. *Patient Educ Couns.* 2002;48(3):207-216.

63. Easter DW, Beach W. Competent patient care is dependent upon attending to empathic opportunities presented during interview sessions. *Curr Surg.* 2004;61(3):313-318.

64. Pollak KI, Arnold RM, Jeffreys AS, et al. Oncologist communication about emotion during visits with patients with advanced cancer. *J Clin Oncol.* 2007;25(36):5748-5752.

65. Morse DS, Edwardsen EA, Gordon HS. Missed opportunities for interval empathy in lung cancer communication. *Arch Intern Med.* 2008;168(17):1853-1858.

66. Johnson Shen M, Ostroff JS, Hamann HA, et al. Structured analysis of empathic opportunities and physician responses during lung cancer patient-physician consultations. *J Health Commun.* 2019;24(9):711-718.

67. van Hoorn BT, Menendez ME, Mackert M, Donovan EE, van Heijl M, Ring D. Missed empathic opportunities during hand surgery office visits. *Hand.* 2019.

68. Goodchild CE, Skinner TC, Parkin T. The value of empathy in dietetic consultations: a pilot study to investigate its effect on satisfaction, autonomy and agreement. *J Hum Nutr Diet.* 2005;18(3):181-185.

69. Alexander SC, Pollak KI, Morgan PA, et al. How do non-physician clinicians respond to advanced cancer patients' negative expressions of emotions? *Support Care Cancer.* 2011;19(1):155-159.

70. Bry K, Bry M, Hentz E, Karlsson HL, Kyllönen H, Lundkvist M, Wigert H. Communication skills training enhances nurses' ability to respond with empathy to parents' emotions in a neonatal intensive care unit. *Acta Paediatrica.* 2016;105(4):397-406.

71. Foster A, Chaudhary N, Kim T, Waller JL, Wong J, Borish M, Buckley PF. Using virtual patients to teach empathy: a randomized controlled study to enhance medical students' empathic communication. *Simul Healthc.* 2016;11(3):181-189.

72. Del Piccolo L, Benpensanti MG, Bonini P, Cellerino P, Saltini A, Zimmermann C. Il Verona-Medical Interview Classification System/Patient VR-MICS/P Presentazione dello strumento e studio di attendibilita. *Epidemiol Psichiatr Soc.* 1999; 8:56–67.

73. Zimmermann C, Del Piccolo L, Mazzi MA. Patient cues and medical interviewing in general practice: examples of the application of sequential analysis. *Epidemiologia e Psichiatria Sociale.* 2003;12:115-123.

74. Goss C, Mazzi MA, Del Piccolo L, Rimondini M, Zimmermann C. The information giving process in general practice consultations. *J Eval Clin Pract.* 2005;11:339-349.

75. Del Piccolo L, Mead N, Gask L, et al. The English version of the Verona Medical Interview Classification System VR-MICS: an assessment of its reliability and a comparative cross-cultural test of its validity. *Patient Educ Couns.* 2005;58:252-263.

76. Stewart M, Brown JB, Weston WW, McWhinney JR, McWilliam C, Freeman TR. *Patient-Centered Medicine: Transforming the Clinical Method.* Thousand Oaks, CA: Sage Publications, Inc.; 1995.

77. Saltini A, Cappellari D, Cellerino P, Del Piccolo L, Zimmermann Ch. Uno strumento per la valutazione dell'intervista medica nel contestodella medicina generale, il VR-MICS/D Verona-Medical Interview Classification System/Doctor. *Epidemiol Psichiatr Soc.* 1998;3:210–23.

78. Del Piccolo L, Mazzi MA, Dunn G, Sandri M, Zimmermann C. Sequence analysis in multilevel models: a study on different sources of patient cues in medical consultations. *Soc Sci Med.* 2007;65:2357-2370.

79. Levinson W, Horawara-Bhat R, Lamb J. A study of patient clues and physician responses in primary care and surgical settings. *JAMA.* 2000;284:1021-1027.

80. Ford S, Hall A, Ratcliffe D, Fallowfield L. The medical interaction process system MIPS: an instrument for analysing interviews of oncologists and patients with cancer. *Social Science and Medicine.* 2000; 50 (4): 553-566.

81. Fallowfield L, Jenkins V, Farewell F, Saul J, Duffy A, Eves R. Efficacy of a cancer research UK communication skills training model for oncologists: a randomized trial. *Lancet.* 2002;359:650-656.

82. Fallowfield L, Jenkins V, Farewell F, Solis-Trapal I. Enduring impact of communication skills training: results of a 12-month follow-up. *Br J Cancer.* 2003;89:1445-1449.

83. Ford S, Hall A. Communication behaviours of skilled and less skilled oncologists: a validation study of the medical interaction process system MIPS. *Patient Educ Couns.* 2004;54(3):275-282.

84. Pawlikowska T, Zhang W, Griffiths F, van Dalen J, van der Vleuten C. Verbal and non-verbal behavior of doctors and patients in primary care consultations — how this relates to patient enablement. *Patient Educ Couns.* 2012;86(1):70-76.

85. Schoenthaler A, Knafl GJ, Fiscella K, Ogedegbe G. Addressing the social needs of hypertensive patients the role of patient-provider communication as a predictor of medication adherence. *Circ Cardiovasc Qual Outcomes.* 2017;10(9):e003659.

86. Butow PN, Dunn SM, Tattersall MH. Communication with cancer patients: does it matter? *J Palliat Care.* 1995;11(4):34-38.

87. Butow PN, Dunn SM, Tattersall MHN, Jones QJ. Computer-based interaction analysis of the cancer consultation. *Br J Cancer.* 1995;71(5):1115-1121.

88. Butow PN, Brown RF, Cogar S, Tattersall MHN, Dunn SM. Oncologists' reactions to cancer patients' verbal cues. *Psychooncology.* 2002;11(1):47-58.

89. Brown RF, Butow PN, Henman M, Dunn SM, Boyle F, Tattersall MHN. Responding to the active and passive patient: flexibility is the key. *Health Expect.* 2002;5(3):236-245.

90. Duric V, Butow P, Sharpe L, Lobb E, Meiser B, Barratt A, Tucker K. Reducing psychological distress in a genetic counseling consultation for breast cancer. *J Genet Couns.* 2003;12(3):243-264.

91. Oguchi M, Jansen J, Butow P, Colagiuri B, Divine R, Dhillon H. Measuring the impact of nurse cue-response behaviour on cancer patients' emotional cues. *Patient Educ Couns.* 2011;82(2):163-168.

92. Butow P, Cockburn J, Girgis A, et al. Increasing oncologists' skills in eliciting and responding to emotional cues: evaluation of a communication skills training program. *Psychooncology.* 2008;17(3):209-218.

93. Del Piccolo L, de Haes H, Heaven C, et al. Development of the Verona coding definitions of emotional sequences to code health providers' responses VR-CoDES-P to patient cues and concerns. *Patient Educ Couns.* 2011;82:149-155.

94. Del Piccolo L, Finset A, Mellblom AV, et al. Verona Coding Definitions of Emotional Sequences VR-CoDES: conceptual framework and future directions. *Patient Educ Couns.* 2017;100(12):2303-2311.

95. Zandbelt LC, Smets EMA, Oort FJ, De Haes HCJM. Coding patient-centred behaviour in the medical encounter. *Soc Sci Med.* 2005;61(3):661-671.

96. Zandbelt LC, Smets EMA, Oort FJ, Godfried MH, de Haes HCJM. Determinants of physicians' patient-centred behaviour in the medical specialist encounter. *Soc Sci Med.* 2006;63(4):899-910.

97. Bensing J, Zandbelt L, Zimmermann C. Introduction: sequence analysis of patient-provider interaction. *Epidemio Psichiatr Soc.* 2003;12:78-80.

98. Del Piccolo L, Danzi O, Fattori N, Mazzi MA, Goss C. How psychiatrist's communication skills and patient's diagnosis affect emotions disclosure during first diagnostic consultations. *Patient Educ Couns.* 2014;96:151-158.

99. Del Piccolo L, Pietrolongo E, Radice D, Tortorella C, Confalonieri P, Pugliatti MT, et al. Patient expression of emotions and neurologist responses in first multiple sclerosis consultations. *PLoS ONE.* 2015;10:e0127734.

100. Heyn L, Finset A, Ruland C. Talking about feelings and worries in cancer consultations. *Cancer Nurs.* 2013;36(2):E20-E30.

101. Vatne TM, Ruland CM, Ørnes K, Finset A. Children's expressions of negative emotions and adults' responses during routine cardiac consultations. *J Pediatr Psychol.* 2012;37:232-240.

102. Del Piccolo L, Mazzi MA, Mascanzoni A, et al. Factors related to the expression of emotions by early-stage breast cancer patients. *Patient Educ Couns.* 2019;102:176-1773.

103. Barracliffe L, Yang Y, Cameron J, Bedi C, Humphris G. Does emotional talk vary with fears of cancer recurrence trajectory? A content analysis of interactions between women with breast cancer and their therapeutic radiographers. *J Psychosom Res.* 2018;106 41-48.

104. Humphris G, Yang Y, Barracliffe L, Cameron J, Bedi C. Emotional talk of patients with breast cancer during review appointments with therapeutic radiographers: effects on fears of cancer recurrence. *Support Care Cancer.* 2019;27:2143-2151.

105. Torre JB, Lieberman MD. Putting feelings into words: affect labeling as implicit emotion regulation. *Emot Rev.* 2018;10:116-124.

106. Kandsberger J, Rogers S, Zhou Y, Humphris G. Using fundamental frequency of cancer survivors' speech to investigate emotional distress in out-patient visits. *Patient Educ Couns.* 2016;99:1971-1977.

107. Drew P. Turn design. In: Sidnell J, Stivers T, eds. *The Handbook of Conversation Analysis.* Chichester: Wiley-Blackwell; 2013:131-149.

108. Finset A. Talk-in-interaction and neuropsychological processes *Scand J Psychol.* 2014;55:212-18.

109. Jefferson G. On the sequential organization of trouble talks in ordinary conversation. *Soc Probl.* 1988;35(4):418-441.

110. Mellblom AV, Lie HC, Korsvold L, Ruud E, Loge JH, Finset A. Sequences of talk about emotional concerns in follow-up consultations with adolescent childhood cancer survivors. *Patient Educ Couns.* 2016;99(1):77-84.

111. Ruusuvuori J. "Empathy" and "sympathy" in action: attending to patients' troubles in Finnish homeopathic and general practice consultations. *Soc Psychol Q.* 2005;68(3):204-222.

112. Ruusuvuori J. Managing affect: integration of empathy and problem-solving in health care encounters. *Discourse Stud.* 2007;9(5):597-622.

113. Pino M, Parry R, Land V, Faull C, Feathers L, Seymour J. Engaging terminally ill patients in end of life talk: how experienced palliative medicine doctors navigate the dilemma of promoting discussions about dying. *PLoS ONE.* 2016;11(5):e0156174.

114. Vinson AH, Underman K. Clinical empathy as emotional labor in medical work. *Soc Sci Med.* 2020; 251.

115. Dean M, Street RL. A 3-stage model of patient-centered communication for addressing cancer patients' emotional distress. *Patient Educ Couns.* 2014;94(2):143-148.

116. Patel S, Pelletier-Bui A, Smith S, et al. Curricula for empathy and compassion training in medical education: a systematic review. *PLoS One.* 2019;14(8):e0221412.

117. Schmitz FM, Schnabel KP, Bauer D, Bachmann C, Woermann U, Guttormsen S. The learning effects of different presentations of worked examples on medical students' breaking-bad-news skills: a randomized and blinded field trial. *Patient Educ Couns.* 2018;101:1439-1451.

118. Ortwein H, Benz A, Carl P, et al. Applying the Verona coding definitions of emotional sequences VR-CoDES to code medical students' written responses to written case scenarios: some methodological and practical considerations. *Patient Educ Couns.* 2017;100(2):305-312.

119. Zhou Y, Collinson A, Laidlaw A, Humphries G. How do medical students respond to emotional cues and concerns expressed by simulated patients during OSCE consultations? A multilevel study. *PLoS One.* 2013;8:e79166.

120. Barbosa M, Del Piccolo L, Barbosa A. Effectiveness of a brief training program in relational/communication skills for medical residents. *Patient Educ Couns.* 2019; 102:1104-1110.

121. Frankel RM, Stein T. Enhancing clinician. Getting the most out of the clinical encounter: the Four Habits Model. *J Med Pract Manage.* 2001;16(4):184-191.

122. Stein T, Frankel RM, Krupat E. Enhancing clinician communication skills in a large healthcare organization: a longitudinal case study. *Patient Educ Couns.* 2005;58(1):4-12.

123. Langewitz W, Heydrich L, Nübling M, Szirt L, Weber H, Grossman P. Swiss cancer league communication skills training programme for oncology nurses: an evaluation. *J Adv Nurs.* 2010;66(10):2266-2277.

124. Tulsky JA, Arnold RM, Alexander SC, Olsen MK, Jeffreys AS, Rodriguez KL, Skinner CS, Farrell D, Abernethy AP, Pollak KI. Enhancing communication between oncologists and patients with a computer-based training program: a randomized trial. *Ann Intern Med.* 2011;155(9):593-601.

125. O'Grady C. Clinical communication training for the general practice of medicine: a case for including discourse analytical findings from real-world practice. *J Applied Linguistics Professional Pract.* 2016;13(1-3):254-275.

126. Gibbon LM, Hurd CJ, Merel SE. Online module builds skills for internal medicine interns in responding to emotions during complex serious illness conversations. *J Pain Symptom Manage.* 2020;59(6):1379-1383.

127. Van Eikenhorst L, van Dijk L, Cords J, Vervloet M, de Gier H, Taxis K. Pharmacists' responses to cues and concerns of polypharmacy patients during clinical medication reviews. *Patient Educ Couns.* 2020;103(5):930-936.

128. Vijfhuizen M, Bok H, Matthew SM, Del Piccolo L, McArthur M. Analyzing how negative emotions emerge and are addressed in veterinary consultations, using the Verona Coding Definitions of Emotional Sequences (VR-CoDES). *Patient Educ Couns.* 2017;100:682-689.

129. Yin L, Yin M, Wang Q, Yan Y, Tang Q, Deng Y, Liu X. Can Verona Coding Definitions of Emotional Sequences (VR-CoDES) be applied to standardized Chinese medical consultations? a reliability and validity investigation. *Patient Educ Couns.* 2019;102:1460-1466.

130. Zhou Y, Humphris G, Ghazali N, Friderichs S, Grosset D, Rogers SN. How head and neck consultants manage patients' emotional distress during cancer follow-up consultations: a multilevel study. *Eur Arch Otorhinolaryngol.* 2015;27(2):2473-2481.

131. Korsvold L, Mellblom A, Finset A, Rund E, Lie HC. A content analysis of emotional concerns expressed at the time of receiving a cancer diagnosis. *Eur J Oncol Nurs.* 2017;26:1-8.

132. Finset A, Heyn L, Ruland C. Patterns in clinicians' responses to patient emotion in cancer care. *Patient Educ Couns.* 2013;93:80-85.

133. Kale E, Skjeldestad K, Finset A. Emotional communication in medical consultations with native and non-native patients applying two different methodological approaches. *Patient Educ Couns.* 2013;92(3):366-374.

134. Park J, Beach MC, Han D, Moore RD, Korthuis PT, Saha S. Racial disparities in clinician responses to patient emotions. *Patient Educ Couns.* 2020;103(9):1736-1744.

135. Graupe T, Fischer MR, Strijbos JW, Kiessling C. Development and piloting of a Situational Judgement Test for emotion-handling skills using the Verona Coding Definitions of Emotional Sequences (VR-CoDES). *Patient Educ Couns.* 2020;103(9):1839-1845.

Emotion Regulation in Patients, Providers, and the Clinical Relationship

Brett Marroquín and Vera Vine

■ INTRODUCTION

Clinical encounters are often emotional events—few situations are more emotionally laden than when a person's health is at stake. But the role of emotion goes beyond patients' emotional experiences and expressions; it also includes the ways in which people respond to and manage the emotions they experience. It is clear that how people regulate their emotions plays an important role in both physical and mental health outcomes.[1-4] Our goal in this chapter is to expose providers and trainees to the most relevant concepts and current thinking about emotion regulation for patient care and the patient–provider relationship, and to encourage awareness of these issues during the clinical encounter. Clinicians' understanding of emotion regulation offers opportunities to improve experiences of both patients and providers in clinical care interaction, and for dynamic interpersonal effects within the patient–provider relationship that improve intervention and treatment outcomes.

This chapter integrates research findings from psychological science to introduce definitions and basic concepts in emotion regulation, describe specific emotion regulation strategies likely to appear in patient care, and address the social and interpersonal contexts of emotion regulation and their relevance to the clinical encounter. It concludes with a discussion of recommendations and challenges for application in clinical care, including assessment and intervention, and a discussion of providers' own emotion regulation and its role in provider and patient outcomes. Throughout the chapter we provide brief case examples illustrating the role of emotion regulation across the range of health professions. Some are fictional cases and some are drawn from our experiences as clinical psychologists, with identifying details changed.

■ WHAT IS EMOTION REGULATION? DEFINITIONS AND BASIC CONCEPTS

James Gross, a prominent scholar in modern emotion regulation research, has summarized the construct as "the processes by which we influence which emotions we have, when we have them, and how we experience and express them."[5,6] Others have defined emotion regulation as including processes involved in monitoring, evaluating, and making sense of emotional reactions before they can be regulated.[7,8] What all definitions of emotion regulation have in common is a focus on the processes by which individuals modulate their own emotional states. Underlying emotion regulation is an intricate set of biological, psychological, and social mechanisms that allow individuals some degree of influence—sometimes intentional and sometimes relatively automatic—over their emotions. This section introduces several key concepts fundamental to understanding the nature and applications of emotion regulation.

Emotion Regulation versus Coping

To grasp the concept of emotion regulation, it is useful to distinguish it from its close relative, coping. The concept of coping was developed before the concept of emotion regulation, and it has a long history in psychology and health care.[9,10] Generally speaking, much of coping is problem-focused; it describes how people respond to the demands of stressors themselves, such as generating, evaluating, and implementing solutions to problems. Other coping efforts are more emotion-focused; responses such as venting, seeking social support, or changing one's emotion address the emotions elicited by the situations. Like emotion-focused coping, emotion regulation has much to do with the individual's responses to internal states made with the aim of rallying resources or decreasing demands to meet the challenge. However, emotion regulation is more squarely focused on changing emotional reactions than coping is.[6]

Consider a case in which, due to severe injury, a patient is forced to face their inability to manage their activities of daily living by themselves. Several potential behaviors would fall under the umbrella of coping: the patient might conduct online searches of home care agencies in the area, problem-solve new ways of getting around their home, or recruit their social network to bring them meals. All of these coping efforts are responses to the situation at hand, but they are not inherently emotional in nature. The patient's emotion regulation efforts, by contrast, would be more specifically targeted at modifying their emotional states. For example, if the patient reacts with sadness to the news that they will be unable to take care of themselves, they might engage in emotion regulation to decrease sadness. They might choose cognitive strategies such as accepting that their sadness makes sense given their temporary loss of independence, focusing repetitively on what has led them to these circumstances, or looking on the bright side. They might also enact behavioral strategies such as venting their emotions to others, hiding their distress by suppressing their facial expressions, or watching TV to distract themselves. These are just a few examples of specific emotion regulation strategies discussed more thoroughly below. These examples also show how emotion regulation can involve regulating emotional experience (i.e., feelings), emotional expression (i.e., external displays), or both.

Upregulating versus Downregulating Emotions

Both positive and negative emotions can be regulated, and emotion regulation can involve either amplifying or decreasing intensity. An example of *upregulating* a positive emotion is savoring: a patient with cancer receives news that their surgery has been effective and takes a moment to revel in or extend their experience of joy. The same patient might then *downregulate* their positive emotion when they return to the clinic waiting room, attenuating their positive feeling and/or its expression out of respect for the anxious patients there. Upregulating *negative* emotion might occur when a patient consciously or unconsciously senses they must emit a stronger behavioral expression to gain their partner's attention, or when becoming angrier will motivate them to advocate better with their insurance company.

Approach-Oriented versus Avoidant Emotion Regulation

Most emotion regulation strategies can be considered either predominantly *approach-oriented* or predominantly *avoidant*. Overall, approach-oriented emotion regulation—involving active engagement with emotions as opposed to avoiding, disengaging, or denying—is associated with better psychological and physical outcomes.[11–14] The approach/avoidance distinction maps onto core motivational systems in humans and key dimensions of emotions themselves.[15–18] Approaching emotions by attending to, processing, and expressing emotional experience tends to result in better psychological adjustment to stressors and negative events, compared with emotional avoidance.[12] However, this effect is moderated by a number of characteristics, including gender, type of stressor, social support availability, and affective traits, arguing against an oversimplified view of emotional approach as "adaptive."[12,19–21]

Momentary versus Habitual Emotion Regulation

When emotions are regulated in daily life, this occurs as a time-limited, relatively momentary response to emotion. An individual instance in which an emotion is regulated is referred to as "state" emotion regulation. By contrast, habitual or "trait" emotion regulation refers to individuals' *tendencies* to regulate emotion in relatively stable, predictable ways from situation to situation. When we say that a patient experienced fear during a clinical interaction and took a deep breath to decrease their internal feelings of fear, or suppressed their expressions to hide their fear from the provider, we are referring to state regulation. If we say that this patient has a general tendency to suppress their negative emotions in many situations—they do this at most appointments; they present bad news to their partner with flat affect; they respond to slights with anger but refuse to let it show—we are referring to trait expressive suppression. In theory, trait emotion regulation can be thought of as an individual difference, like a personality characteristic that varies from person to person but is fairly stable across situations. Recent findings suggest people display less consistency in their emotion regulation than traditionally presumed,[22,23] but the distinction can be useful for interpreting existing research. While most experiments on emotion regulation processes have examined state emotion regulation, much of the research linking emotion regulation to health and healthcare settings has examined trait regulation.

"Adaptive" versus "Maladaptive" Emotion Regulation

Research on emotion regulation has shown that habitual use of some strategies is associated with better mental and physical health outcomes, and overuse of others is associated with negative outcomes.[1-3] This pattern has led to frequent characterizations of strategies as either "adaptive" or "maladaptive." For example, as we discuss later, habitually engaging in a ruminative emotion regulation style is a robust predictor of developing or remaining stuck in depressive episodes,[24] and rumination is often considered maladaptive. These characterizations are frequently useful and empirically supported; rumination is in fact reliably positively associated with many different psychopathologies, negatively associated with healthy outcomes, and also associated with other "maladaptive" strategies.[1,24] However, it is important to understand that no one strategy for emotion regulation is definitively "good" or "bad." Newer approaches instead characterize emotion regulation attempts as suitable or unsuitable for certain situations, successful or unsuccessful in achieving their objectives, and helpful or unhelpful in their short- or long-term consequences.[25,26]

The purpose of emotion regulation can vary, but often emotions are regulated in the service of objectives like feeling better, being socially appropriate, or achieving goals.[27] Ultimately, much of what determines the helpfulness or unhelpfulness of emotion regulation attempts is not the specific strategy on its own, but rather other factors like the degree of fit between the emotion regulation strategy and the situation.[23] Emotion scientists increasingly recognize the importance of flexibly applying an expansive repertoire of emotion regulation strategies in context-sensitive ways.[28,29] A person who "approaches" emotions too much, returning over and over to analyze a long-ago loss in a passive way, or while ignoring other situational demands, is at risk of negative outcomes. Similarly, a person who unfailingly engages in problem solving, generating and analyzing solutions for every challenge without acknowledging or expressing emotional experience, may lose opportunities for learning, insight, or social connection. People have repertoires of emotion regulation strategies, which they draw from with varying levels of flexibility and skill, and the strategies have different effects depending on features of the situation at hand, such as the emotional intensity and controllability of the situation.[28,30] In the context of patient–provider interactions, therefore, it is critical to be aware that observing a single-emotion regulation strategy in a patient (or in oneself) is not enough information to construe it as adaptive or maladaptive. Just as when applying knowledge derived from medical research, assessing or intervening on emotion regulation in any single person or in any single situation requires a flexible, contextual, person-centered perspective on the clinical encounter.

▓ INDIVIDUAL EMOTION REGULATION STRATEGIES

Here we describe key features of specific strategies from theoretical and empirical work on emotion regulation and provide clinical applications of them. These strategies include problem solving, reappraisal, expressive suppression, rumination, worry, catastrophizing, behavioral avoidance, cognitive and experiential avoidance, distraction, and acceptance. This selection of strategies is by no means exhaustive. Rather, we focus on the strategies most examined in the research literature and most relevant to patient–provider interactions. Given the types of issues that arise in clinical practice, as well as the field's emphasis on regulating *negative* emotion, we will also emphasize such situations. However, people can use many of these strategies when they upregulate or downregulate positive emotion as well.

Problem Solving

This strategy refers to taking active steps of generating, evaluating, and implementing solutions to the situation. We will not cover problem solving in detail here because it is frequently considered more of a coping strategy. However, problem solving is often prompted by emotion and regulates emotion. Engaging in other emotion regulation strategies first can also pave the way toward problem solving; generating and selecting problem solving strategies can be made easier by first getting a handle on the emotion itself.[31]

Reappraisal

Reappraisal (sometimes "cognitive reappraisal" or "positive reappraisal") involves modifying the initial interpretation (appraisal) of the situation, its demands, or the individual's ability to meet those demands, in order to change the resulting emotion. Appraisals are considered by many emotion theorists to be key determinants of emotion—appraising a stimulus as threatening prompts fear, for example, whereas appraising the same stimulus as entertaining prompts pleasure.[32] *Reappraisal* is changing one's interpretation of the stimulus in a way that reframes the situation to prompt a different emotion. A horror movie aficionado may initially construe a monster as a sudden threat and feel a rush of fear, but quickly reframe it as "it's just a movie" and downregulate the fear, or think, "What an absurd costume!" and laugh with enjoyment. Reappraisal can involve distancing oneself from the emotional stimulus in this way, or more actively engaging in reinterpretation of the stimulus based on rationality and accuracy of the appraisal, as emphasized in cognitive psychotherapies.[33] Reappraisal would be considered approach-oriented, and it has positive psychological and social outcomes across multiple studies.[1,34,35] Although reappraisal has a reputation for being adaptive, it can have negative consequences when it does not fit the context, such as when the situation limits the capacity for reappraisal (e.g., it is uncontrollable or very intense), or when the original emotion would lead to more adaptive action (e.g., anger motivating social action against injustice, or fear motivating flight from an abusive partner).[30]

Clinical Application

A family practice physician delivers the news that her patient Nora's blood pressure is extremely high and will require medication to control. Nora's initial interpretation of the news—"There's nothing I can do about this; this is just like what my father had before he died at a young age"—may register as fear, sadness, or shame. By distancing herself from this influential thought, perhaps replacing it with the thought "This news is concerning, but it sounds like if I take my medication I'll be safer," Nora may experience reduced negative emotion and/or an increase of relief and hope. Nora may or may not vocalize either of these alternative appraisals—or even be consciously aware of them—but as discussed later in this chapter, the clinician can nevertheless exert significant influence on patient appraisals of medical events and information.

Expressive Suppression

This strategy refers to the individual's management of outward emotional expression, which is separable from internal experience. Many studies have examined individuals' tendencies to suppress emotions, finding that suppressing negative emotional expression ironically increases subjective experience of the emotion, increases physiological arousal, negatively impacts social interactions and relationships, and impairs memory and cognitive capacity.[6,36,37] Overall, suppression has been approached as a generally maladaptive strategy, but again evidence suggests that this depends on contextual factors. This strategy is particularly relevant to the clinical encounter in that suppression modifies one of the primary "channels" through which clinicians can access patients' emotional experience: the patient's expressions. Dampening emotional expression may not only negatively impact the patient-provider relationship, as it does other types of relationships, but may also conceal the signals that clinicians could use to gauge patients' emotional states.

Clinical Application

Adrian, a teenager in a dentist's office, is unhappy at school, embarrassed by his uneven smile, and bullied by his classmates. The dentist, recognizing a potential need for braces, asks what Adrian thinks about his teeth. Feeling sadness and embarrassment, but believing that hiding these feelings will reduce them or make the dentist think better of him, Adrian clams up, mumbling "I don't care" with a blank face. This use of expressive suppression is likely to backfire internally, by increasing negative emotion, and externally, by leading the dentist to either think that Adrian is content with his smile, or perceive him as uncooperative in his treatment. An empathically attuned dentist might consider asking more direct follow-up questions or normalizing the experience of discomfort with one's smile, or at least not taking the lack of expression as evidence of lack of discomfort.

Rumination

Rumination falls within a broader category of typically maladaptive emotion regulation strategies characterized by unproductive repetitive thought. These include worry (common in generalized anxiety, and discussed below) and post-event processing (common in social anxiety).[38] Rumination is characterized by passive, repetitive thinking about the situation or emotion that is not directed toward active processing or problem solving.[24] Instead, individuals become mentally "stuck" on something negative (the situation, mood, or memory) and slip into a spiral of unanswerable questions such as "Why me?" or "What did I do to deserve this?" rather than active thinking like "What can I change about my current situation?" or "What can I learn from how I'm feeling right now?" Rumination is strongly implicated in depression, and is associated with a range of other psychopathology, poor psychological well-being, and physical health outcomes.[1,24] People who engage in rumination often believe it will be effective in solving problems, finding meaning, or regulating emotion,[39,40] but ample research shows that ruminating in negative mood states exacerbates those moods, impairs problem solving, strengthens maladaptive cognition, and reduces distress tolerance.[14,24]

Watkins and others have emphasized the passive, abstract, and self-focused characteristics of rumination as its most problematic elements.[38] "Rumination" (also known as "brooding") typically refers to this passive type of thinking.[41] However, some forms of self-reflective, even repetitive, thinking can be helpful or benign, especially when they are more active, concrete, and solution-oriented,[41–43] or when they are coupled with active coping behavior.[44,45] Many researchers consider brooding to be avoidant emotion regulation, whereas engaging in active cognitive processing of one's emotions is a more approach-oriented regulation strategy associated with insight and understanding of one's own emotion and more positive mental and physical health outcomes.[12,42] The notion that repetitive cognitive processing is not inherently maladaptive is also bolstered by findings that ruminating on *positive* content can cause an "upward" spiral of positive emotion.[46]

Clinical Application

Maggie, a patient in treatment for colon cancer, is experiencing marked decreases in activity, quality of life, and psychological well-being. Her oncologist provides an array of resources for activity and support, recommending ways that Maggie's family can help her cope. But Maggie continues to mentally rehash the past in a self-blaming or self-pitying way, spending hours on the couch thinking "Why didn't I get screened sooner? … Why do bad things always happen to me? … I should have eaten better or exercised more to prevent the cancer …." The physician may find that this unending, circular brooding exacerbates declines in Maggie's well-being, impairs her ability to capitalize on social support resources, and reduces her engagement in and compliance with treatment until the cycle is interrupted.

Worry and Catastrophizing

Worry is similar to rumination, in that it involves repetitive, unproductive, often uncontrollable thought that rarely leads to adaptive outcomes. Worry is best distinguished from rumination by its focus on the future rather than the past; a person engaging in worry imagines a universe of possible future negative outcomes of varying probability ("What if X? What if Y?"). Worry is considered an avoidant regulation strategy. As in rumination, people who worry often believe they are making progress toward problem solving or preparing proactively to cope, but the repetitive cognitive processing removes focus from concrete aspects of the situation toward abstract thought about the future, thereby avoiding emotion in the present and impairing active problem solving.[38,47] Cognitive models of generalized anxiety argue that even though worry fuels anxious distress, the avoidance of deeper fear or other emotions (e.g., shame, guilt) reinforces worry as a strategy over time and blocks more approach-oriented regulation of those emotions.[47] While worry focuses on repetitively generating an array of possible negative future outcomes, *catastrophizing* involves more actively "endorsing" the imagined worst case, or the worst possible *consequences* of that case. Especially if these are irrational interpretations of the objective situation, people's construals of the situation as catastrophic, rather than merely as painful or difficult, may serve an avoidant function. As an interpretive bias, catastrophic thinking is often a function of past experience and well-worn thinking patterns. It may also function to reduce distress related to the uncertainty of future outcomes. Ironically, assuming the worst possible outcome can, in the short term, decrease anxiety caused by uncertainty—the person "chooses" certain doom over looming threat.[48]

Clinical Application

Worry is extremely common in medical settings, where uncertainty abounds, stakes are high, and control is low. Naturally, patients seek to identify and prepare for potential negative outcomes, but when this becomes excessive, uncontrollable, and uncoupled from engaged coping, worry can become maladaptive. For example, Jamil is a primary care patient whose physician recommends routine preventative screening for sexually transmitted infections. A worry reaction would sound something like this: "What if I have something? Could I die? How will my parents react? Will my partner break up with me if I tell them? What would happen if I don't tell them? What if the test is negative but it's a mistake? How would I ever know? What if I infect my partner? What if they think I knew but I didn't?" Such thinking is well beyond what is indicated for the situation, and its abstract nature is unlikely to lead to positive action. Catastrophizing would be evident if Jamil assumes that his test *will* be positive, and is certain that his partner will leave him and he will be unable to find a place to stay. Such conclusions might cause him to refuse the test altogether, to decline the call when the results come in, or even to break up with his partner preemptively.

Worry is normative in situations with high uncertainty, and providers should be prepared to encounter it often. Some people, though, are more prone to worry than others and may use the strategy all the time, or in ways that seem out of proportion to the situation. In Jamil's case, certainty may (or may not) be regained within a few days, and catastrophic conclusions may (or may not) be contradicted by facts. But in many other cases worry will loom longer, such as in the month-to-month anxieties during fertility treatment, or the years of open-ended uncertainty in cancer survivorship or neurodegenerative disease. Clinical attention to the underlying emotion, including validation of fear or anxiety, encouragement of active problem solving, or acceptance of distress (discussed later in this chapter), can decrease the maladaptive spirals that such regulatory efforts generate.

Behavioral Avoidance

Behavioral avoidance refers to actions people take to eliminate exposure to situations or stimuli that cause emotional distress. The efficacy of avoidant behavior lies in the fact that the emotion-eliciting stimulus is not present, so it cannot produce the perceptual and cognitive content that drives the undesired emotion. For example, a person who feels shame or embarrassment when working out at the gym finds that by avoiding the gym she preempts these emotions, with the unfortunate byproduct of moving further away from her identified health goals. Avoidance can interfere with approach-oriented emotion regulation strategies that might be more helpful. For example, if avoidance becomes this person's preferred strategy for regulating distress, she will cut short her opportunities to engage in reappraisal of the thoughts underlying her emotions (e.g., "Well here I am working out; it's not so bad after all"). As with all strategies, behavioral avoidance need not be inherently maladaptive. The same person may decide to minimize exposure to cues that are inconsistent with her health goals by avoiding the block with the ice cream parlor, to decrease the likelihood of triggering feelings (e.g., craving) that threaten her goal.

Clinical Application

Behavioral avoidance is common in clinical settings and can be problematic. As in the example above, avoidance of difficult emotions can lead patients to poor health behaviors inconsistent with their health or treatment recommendations. Treatment nonadherence, including noncompliance with essential medication, is also often a form of behavioral avoidance. For example, Surya, a patient with breast cancer, is taking hormone therapy as adjuvant treatment following surgery. She experiences the physical discomfort of fatigue and hot flashes, but also the anxiety of potential recurrence and grief over lost health, all especially salient to her when she takes her medication. The fact that Surya can avoid such cues and emotions by skipping medication leads her to skip more and more, making her hormone therapy ineffective. In clinical settings, uses of avoidance to regulate distress can also manifest as avoidance of clinical encounters altogether. Patients struggling with negative emotions related to their use of clinical services are more likely to dismiss telephone calls or written communications from providers, or to cancel or no-show to appointments. Surya may continually reschedule her checkups, avoiding the anxiety of the reminder that recurrence is possible, or the shame she might feel reporting her medication noncompliance.

Cognitive and Experiential Avoidance

While behavioral avoidance involves taking actions to disengage from stressors or emotional situations, cognitive and experiential forms of avoidance are internal in nature. Strategies such as *denial* or *minimization* represent forms of cognitive avoidance; they involve imagining or construing the situation as if it does not exist or is of little consequence. *Thought suppression* is more active: it involves mental efforts to tamp down distressing thoughts, such as when a driver experiences a momentary fantasy of crashing into the car that just cut them off, and pushes the uncomfortable thought away. Thought suppression can be quite ineffective, especially when used chronically; ironically, it often causes increases in the frequency or strength of the thought one is attempting to eliminate.[49] *Experiential avoidance* is an overarching term for detaching oneself from uncomfortable experience by avoiding thoughts, sensations, memories, and emotions by suppressing or avoiding these internal experiences.[50,51] A similar strategy called "*nonacceptance*" also involves mental rejection of the situation or the emotions it elicits.[8]

Clinical Application

Clinicians encounter cognitive avoidance frequently. The patient who responds to a warning about an unhealthy diet with "Nah, it'll be fine" is dismissing the cognitive content that would cause them anxiety or regret. So is the patient who notices a new, oddly shaped mole, thinks "Could this be cancer?" and then pushes the scary thought away. These emotion regulatory efforts can decrease positive health behaviors and treatment-seeking, and the short-term emotional gain—which reinforces the avoidance and causes it to reoccur—is likely to come at long-term physical and emotional cost. Cognitive avoidance also interferes with intervention. For example, a patient with chronic back pain may find themselves frustrated, depressed, and angry about their inability to escape from pain. A physical therapist working with this patient will likely note that an inordinate amount of time spent "wishing away" or "arguing with" pain that cannot go away improves neither the physical pain nor the emotional distress, and makes active engagement in therapy less likely. In the section on clinical challenges and recommendations below, we discuss how cognitive avoidance can be addressed in the context of intervention.

Distraction

This strategy involves modifying or reducing emotional response by modifying the content being held in attention (as opposed to one's appraisals of it). Distraction can take many forms, as it can be achieved with any absorbing mental activity. In daily life it may involve coping with a stressful workday by zoning out with the TV, counting to 10 in the middle of an argument to control anger, or humming to calm one's nerves while walking through a dark alley. In a doctor's office, patients might distract themselves by reciting the alphabet backwards, counting the number of cotton swabs visible through a transparent jar, reciting a favorite poem, visualizing a mental scene, and so on. Distraction may be among the most frequently used emotion regulation strategies for negative affect in daily life[52] and it is often a preferred strategy to cope with intense affect.[53] As an emotion regulation strategy, distraction is not likely to drastically improve a negative mood, but empirical studies show that it is effective for preventing a negative mood from spiraling out of control[24] and can be deployed early in the emotion regulatory process.[53] These features can make it useful for increasing distress tolerance.[54] In some ways, distraction is similar to cognitive avoidance, but it is more neutral; distraction involves temporarily turning attention to something else, as opposed to denying, minimizing, or pushing away distressing thoughts. Although distraction can be effective and helpful in the short term, if overused over the long term, distraction can become cognitive avoidance.

Clinical Application

In a medical setting, distraction can help patients tolerate short-term discomfort that may be necessary for complying with treatment. Pediatric providers, for instance, frequently use attention-grabbing strategies (e.g., funny faces, a TV set streaming cartoons) to occupy youngsters during painful or uncomfortable exams or procedures (see Chapter 8, Managing Emotion in Medical Encounters with Children). Adult patients, too, can benefit from using mental distraction to help tolerate unpleasant portions of the medical visit, which can range from the mild suspense of the waiting room, to the social awkwardness of the routine gynecological exam, to the existential dread of life-threatening surgery. Giving patients sensory objects to anchor their attention—perhaps captivating wall art, or a stream of lively chit chat, or a wall-mounted TV—provides a strategic distraction to temper the discomfort of awkward, painful, or otherwise unpleasant aspects of receiving medical care. On the other hand, when the provider believes the patient is distracting themselves at a time when attention is required despite distressing content (such as when reviewing potential side effects of medication, or onerous follow-up instructions), long-term implications should be prioritized and distraction discouraged.

Acceptance

Acceptance is an approach-oriented strategy that can be thought of as an opposite of cognitive avoidance and distraction. It involves acknowledging the emotion and/or the prompting situation for what they are, as opposed to rejecting or pushing away thoughts, emotions, and sensations. The term "acceptance" can sound cheesy or "new age" to some empirically-minded providers or patients, so it is important to underscore that acceptance is both a fairly straightforward mental stance, and effective for improving clinical outcomes. Acceptance means acknowledging unchangeable realities as true. Such realities include situations themselves, or facts "on the ground" (such as a long-term diagnosis), as well as unwanted emotions that the situations may elicit (such as terror or sadness). Acceptance does not mean "agreeing with" or "endorsing" the distress as a positive thing, or necessarily finding benefit or value in it. Instead, acceptance is what allows a patient or provider to name facts, such as "I have multiple sclerosis" or "I'm scared." Acceptance is a key element of several modern psychotherapeutic approaches, such as dialectical behavior therapy[54] and acceptance and commitment therapy,[50] as well as philosophical and spiritual traditions like Zen Buddhism.

The goal of these approaches, and of the acceptance strategy, is not to eliminate pain or negative emotions. Rather, it is to relieve oneself of an additional layer of distress that comes with fighting the unwinnable fight of denying unpleasant realities. One concrete reason acceptance may work to relieve discomfort is that applying verbal labels to emotional states (e.g., "I'm scared") engages the prefrontal cortex of the brain and reciprocally inhibits activity in the limbic system, thereby taking the "edge off" the intensity of emotional activation.[55,56] A significant benefit to acceptance is that the patient may be able to engage in *other* emotion regulation strategies once the situation or the emotion is accepted. Instead of falling into a hopeless, angry, depressive state because of their pain, they might recognize that their pain will be an unfortunate but ongoing feature of experience, and so they can find ways to move forward in life with pain. Problem solving and emotional processing, for example, are much easier when the existence of the problem and emotion is accepted.

Clinical Application

In clinical practice, the provider can help the patient identify which ideas are facts that may need to be accepted, and which ideas are not facts to be accepted—perhaps because they are highly subjective ("I just know I won't get better"), or because they are too far into the future to be known ("None of these treatment options will work"). Misapplying acceptance to an idea not based on here-and-now facts can backfire and promote demoralization and passivity. In general, one useful rule of thumb is that it is more useful to accept facts than opinions: for instance, "I had my arm amputated" versus "I am useless without my arm." Another rule of thumb is that it is more useful to accept the here-and-now than the future: "I have COPD" versus "I'm never going to live a good life again." An exception to this rule comes in cases when a patient's prognosis is terminal (such as when a patient is referred to hospice care), or other cases with a firm scientific basis for making strong predictions about the future. Critically, when the phenomenon to be accepted is not the situation but the *emotion*, it is not necessary that the emotion be objectively "appropriate" or fact-based. A patient can *accept* that they are feeling anger simply because they *are* feeling anger.

Other Behavioral Strategies

Many of the strategies we have discussed take place mentally, but a variety of other strategies involve overt behavior. These are too plentiful to discuss in great detail, so here we provide a few examples. For instance, behavioral activation (i.e., engaging in any active behavior, such as going to the store, seeing friends, taking a walk) is a key ingredient of many treatments for depression, directly countering behavioral tendencies like withdrawal that are prompted by depressive emotional states,[57] and can be used to address behavioral withdrawal or passivity outside of depression as well. Using targeted behaviors to tangibly alter the physical state of the body can be effective in diverting attention away from distress, downregulating distress, and upregulating pleasant feelings. These could include sense-oriented or "self-soothing" behaviors like splashing cold water on one's face or running one's fingers over a pleasant texture like a smooth stone, or more structured behaviors like paced breathing and progressive muscle relaxation.[54,58] An additional behavioral approach to regulating emotions involves changing one's feelings by emitting behaviors that contrast with the current emotion. Experimental evidence suggests that engaging in behaviors that are typically elicited by a particular emotion can trick the brain into actually upregulating that emotion; for instance, the mere act of engaging smile muscles may cause a modest uptick in positive feelings.[59] Related strategies involve the strategic use of humor (e.g., watching a funny movie when one is sad, or appreciating the absurd in a negative situation), and "opposite action," which means engaging in any behavior that opposes the urge associated with a given emotion (e.g., anger creates an urge to attack someone, so opposite action might be paying them a compliment).[54]

Clinical Application

Behavioral strategies such as self-soothing and opposite action can be especially useful when patients' main regulatory goal is to tolerate distress in the short term, or when active engagement in cognitive regulation is difficult (either due to the overwhelming nature of the situation, or the cognitive capacities of the patient). An ophthalmologist, for example, may find that asking a patient to squeeze a stress ball and focus on the sensations is more effective than encouraging them to reappraise the perceived threat of the assessment instruments. Clinicians and treatment settings can build in structural opportunities for patients to self-soothe by engaging the senses, such as by including uplifting music or warm lighting in waiting rooms. For pediatric patients, allowing them to bring comfort objects if possible—e.g., a favorite blanket or stuffed animal—offers them resources to engage in these regulation strategies with which they are most practiced (see Chapter 8, Managing Emotion in Medical Encounters with Children). Clinicians can also give breaks for behavioral regulation during challenging procedures, such as when a physical therapist interrupts a session to allow the patient to step outside for a breath of cold air. Providing instruction in relaxation exercises like paced breathing, either verbally or with a well-placed poster on the wall, can help patients regulate during the encounter, and brief training or a handout at the end of an appointment can help them deploy skills at home. Lastly, clinicians can consider appropriate ways to engage the patient in acting opposite to their distress or anxiety, such as by using humor, smiling, and projecting confidence in the face of challenge. These can be tricky, however: as we discuss in the sections below, aspects of the patient–provider relationship and the clinical situation determine whether and when such strategies are indicated.

■ SOCIAL FACTORS IN EMOTION REGULATION

Most approaches to emotion regulation, as in the above discussion, take an intrapersonal approach, that is, they focus on processes within the individual for modifying their own emotions. In Fig. 7-1, we present an integrated model of relations among patients' emotion regulation, providers' emotion regulation, patient–provider interconnections within the clinical encounter, and clinical outcomes. In this model, *intrapersonal* emotion regulation corresponds to processes occurring within the patient and provider boxes. The study of *interpersonal* emotion regulation recognizes that people also synchronize or coregulate emotions and influence one another's emotional states, emotion regulation strategy use, and strategy effectiveness.[60-64] In the figure, these links are depicted with the reciprocal arrow between patient and

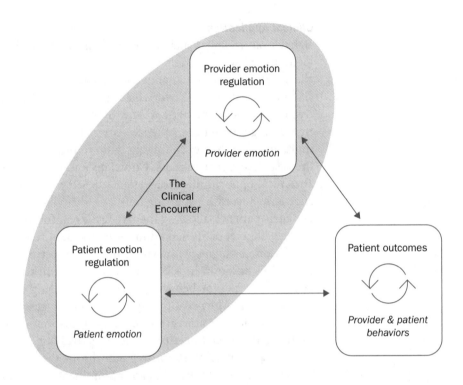

FIGURE 7-1. Integrated Intrapersonal-Interpersonal Model of Emotion Regulation in the Clinical Encounter. Boxes represent intrapersonal processes in patients, providers, and clinical outcomes. Shaded oval represents the social context of the clinical encounter in which intrapersonal processes are embedded. Arrows represent reciprocal influences, including interpersonal influences in the patient–provider relationship.

provider, within the shaded bubble representing the social context of the clinical encounter.

The Social Nature of Emotion Regulation

Developmental psychology research has shown that from the earliest stages of childhood, emotion regulation depends on social context. Relationships between children and caregivers, and later between children and peers, form the foundation of emotion regulation throughout life.[7,65,66] This powerful role of social input continues into adulthood. People commonly address negative emotion by sharing with others, which can soothe distress and solidify social bonds,[67] and in laboratory studies, responses by supporters that encourage emotion regulation—such as cognitive reappraisal—influence recipients' cognition and emotion.[68–70] The neural substrates of cognition and emotion, which evolved within social contexts, may depend on social resources in adulthood as they do in childhood.[71] In fMRI studies, people under the threat of electric shock show attenuated activation of neurobiological threat systems when holding the hands of others, and attenuation is greater with increased relationship closeness (i.e., marital partners vs. friends vs. strangers) and relationship quality.[72]

Overall, the interpersonal aspects of emotion regulation can be summarized by considering three forms of influence. First, the ways in which individuals regulate their own emotion has *social consequences.* Clinical encounters are, at their core, social encounters, and thus the interpersonal consequences of patients' emotion regulation can affect clinical care. Patients' use of strategies that either exacerbate negative emotion or tax the clinician's capacities are liable to prompt negative affective reactions from clinicians, which may result in less motivation or attention in the encounter, or decreased reward. For example, in social relationships expressive suppression negatively affects interaction quality, relationship formation, close relationship quality, and evaluations by others.[36,37,73,74] Similarly, rumination can frustrate others and decrease social support, such as when individuals' constant sharing of passive, negative thinking and refusal to engage in more active regulation exhausts friends and family and leads them to give up trying to help.[75]

Second, individuals' emotion regulation repertoires, strategy deployment, and outcomes are *affected by* social interactions. Outside resources can directly influence individuals' emotion regulation strategy use by encouraging use of particular strategies (e.g., prompting positive reappraisals), counteracting particular strategies (e.g., asking the individual to express rather than suppress their emotions), or introducing strategies that are not part of the individual's own repertoire (e.g., modeling acceptance of distress). This is especially relevant to clinical care because it offers a window through which clinicians can affect patients' emotion regulation. Third, social resources can buffer or magnify *effects or outcomes* of individuals' emotion regulation. For example, a patient brooding about the causes of their misfortune may experience less negative emotion if their social environment demands attention or action that dilutes the impact of rumination even when it is engaged in.

The clinical encounter is a complex social and interpersonal interaction, embedded in wider social systems including social networks, health care systems, and culture, and thus includes the factors involved in interpersonal emotion regulation. Moreover, social resources and interpersonal emotion regulation are associated with physical and mental health, including in depression, anxiety, personality disorder, general psychological well-being, and coping with acute and chronic illness.[3,4,62,76,77] For the present purposes, it is most important to emphasize that individuals' emotion regulation does not play out in a vacuum: patients' emotion regulatory resources include others in their social environment—especially their closest relationships, but also their day-to-day social interactions in less close relationships and their interactions with their healthcare providers. The primary outcome of the interplay between intra- and interpersonal emotion regulation, in the health-care context, is the effectiveness of clinical care itself, including patient and provider behaviors and health outcomes (represented in the rightmost box in Fig. 7-1).

Dyadic and Relational Factors

Interpersonal emotion regulation and the role of social context are increas-ing areas of research focus, but little of that work involves patient–provider interactions. Rather, interpersonal emotion regulation has been studied in the context of overall social resources, social support provision, and close relationships with parents, romantic partners, or friends. One implication for clinical practice, then, is to consider the social and relational contexts in which patients are embedded. Even when a partner, family member, or care-giver is not present during the clinical encounter (and especially when they are present), the patients' emotional state and regulation are likely determined partly by these social resources, for better or worse.

Research on social support and on close relationships suggests particular relationship characteristics that moderate interpersonal influences in emotion regulation. The presence of social supporter figures should not be assumed to be "positive"—we all know from experience that even well-meaning family members can cause more emotional distress. Indeed, empirical work shows that social support can have positive, negative, or null consequences in affect-ing emotion, largely dependent on characteristics of the supporter and the relationship.[78,79] Interpersonal influences tend to be stronger and more posi-tive when relationships are closer, more trusting, and more intimate,[62] more supportive of emotional expression,[12,80] more satisfying,[78] and when relation-ship partners are perceived as more responsive (i.e., understanding, validat-ing, and caring).[81] Emotional validation—communicating that the person's distress is real, genuine, understandable, and/or appropriate—appears to be particularly important. Validating responses to distress directly reduce the distress, are evaluated by recipients as more helpful than other responses, and facilitate the effectiveness of other interpersonal influences (such as problem solving or cognitive change).[82–85] When these various relational characteris-tics are more present in the patient's life, as assessed by either patient report or provider observation, the provider can expect more interpersonal influence on regulation and patients to have more available resources to draw on. When these characteristics are less present, or when patients are relatively socially isolated, providers can expect patients' own intrapersonal emotion regulation tendencies to hold sway.[62,86]

This research not only points to the role of patients' social environments in their emotion regulation, but also has implications for patient–provider relationships. Since the earliest ideas of Freud (although he did not use the term "emotion regulation"), theory and empirical research in psychotherapy support the idea of a clinical provider as a conduit of emotion regulatory influence. Although formal intervention on emotion regulation is inappropriate for untrained clinical providers, it is important for clinicians in nonmental health disciplines to be aware of the emotional and relational dimensions discussed here, which are naturally at play in all types of social relationships, including patient–provider relationships. Providers who establish closer and more trusting relationships with patients, and who are more emotionally responsive, caring, and validating during encounters with patients, can likely gain more insight into patients' emotional experiences and exert more supportive influence on their regulatory processes. In the next section, we turn to how clinical providers, even those without a mental health background or mental health role, can incorporate knowledge of emotion regulation into their interactions with patients.

■ CHALLENGES AND RECOMMENDATIONS FOR PRACTICE

To varying degrees, the medical issues that motivate encounters can be intensely personal, and patients may have a lot at stake—the excitement of a first ultrasound in pregnancy, the awkward discomfort of a colonoscopy, the looming threat of test results. Because how individuals regulate emotion is linked with mental health, physical health, and general well-being, in this section we consider how providers might apply knowledge about emotion regulation in clinical practice. First, we address how providers can recognize and assess emotion regulation in patients. Second, we briefly discuss resources and tools for intervening on emotion regulation when indicated, including the role of mental health providers and consultation. Finally, in line with our emphasis on dyadic processes and social contexts, we consider the role of emotion regulation taking place in providers themselves.

Recognizing and Assessing Emotion Regulation

Emotion regulation depends largely on internal processes of emotion and cognition, and even when it occurs within an interpersonal context, it unfolds largely invisible to the naked eye. This is perhaps especially true in patient–provider encounters, which can be brief and task-oriented, and are embedded in contexts of authority, professionalism, and interpersonal distance.

Patients are unlikely to volunteer, "I'm having trouble with acceptance, so I find myself suppressing my emotions." And few clinicians outside of psychotherapy seek to (or have the time to) deeply explore the emotional processes happening within patients. How is a provider meant to recognize and assess emotion regulation under these constraints? And when is it even important to do so?

Emotion regulation can be viewed as an ongoing, continuously operating system, constantly responding to emotional states and "creating" new emotional states (represented in Fig. 7-1 as round arrows cycling between emotions and their regulation). In this way it is like the immune system—a set of interlinked processes constantly scouting for signals and modifying them as necessary. Clinicians can assume the immune system is functioning without visible indicators, and they can assume that to some degree, patients are constantly regulating emotions. Still, emotion regulation as we have discussed it here is most relevant under conditions of significant emotional provocation, just as immune system activation is most relevant under conditions of infection. Providers can assume that when they are delivering bad news, taking sensitive histories, assessing pain, or even describing promising treatments, their patients will likely experience emotion. From the patient perspective, providers themselves are part of the situation; providers' styles of interaction, regardless of the content of the conversation or procedure, can provoke positive or negative emotions in patients.

The provider can also assume that the patient will probably then engage in conscious or unconscious attempts to regulate that emotion, whether to mitigate distress, manage their self-presentation, or meet a treatment goal. Patients vary in how much feedback they feel capable of giving the provider (e.g., they may fear that revealing emotional distress will displease or disappoint the provider), but behaviors that occur in proximity to likely emotional events, or soon after patients' displayed emotion, should be considered as potentially serving emotion regulatory functions. Such responses can be helpful or unhelpful, but they may be especially consequential if they form a consistent pattern across multiple clinical encounters, or in the patient's life. A patient who lightens the mood by making a few jokes with their nurse may be engaging in harmless—even helpful—avoidant regulation in the moment, but if every clinical visit is dominated by comedic banter, or if the nurse learns the patient never treats their condition seriously, the behavior may represent more clinically concerning avoidance.

Many of the clinical examples in earlier sections provide a sense of the behaviors that can reveal the existence of significant emotion regulation, or of the specific strategies being deployed. Some of these are nonverbal and accessible to the provider through observation, such as when a patient strokes their arm throughout a visit to self-soothe. Many, however, are most detectable through verbal behavior, as our communication of internal thoughts and feelings depends so heavily on language as a vehicle. For example, unless verbalized, it is hard for a provider to detect the fundamentally cognitive strategies of rumination or reappraisal. Luckily, there are several ways to assess emotion regulation strategies from the "outside."

Emotion regulation researchers have developed and psychometrically validated a number of relatively brief self-report questionnaires measuring both intrapersonal and interpersonal emotion regulation.[8,34,41,76,87–91] These standardized, validated assessments of emotion regulation can provide suggestive information to guide further assessment, promote effective patient–provider communication, and perhaps suggest possible follow-up with counseling, psychotherapy, or support group resources. These measures were developed for use in the general population, and their standard versions measure people's perceptions of their *trait* emotion regulation tendencies. They are not diagnostic tools. Without clinical norms, an individual's particular score cannot be interpreted as inherently adaptive or maladaptive, but rather as an estimate of their relative use of a strategy. Just as a primary care physician might administer a self-report screening tool to guide more thorough evaluation of symptoms or complaints, they might also assess emotion regulation in this way. Still, in most clinical contexts, for practical and other reasons, the provider is unlikely to regularly administer these assessments. Instead, they might choose to administer them under specific conditions in targeted ways. If necessary, standard general-population instructions can be modified to particular healthcare situations (e.g., "When I feel down…" can be modified to "In dealing with my cancer diagnosis, when I feel down…"), and general trait wording can be modified to specify a more constrained time period ("In the last month…" or "Today…" or "Since my last appointment…"). Each such change moves the measure further away from the psychometrically validated version, but such changes can be clinically useful.

In the end, however, probably the most clinically effective way to assess emotion regulation is to ask. People are not unbiased or perfectly objective reporters of their own emotional states or regulation, but they are usually more knowledgeable about their emotional tendencies than their providers are. Moreover, the communication process itself gathers unique information and can even act as intervention. For example, an occupational therapist notices a stroke patient seemingly frustrated with his fine motor skills during a task, welling up briefly with tears, then plastering on a smile, saying "It's fine," and continuing. The therapist concerned that expressive suppression or low levels of acceptance might be impeding progress might ask, at a very general level, "I noticed you seemed frustrated just then. Is that what was going on?" and either use the interaction as an assessment tool, or go on to engage in discussion that develops emotional processing and acknowledgment of distress. A more targeted communication might be "Hey, why don't we take a break for a minute? I think it's important to talk about what you were feeling just now."

For recognizing emotion regulation and specific strategies, as well as for intervening, the roles of clinician empathy and awareness are key. The relationship variables that influence emotion regulation in other social relationships (e.g., closeness, trust) also vary across patient–provider relationships. Some providers encounter a patient once a year for a physical and have positive but relatively superficial relationships; emergency medicine providers may see a patient for 5 minutes and never again. Psychotherapists often see patients for months or years, building a close (although not reciprocal) relational bond. In between these endpoints fall many other patient–provider pairings—physical therapists working with some patients for 2 weeks, and others for a year; infertility specialists spending repeated, highly charged appointments with patients; oncologists tapering off in frequency of contact over the course of survivorship. Assessing and intervening on emotion regulation will differ widely among these contexts, and also by the providers' and patients' unique personalities; relatively closer patient–provider relationships and more frequent interaction facilitate more assessment and intervention opportunities.

Across these contexts, however, it is important to return to the dyadic processes of emotional expression, empathy, and validation. Even in brief encounters, an empathic provider who displays openness to patients' emotional experience will encourage disclosure from the patient and will be more effective in exploring patients' regulation and its role in their care. For example, unlike the provider delivering bad diagnostic news, the patient receiving the news is not expecting this information, does not have the training or experience to accurately understand it, and is forced to respond to a murky stressor with implications—either real or perceived—for their life. There is always an inherent gap between the provider's appraisals and emotion and the patient's appraisals and emotion. Empathy comes when providers put themselves in the patient's shoes by attending to the patient's emotional expression (whether verbal or nonverbal), allow themselves to feel some of this emotion if possible, accept the patient's emotional experience as valid (even when the provider themselves would not share it, or when it seems unusual or extreme), and clearly communicate this understanding. In these ways, empathy facilitates an effective interaction that capitalizes on emotion, rather than being impeded by it, in part by facilitating the processes of emotion regulation discussed in this chapter. Although we hope this chapter helps providers understand the processes and strategies of emotion regulation, probably the most essential action providers can take in this aspect of the clinical encounter is to listen to, empathize with, and validate patients' experiences.

Intervening on Emotion Regulation

The literature on interpersonal emotion regulation, social support, and psychotherapy suggests multiple ways in which providers can intervene on patients' emotion regulation. Such intervention may only be necessary when the patients' emotional state or regulatory efforts are causing problems, such as when avoidance is extreme enough to affect treatment adherence, or positive reappraisal is leading to denial of the realities of the situation or leading to inaction when action is possible. Even in brief encounters, clinicians can intervene by (1) assessing emotional states and emotion regulation efforts as described in this chapter, (2) examining whether these efforts are leading to helpful or unhelpful outcomes, (3) providing advice or education to encourage helpful strategies and discourage unhelpful strategies given the person and the situation, (4) addressing aspects of the patient's social environment, especially close relationships and caregiver relationships, and (5) presenting themselves as available, knowledgeable resources for regulation.

Clinicians are used to providing information and encouragement within their area of expertise, and strategies for effective communication are readily adaptable to include attention to emotion regulation. For example, topics typically addressed in conversation regarding current symptoms and how patients have been following through on treatment recommendations can include additional follow-up focused on emotion. Consider a patient who reports not taking her medication as prescribed because she keeps forgetting. A provider might respond simply by showing disapproval or emphasizing the medication's benefits; more effectively, the provider might suggest getting a pill organizer or placing sticky notes on the bathroom mirror. The provider here might also consider the possibility that the patient is avoiding emotional distress associated with the medication ("forgetting" or "being too busy" often means "avoiding"), and introduce tools to counter avoidance. These might simply include an open, expressive discussion of the underlying distress and thoughts, or education about acceptance as a strategy. As discussed, fostering a trusting, validating relationship with the patient almost always maximizes the power of such interventions. When close others are part of the interaction, this can also be taken advantage of—friends and family can be educated about emotion regulation and encouraged to support the patient in specific ways that influence or contextualize the patient's efforts. When close others are unavailable—such as among socially isolated patients—encouraging positive, caring social relationships, such as by reconnecting with dormant relationships or accessing community resources and social activities, can be part of an empirically grounded treatment plan that simultaneously targets physical and emotional health.

Collaboration with Mental Health Providers

Interpersonal aspects of emotion regulation are natural phenomena; providers across disciplines are capable of addressing emotion regulation in patients, and most do so intuitively or by using lay theories of emotion regulation. Still, providers' focus during the clinical encounter is necessarily on their area of expertise, and lay theories do not always line up with evidence. Many issues of emotion regulation in health care settings—especially situations when emotion is dysregulated enough to pose significant problems or appears due to psychopathology—benefit from consultation with specialists and a team treatment approach that includes mental health providers. Providers who feel more formal assessment or intervention is indicated should refer to psychologists, clinical social workers, or other mental health professionals who have more concentrated expertise in affective processes and tools for how to address them.

For example, one of us consulted on a primary care case in which specialist knowledge of emotion regulation was necessary to enable medical treatment to occur. A primary care physician, who was referring a middle-aged male patient for a colonoscopy to assess suspected colon cancer, noticed that the patient repeatedly disregarded recommendations and missed colonoscopy appointments (i.e., cognitive and behavioral avoidance). The physician consulted with the psychologist (and author of this chapter), who was integrated in the primary care clinic. The psychologist met with the patient and was able to determine that his avoidance of the colonoscopy was explained by posttraumatic stress disorder from a history of sexual assault. The psychologist delivered a brief psychological intervention to give the patient other ways to regulate his fears of the colonoscopy, and collaborated with physicians to assist the patient through the necessary medical procedure.

This consultative relationship works both ways. The other of us treated a young woman for severe generalized anxiety disorder and health anxiety who had a diagnosis of a slow-growing cancer. She was paralyzed by worry and rumination that led her to avoid all meaningful social relationships and career opportunities because of the possibility that she could die at any time, so there was "no use" pursuing them. While intervening on the patient's use of worry, rumination, and catastrophizing as avoidant emotion regulation, the psychologist consulted with the patient's oncologist to learn that the cancer was unlikely to pose any realistic threat for decades, improving acceptance-based psychological treatment. Psychotherapists regularly confer with cardiology colleagues when treating patients with panic disorder, to separate psychological processes from physical symptoms and to guide behavioral interventions that counter the avoidant emotion regulation that sustains the disorder. In these ways, collaboration between mental health specialists and nonmental health providers benefits a comprehensive treatment plan that capitalizes on diverse areas of expertise.

Ideally such collaborative resources are available in team treatment settings (e.g., in consultation/liaison services, or comprehensive care models), but in many cases, this will involve consultation with or referral to other community providers. Maintaining some degree of consultative communication with these providers fosters the patient's sense of an individualized treatment team and makes comprehensive treatment more effective. In cases of suspected psychopathology, specialists in treatments that explicitly target emotion regulation may be ideal (e.g., dialectical behavior therapy, acceptance and commitment therapy, emotion regulation therapy), but therapists from all orientations address emotion regulation to some degree. Other, less formal interventions may include referral to empirically grounded self-help books focused on emotion regulation and coping, or lay support groups that can strengthen the individual's regulation in its social context (such as Alcoholics Anonymous, cancer support groups, or bereavement groups).

Emotion Regulation in Providers

Of course, providers experience emotions, too. Note that in Fig. 7-1, patient and provider are depicted identically, each containing a steady stream of emotions and their continual regulation. Consistent with dyadic views of emotion regulation, providers' own emotion regulation plays a role in clinical care, both for their own sake and for patient care. Medical staff who report higher tendencies to use reappraisal also report higher job satisfaction,[92] and providers' emotional reactions on the job can at times compromise their decision making.[93] Here we consider several examples of how emotion regulation, including up- and downregulation of negative and positive emotions, may be usefully enacted to modify providers' emotions during patient–provider interactions.

Regulating Negative Provider Emotions

Any provider's workday is rife with potential emotional upsets. Negative emotional provocations may come from the organizational setting—as in any workplace, administrative hassles and tensions arising from workplace hierarchy can provoke negative emotions. Clinical workplaces are usually hierarchical, and trainees often report anxiety and other negative emotions related to frequent evaluation by peers and supervisors (see Chapter 15, Changing Medical Education to Support Emotional Wellness).[94] There are also provocations related to the nature of working with medical conditions—for instance, in treating serious illnesses providers witness traumatic injuries, significant losses (e.g., deaths, declines in patient function), and tragic stories of how their patients' lives are affected. Working in medical and related helping professions is well known to carry emotional risks of burnout and compassion fatigue (see Chapter 16, Striving and Thriving: Challenges and Opportunities for Clinician Emotional Wellness).[95,96]

There are also provocations related to interactions with patients themselves, who are often stressed and frustrated by their symptoms and their experiences of medical help-seeking; patients may be testy, dismissive, or behave angrily with medical staff and providers. They may behave in these ways out of fears or frustrations they encounter in the moment, or for reasons happening outside of view, like financial impacts or unrelated problems in their own workplaces and relationships. No matter the patient's reasons, interactions with angry patients present an emotion regulatory challenge for providers. Angry patient interactions in emergency departments, for instance, have been associated not only with provider stress, but also riskier medical decision making (see Chapter 13, Emotion and Decision Making in the Clinical Encounter).[93] Providers are encouraged to practice the strategies discussed above to mitigate their own negative emotions on the job. Importantly, the physical drain of providing care—long hours, sleep deprivation, rushed meals, and limited time for self-care—can exacerbate any negative emotional state and shorten a person's emotional fuse, making regulation harder.[97–100] Ameliorating some of these vulnerability factors through providers' physical health and health behaviors can go a long way toward supporting provider downregulation of negative emotions.

At times it may even be useful for providers to upregulate—yes, increase—negative emotions in order to provide better care. Negative mood has known effects on cognition (e.g., attention, memory, decision making), and while these effects are subtle and vary from context to context, in some situations negative emotions can facilitate concrete focus on details of the here-and-now.[101,102] Specific negative emotions have a function of motivating and coordinating goal-oriented behaviors,[18] which means that sometimes dialing up their intensity can help achieve some goals. Fear can help motivate cautious or defensive behaviors, which may be important during a high-stakes surgery, where a small misstep could have disastrous consequences. Anger can help mobilize assertive action, including corrective responses to injustice; this might be useful if a provider needs to advocate to a colleague or superior that a patient needs better or different treatment. Guilt, although unpleasant, is essential for repairing mistakes and learning enhanced behaviors for the future. Sadness, although draining on the provider, may build empathy for a patient receiving negative news. All of this is to say that emotional neutrality, or the absence of negative emotion, is not necessarily the goal. Instead, flexibly and selectively attending to, and perhaps sometimes dialing up the presence of negative emotions, can make for more effective practitioners.

Regulating Positive Provider Emotions

Perhaps somewhat counterintuitively, regulating positive emotions may also be useful in clinical settings. Often positive emotions in the provider are helpful, but sometimes they are an obstacle. For example, a positive social interaction with a colleague may produce a feeling of joy or entertainment, but the clinician may need to attenuate or suppress its expression upon entering an exam room to resume a serious interaction with a patient. A provider whose positive expression is mismatched to the negative emotion of a patient—perhaps a patient anxious to learn a diagnosis, or frustrated with the long wait—risks insulting or invalidating the patient, which could ultimately threaten the quality of care. Other positive emotions in providers that may cause problems if unchecked include pride and related feelings like self-satisfaction and confidence. At some point in their career, most providers will feel a pleasant, gratifying sense of flow that comes from increasing mastery of their work activities. At the same time, patients may be highly sensitive to provider displays of confidence and related emotions. Expressions of these emotions signal power, status, and sometimes threat in human social interactions, and so may compound inequalities already embedded in the patient–provider exchange (e.g., in terms of implicit social hierarchies or discrepant medical knowledge). Moreover, in some cultures (e.g., East Asian), marked displays of positive emotion are considered inappropriate or are less valued than in dominant American or Western cultures.[103] Providers are encouraged to be cognizant of their verbal and nonverbal displays of confidence, pride, and related emotions, and to practice downregulating these flexibly and responsively.

Lastly, we encourage providers to be on the lookout for opportunities to upregulate positive emotions in themselves during the course of clinical encounters. Put simply, this means looking for opportunities to create a positive feeling when there is little or no positive emotion happening. Perhaps a provider is engaged in a few routine appointments at the end of a long week. The provider's default emotion might be neutral to slightly negative—perhaps there is boredom or dissatisfaction, or mild frustration with needing to still be at work. Finding even a small moment in which to upregulate or give rise to a positive emotion might be far from the provider's mind, but it could have profound effects on the quality of the encounter. Behavioral strategies to use in this case might include opposite action (e.g., smiling, despite neutral-to-negative feelings), using humor, or savoring a brief flicker of connection between the provider and patient. In light of the dyadic emotion regulation framework we have emphasized, and the reciprocal influence partners in social encounters have on one another's emotions,[60,61,64,104] the provider in moments like these can think of their own emotion regulation as an intervention in the emotional tenor of the entire encounter. In the long run, this change in tone could have benefits for patient and provider alike: the patient has a more positive experience, and perhaps engages more fully in their treatment or health maintenance behaviors as a result; the provider finds that the afternoon passes just a bit more quickly, and some burnout is forestalled. Outside of the moment itself, providers' self-care and attention to emotional health—including diet, exercise, sleep, positive social relationships, and engagement in pleasurable activities outside of work—not only promote positive emotional experience, but also set the stage for flexible, skilled, and effective regulation when it is needed to serve patients.

■ CONCLUSION

Emotion regulation is an essential component of human functioning—it enables us to adaptively navigate the challenges and joys of life in the service of our many goals. Healthcare interactions are almost always emotionally relevant events for both patients and providers: with the most important concerns of health and life at stake, the very nature of clinical encounters brings fear, despair, joy, anger, or any number of other emotions. In this chapter, we have emphasized the basic processes of emotion regulation in patients and providers, the unique dyadic setting of the patient–provider relationship, and potential applications of emotion regulation in clinical care. Providers armed with knowledge and understanding of emotion regulation have one more tool for addressing the complex emotional processes underlying the clinical encounter, and for optimizing outcomes for patients, providers themselves, and the complex and essential patient–provider relationship.

REFERENCES

1. Aldao A, Nolen-Hoeksema S, Schweizer S. Emotion-regulation strategies across psychopathology: a meta-analytic review. *Clin Psychol Rev.* 2010;30(2):217-237.

2. Sheppes G, Suri G, Gross JJ. Emotion regulation and psychopathology. *Annu Rev Clin Psychol*. 2015;11:379-405.

3. DeSteno D, Gross JJ, Kubzansky L. Affective science and health: the importance of emotion and emotion regulation. *Health Psychol*. 2013;32(5):474-486.

4. Marroquín B, Tennen H, Stanton AL. Coping, emotion regulation, and well-being: intrapersonal and interpersonal processes. In: Robinson MD, Eid M, eds. *The Happy Mind: Cognitive Contributions to Well-Being*. Cham, Switzerland: Springer; 2017:253-274.

5. Gross JJ. Emotion regulation: affective, cognitive, and social consequences. *Psychophysiology*. 2002;39(3):281-291.

6. Gross JJ. Emotion regulation: current status and future prospects. *Psychol Inq*. 2015;26(1): 1-26.

7. Thompson RA. Emotion regulation: a theme in search of definition. *Monogr Soc Res Child Dev*. 1994;59(2-3):25-52.

8. Gratz KL, Roemer L. Multidimensional assessment of emotion regulation and dysregulation: development, factor structure, and initial validation of the Difficulties in Emotion Regulation Scale. *J Psychopathol Behav Assess*. 2004;26(1):41-54.

9. Lazarus RS, Folkman S. *Stress, Appraisal, and Coping*. New York, NY: Springer; 1984.

10. Taylor SE, Stanton AL. Coping resources, coping processes, and mental health. *Annu Rev Clin Psychol*. 2007;3:377-401.

11. Carver CS, Vargas S. Stress, coping, and health. In: Friedman HS, ed. *Oxford Handbook of Health Psychology*. New York, NY: Oxford University Press; 2011:162-188.

12. Moreno PI, Wiley JF, Stanton AL. Coping through emotional approach: the utility of processing and expressing emotions in response to stress. In: Snyder CR, Lopez SJ, Edwards LM, Marques SC, eds. *Oxford Handbook of Positive Psychology*. 3rd ed. New York, NY: Oxford University Press; Published online 2017 ahead of print.

13. McMahon TP, Naragon-Gainey K. The multilevel structure of daily emotion-regulation-strategy use: an examination of within- and between-person associations in naturalistic settings. *Clin Psychol Sci*. 2019;7(2):321-339.

14. Naragon-Gainey K, McMahon TP, Chacko TP. The structure of common emotion regulation strategies: a meta-analytic examination. *Psychol Bull*. 2017;143(4):384-427.

15. Carver CS. Approach, avoidance, and the self-regulation of affect and action. *Motiv Emot*. 2006;30(2):105-110.

16. Corr PJ. Approach and avoidance behaviour: multiple systems and their interactions. *Emot Rev*. 2013;5(3):285-290.

17. Eder AB, Elliot AJ, Harmon-Jones E. Approach and avoidance motivation: issues and advances. *Emot Rev*. 2013;5(3):227-229.

18. Frijda NH. *The Laws of Emotion*. New York, NY: Lawrence Erlbaum Associates; 2007.

19. Baker JP, Berenbaum H. Emotional approach and problem-focused coping: a comparison of potentially adaptive strategies. *Cogn Emot*. 2007;21(1):95-118.

20. Holahan CJ, Holahan CK, Moos RH, Brennan PL. Psychosocial, adjustment in patients reporting cardiac illness. *Psychol Health*. 1997;12(3):345-359.

21. Lepore SJ. A social–cognitive processing model of emotional adjustment to cancer. In: Baum A, Anderson BL, eds. *Psychosocial Interventions for Cancer*. Washington, D.C.: American Psychological Association; 2001:99-116.

22. Daros AR, Daniel KE, Boukhechba M, Chow PI, Barnes LE, Teachman BA. Relationships between trait emotion dysregulation and emotional experiences in daily life: an experience sampling study. *Cogn Emot*. 2020;34(4):743-755.

23. Haines SJ, Gleeson J, Kuppens P, et al. The wisdom to know the difference: strategy-situation fit in emotion in daily life is associated with well-being. *Psychol Sci*. 2016;27(12):1651-1659.

24. Nolen-Hoeksema S, Wisco BE, Lyubomirsky S. Rethinking rumination. *Perspect Psychol Sci*. 2008;3(5):400-424.

25. Aldao A, Sheppes G, Gross JJ. Emotion regulation flexibility. *Cognit Ther Res*. 2015; 39(3):263-278.

26. Aldao A. The future of emotion regulation research: capturing context. *Perspect Psychol Sci*. 2013;8(2):155-172.

27. Tamir M. Why do people regulate their emotions? A taxonomy of motives in emotion regulation. *Pers Soc Psychol Rev*. 2016;20(3):199-222.

28. Bonanno GA, Burton CL. Regulatory flexibility: an individual differences perspective on coping and emotion regulation. *Perspect Psychol Sci*. 2013;8(6):591-612.

29. Ford BQ, Gross JJ, Gruber J. Broadening our field of view: the role of emotion polyregulation. *Emot Rev*. 2019;11(3):197-208.

30. Ford BQ, Troy AS. Reappraisal reconsidered: a closer look at the costs of an acclaimed emotion-regulation strategy. *Curr Dir Psychol Sci*. 2019;28(2):195-203.

31. Vine V, Bernstein EE, Nolen-Hoeksema S. Less is more? Effects of exhaustive vs. minimal emotion labelling on emotion regulation strategy planning. *Cogn Emot*. 2019;33(4):855-862.

32. Moors A, Ellsworth PC, Scherer KR, Frijda NH. Appraisal theories of emotion: state of the art and future development. *Emot Rev*. 2013;5(2):119-124.

33. Leahy RL. *Cognitive Therapy Techniques, Second Edition: A Practitioner's Guide*. New York, NY: Guilford; 2017.

34. Gross JJ, John OP. Individual differences in two emotion regulation processes: implications for affect, relationships, and well-being. *J Pers Soc Psychol*. 2003;85(2):348-362.

35. Webb TL, Miles E, Sheeran P. Dealing with feeling: a meta-analysis of the effectiveness of strategies derived from the process model of emotion regulation. *Psychol Bull*. 2012;138(4):775-808.

36. Richards JM, Butler EA, Gross JJ. Emotion regulation in romantic relationships: the cognitive consequences of concealing feelings. *J Soc Pers Relat*. 2003;20(5):599-620.

37. Butler EA, Egloff B, Wilhelm FH, Smith NC, Erickson EA, Gross JJ. The social consequences of expressive suppression. *Emotion*. 2003;3(1):48-67.

38. Watkins ER. Constructive and unconstructive repetitive thought. *Psychol Bull*. 2008; 134(2):163-206.

39. Papageorgiou C, Wells A. Metacognitive beliefs about rumination in recurrent major depression. *Cogn Behav Pract*. 2001;8(2):160-164.

40. Vine V, Aldao A, Nolen-Hoeksema S. Chasing clarity: rumination as a strategy for making sense of emotions. *J Exp Psychopathol*. 2014;5(3):229-243.

41. Treynor W, Gonzalez R, Nolen-Hoeksema S. Rumination reconsidered: a psychometric analysis. *Cognit Ther Res*. 2003;27(3):247-259.

42. Joormann J, Dkane M, Gotlib IH. Adaptive and maladaptive components of rumination? diagnostic specificity and relation to depressive biases. *Behav Ther.* 2006;37(3):269-280.

43. Trapnell PD, Campbell JD. Private self-consciousness and the five-factor model of personality: distinguishing rumination from reflection. *J Pers Soc Psychol.* 1999;76(2):284-304.

44. Marroquín BM, Fontes M, Scilletta A, Miranda R. Ruminative subtypes and coping responses: active and passive pathways to depressive symptoms. *Cogn Emot.* 2010;24(8): 1446-1455.

45. Wang AW-T, Chang C-S, Hsu W-Y. The double-edged sword of reflective pondering: the role of state and trait reflective pondering in predicting depressive symptoms among women with breast cancer. *Ann Behav Med.* 2020. [Published ahead of print August 20, 2020].

46. du Pont A, Welker K, Gilbert KE, Gruber J. The emerging field of positive emotion dysregulation. In: Vohs KD, Baumeister RF, eds. *Handbook of Self-Regulation: Research, Theory and Applications.* New York, NY: Guilford; 2016:364-379.

47. Behar E, DiMarco ID, Hekler EB, Mohlman J, Staples AM. Current theoretical models of generalized anxiety disorder (GAD): conceptual review and treatment implications. *J Anxiety Disord.* 2009;23(8):1011-1023.

48. Riskind JH, Rector NA. *Looming Vulnerability: Theory, Research and Practice in Anxiety.* New York, NY: Springer; 2018.

49. Wenzlaff RM, Wegner DM. Thought suppression. *Annu Rev Psychol.* 2000;51:59-91.

50. Hayes SC, Strosahl KD, Wilson KG. *Acceptance and Commitment Therapy, Second Edition: The Process and Practice of Mindful Change.* New York, NY: Guilford; 2011.

51. Hayes-Skelton SA, Eustis EH. Experiential avoidance. In: Abramowitz JS, Blakey SM, eds. *Clinical Handbook of Fear and Anxiety: Maintenance Processes and Treatment Mechanisms.* Washington, DC: American Psychological Association; 2020:115-131.

52. Brans K, Koval P, Verduyn P, Lim YL, Kuppens P. The regulation of negative and positive affect in daily life. *Emotion.* 2013;13(5):926-939.

53. Sheppes G, Scheibe S, Suri G, Radu P, Blechert J, Gross JJ. Emotion regulation choice: a conceptual framework and supporting evidence. *J Exp Psychol Gen.* 2014;143(1):163-181.

54. Linehan MM. *Cognitive-Behavioral Treatment of Borderline Personality Disorder.* New York, NY: Guilford; 1993.

55. Torre JB, Lieberman MD. Putting feelings into words: affect labeling as implicit emotion regulation. *Emot Rev.* 2018;10(2):116-124.

56. Lieberman MD, Inagaki TK, Tabibnia G, Crockett MJ. Subjective responses to emotional stimuli during labeling, reappraisal, and distraction. *Emotion.* 2011;11(3):468-480.

57. Dimidjian S, Martell CR, Herman-Dunn R, Hubley S. Behavioral activation for depression. In: Barlow DH, ed. *Clinical Handbook of Psychological Disorders: A Step-by-Step Treatment Manual.* 5th ed. New York, NY: Guilford; 2014:353-393.

58. Grossman P, Niemann L, Schmidt S, Walach H. Mindfulness-based stress reduction and health benefits. a meta-analysis. *J Psychosom Res.* 2004;57(1):35-43.

59. Coles NA, Larsen JT, Lench H. A meta-analysis of the facial feedback literature: effects of facial feedback on emotional experience are small and variable. *Psychol Bull.* 2019;145(6):610-651.

60. Barthel AL, Hay A, Doan SN, Hofmann SG. Interpersonal emotion regulation: a review of social and developmental components. *Behav Change*. 2018;35(4):203-216.

61. Butler EA, Randall AK. Emotional coregulation in close relationships. *Emot Rev*. 2013;5(2):202-210.

62. Marroquín B, Nolen-Hoeksema S. Emotion regulation and depressive symptoms: close relationships as social context and influence. *J Pers Soc Psychol*. 2015;109(5):836-855.

63. Niven K. The four key characteristics of interpersonal emotion regulation. *Curr Opin Psychol*. 2017;17:89-93.

64. Zaki J, Williams WC. Interpersonal emotion regulation. *Emotion*. 2013;13(5):803-810.

65. Cassidy J. Emotion regulation: influences of attachment relationships. *Monogr Soc Res Child Dev*. 1994;59(2-3):228-249.

66. Spinrad TL, Morris AS, Luthar SS. Introduction to the special issue: socialization of emotion and self-regulation: understanding processes and application. *Dev Psychol*. 2020;56(3):385-389.

67. Rimé B, Bouchat P, Paquot L, Giglio L. Intrapersonal, interpersonal, and social outcomes of the social sharing of emotion. *Curr Opin Psychol*. 2020;31:127-134.

68. Levy-Gigi E, Shamay-Tsoory SG. Help me if you can: evaluating the effectiveness of interpersonal compared to intrapersonal emotion regulation in reducing distress. *J Behav Ther Exp Psychiatry*. 2017;55:33-40.

69. Marroquín B, Nolen-Hoeksema S, Clark MS, Stanton AL. Social influences on cognitive processing in enacted social support: effects on receivers' cognitive appraisals, emotion, and affiliation. *Anxiety Stress Coping*. 2019;32(4):457-475.

70. Nils F, Rimé B. Beyond the myth of venting: social sharing modes determine the benefits of emotional disclosure. *Eur J Soc Psychol*. 2012;42(6):672-681.

71. Coan JA, Maresh EL. Social baseline theory and the social regulation of emotion. In: Gross JJ, ed. *Handbook of Emotion Regulation*. 2nd ed. New York, NY: Guilford; 2014:221-236.

72. Coan JA, Schaefer HS, Davidson RJ. Lending a hand: social regulation of the neural response to threat. *Psychol Sci*. 2006;17(12):1032-1039.

73. Lopes PN, Salovey P, Coté S, Beers M. Emotion regulation abilities and the quality of social interaction. *Emotion*. 2005;5(1):113-118.

74. Srivastava S, Tamir M, McGonigal KM, John OP, Gross JJ. The social costs of emotional suppression: a prospective study of the transition to college. *J Pers Soc Psychol*. 2009;96(4):883-897.

75. Nolen-Hoeksema S, Davis CG. "Thanks for sharing that": ruminators and their social support networks. *J Pers Soc Psychol*. 1999;77(4):801-814.

76. Dixon-Gordon KL, Haliczer LA, Conkey LC, Whalen DJ. Difficulties in interpersonal emotion regulation: initial development and validation of a self-report measure. *J Psychopathol Behav Assess*. 2018;40(3):528-549.

77. Hofmann SG. Interpersonal emotion regulation model of mood and anxiety disorders. *Cognit Ther Res*. 2014;38(5):483-492.

78. Frazier PA, Tix AP, Barnett CL. The relational context of social support: relationship satisfaction moderates the relations between enacted support and distress. *Pers Soc Psychol Bull*. 2003;29(9):1133-1146.

79. Schoebi D, Randall AK. Emotional dynamics in intimate relationships. *Emot Rev.* 2015;7(4):342-348.

80. Hoyt MA. Gender role conflict and emotional approach coping in men with cancer. *Psychol Health.* 2009;24(8):981-996.

81. Maisel NC, Gable SL. The paradox of received social support: the importance of responsiveness. *Psychol Sci.* 2009;20(8):928-932.

82. Shenk CE, Fruzzetti AE. The impact of validating and invalidating responses on emotional reactivity. *J Soc Clin Psychol.* 2011;30(2):163-183.

83. Pauw LS, Sauter DA, van Kleef GA, Fischer AH. Sense or sensibility? Social sharers' evaluations of socio-affective vs. cognitive support in response to negative emotions. *Cogn Emot.* 2018;32(6):1247-1264.

84. Dixon-Gordon KL, Whalen DJ, Scott LN, Cummins ND, Stepp SD. The main and interactive effects of maternal interpersonal emotion regulation and negative affect on adolescent girls' borderline personality disorder symptoms. *Cognit Ther Res.* 2016;40(3):381-393.

85. Fruzzetti AE, Worrall JM. Accurate expression and validating responses: a transactional model for understanding individual and relationship distress. In: Sullivan K, Davila J, eds. *Support Processes in Intimate Relationships.* New York, NY: Oxford University Press; 2010:121-150.

86. Marroquín B, de Rutte J, May CL, Wisco BE. Emotion regulation in context: social connectedness moderates concurrent and prospective associations with depressive symptoms. *J Soc Clin Psychol.* 2019;38(7):605-626.

87. Nolen-Hoeksema S, Morrow J. A prospective study of depression and posttraumatic stress symptoms after a natural disaster: the 1989 Loma Prieta earthquake. *J Pers Soc Psychol.* 1991;61(1):115-121.

88. Bond FW, Hayes SC, Baer RA, et al. Preliminary psychometric properties of the Acceptance and Action Questionnaire–II: a revised measure of psychological inflexibility and experiential avoidance. *Behav Ther.* 2011;42(4):676-688.

89. Garnefski N, Kraaij V. The Cognitive Emotion Regulation Questionnaire. *Eur J Psychol Assess.* 2007;23(3):141-149.

90. Hofmann SG, Carpenter JK, Curtiss J. Interpersonal Emotion Regulation Questionnaire (IERQ): scale development and psychometric characteristics. *Cognit Ther Res.* 2016;40(3):341-356.

91. Williams WC, Morelli SA, Ong DC, Zaki J. Interpersonal emotion regulation: implications for affiliation, perceived support, relationships, and well-being. *J Pers Soc Psychol.* 2018;115(2):224-254.

92. Wang M, Hu C, Huang M, Xie Y, Zhu W. The effect of emotional clarity and attention to emotion on job satisfaction: a mediating role of emotion regulation among Chinese medical staff. *Asian J Soc Psychol.* 2019;22(3):316-324.

93. Isbell LM, Tager J, Beals K, Liu G. Emotionally evocative patients in the emergency department: a mixed methods investigation of providers' reported emotions and implications for patient safety. *BMJ Qual Saf.* 2020;29:803-814.

94. Dyrbye LN, Thomas MR, Shanafelt TD. Systematic review of depression, anxiety, and other indicators of psychological distress among U.S. and Canadian medical students. *Acad Med.* 2006;81(4):354-373.

95. Kumar S. Burnout and doctors: prevalence, prevention and intervention. *Healthcare (Basel).* 2016;4(3):37.

96. Potter P, Deshields T, Divanbeigi J, et al. Compassion fatigue and burnout: prevalence among oncology nurses. *Clin J Oncol Nurs.* 2010;14(5):E56-E62.

97. Franzen PL, Buysse DJ, Dahl RE, Thompson W, Siegle GJ. Sleep deprivation alters pupillary reactivity to emotional stimuli in healthy young adults. *Biol Psychol.* 2009;80(3):300-305.

98. Gujar N, Yoo S-S, Hu P, Walker MP. Sleep deprivation amplifies reactivity of brain reward networks, biasing the appraisal of positive emotional experiences. *J Neurosci.* 2011;31(12):4466-4474.

99. Macht M. Effects of high- and low-energy meals on hunger, physiological processes and reactions to emotional stress. *Appetite.* 1996;26(1):71-88.

100. Gibson EL, Green MW. Nutritional influences on cognitive function: mechanisms of susceptibility. *Nutr Res Rev.* 2002;15(1):169-206.

101. Huntsinger JR. Does emotion directly tune the scope of attention? *Curr Dir Psychol Sci.* 2013;22(4):265-270.

102. Huntsinger JR, Isbell LM, Clore GL. The affective control of thought: malleable, not fixed. *Psychol Rev.* 2014;121(4):600-618.

103. Matsumoto D, Yoo SH, Nakagawa S. Culture, emotion regulation, and adjustment. *J Pers Soc Psychol.* 2008;94(6):925-937.

104. Parkinson B. Interpersonal emotion transfer: contagion and social appraisal. *Soc Personal Psychol Compass.* 2011;5(7):428-439.

Managing Emotion in Medical Encounters with Children

CHAPTER 8

Benjamin A. Krauss, Piet L. Leroy, and Baruch S. Krauss

> *"I see no more than you, but I have trained myself to notice what I see."*
>
> – Sir Arthur Conan Doyle[1]

■ INTRODUCTION

Medical encounters can be frightening for children, who, when afraid, may resist cooperating, inhibiting assessment and treatment. When trust is established, children cooperate, making it easier to obtain accurate and complete diagnostic information and perform a physical examination or procedure. Understanding and effectively managing a child's emotional state during medical encounters are essential to building trust, eliciting cooperation, and creating a positive experience for the child and their family.[2-5] While negative medical experiences can be emotionally traumatic for children, leading to apprehension of medical treatment and personnel,[6-15] positive medical experiences favorably influence future medical encounters for children and their families.[16-20]

This chapter defines and examines the elements of establishing trust with children and describes a methodology for managing a child's emotional state during medical encounters.

■ METHODOLOGY

This methodology involves a cyclical practice of observation, assessment, and engagement based on perceiving, accurately interpreting, and appropriately responding to a child's verbal and nonverbal cues. This process facilitates management of the child's emotional state and formation of trust.[2,3] Here, clinical observation is used to gather, analyze, and interpret data from the child's cues, leading to assessment of their emotional state and positioning on the Fear-to-Trust Axis (Fig. 8-1).[21] The provider then employs a set of engagement methods to alleviate fear and establish trust, while continuously observing and adapting to the child's responses (Fig. 8-2). This process is not formulaic; it is iterative, individualized, and—importantly—inductive. Verbal and nonverbal data from the provider–child–parent interaction are used to inform and guide the interaction toward trust. Formulaic approaches inconsistently engage children and establish trust because they employ the same methods irrespective of the child's cues (e.g., blowing bubbles to engage every 2-year-old).

This methodology parallels how we might approach a dog, something we all know how to do intuitively. We would not approach a dog without assessing its "emotional state," for fear of being bitten or attacked. Our approach might follow a specific methodology:

1. We observe the dog's initial cues and response to our presence, noting facial expressions (is the dog baring its teeth? Are its ears tense and elevated or relaxed?) and posture and gestures (is its fur standing on end or flat? Is its tail wagging? Is it growling?).
2. We might begin interacting with the dog from a distance, adjusting our posture, gestures, and eye contact so as not to startle or threaten it.
3. We may use distinct speech, as if talking to a child, which contains simple statements conveyed in high-pitched tones: "*Nice doggie. Good doggie.*"
4. We monitor the dog's response to our actions, whether positive (e.g., softening of facial expression, fur and ears down, tail wagging) or negative (no change or worsening features), and adjust our approach accordingly. With positive responses, we might move closer until we assess that it's safe to stand next to the dog and apply touch.

This process of reading and responding to the dog's verbal and nonverbal cues is a useful model for thinking about interactions with children in medical settings. Moreover, this example shows how natural, even innate, it is to read and respond to emotions in other living beings.

In this chapter, we deconstruct the provider–child interaction in order to elevate it from an intuitive and unstructured practice to a set of skills that providers can learn to apply intentionally and systematically.

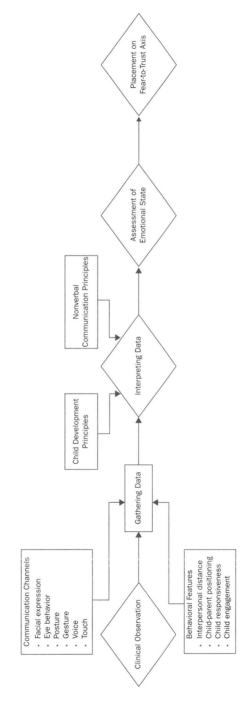

FIGURE 8-1. Observing and assessing.

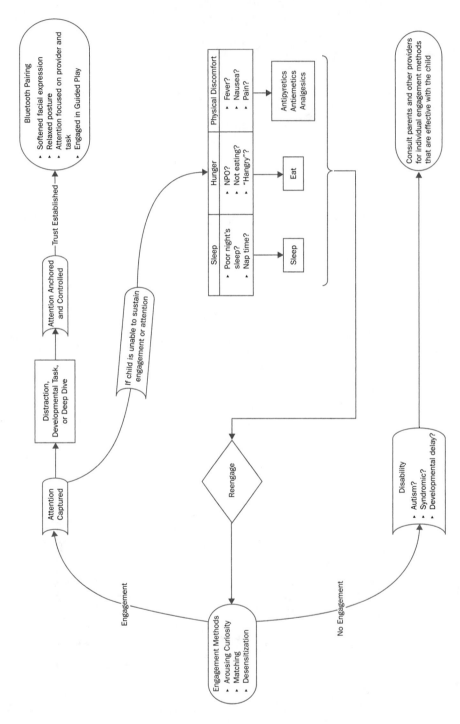

FIGURE 8-2. Engaging and monitoring.

■ OBSERVING AND ASSESSING

Gathering Data

In clinical observation, specific patient features are distinguished, bringing them to the foreground of awareness, where they can be organized into distinct patterns used to assess a patient's emotional state.[22,23] These features include the communication channels (facial expression, eye behavior, posture, gesture, voice, touch) and specific behavioral features (interpersonal distance, child–parent positioning, child engagement and responsiveness), along with environmental factors (e.g., objects in the room, examination room layout, number and arrangement of people in the room, ambient light and noise, level of other sensory stimuli).[2,3,5,21]

Communication Channels

Facial Expression, Eye Behavior, Posture, and Gestures Facial expression, eye behavior, posture, body orientation relative to the provider, and gestures are all readily observable and can be used to assess the child's emotional state.[21,24–26] This is especially clear in infants and young children, who have not yet been socially conditioned to mask their emotions.[23,24]

Voice Voice characteristics affect mood and emotion.[27,28] Modulation of vocal response through changes in cadence, rhythm, tone, tempo, and intonation can be used to create specific speech patterns that are familiar and calming to children. The distinctive way parents speak to young children, termed parentese, is characterized by speech that is clear, simple, attention maintaining, and has longer pauses.[29–32] Infants respond to vocal tones that are ascending, high-pitched, rhythmic, and repetitive (see Language).[33,34]

Touch Touch can influence perception, mood, and behavior by both conveying discrete emotion (tactile communication) and acting as a physiologic stimulus, which calms children when expected or arouses fear (increased heart rate and galvanic skin response) when unexpected.[35,36] Using information gathered on the child's emotional state, providers can determine when and how to initiate touch (e.g., the location and duration of touch, the degree of pressure applied, whether the touch is still or moving). Different kinds of touch denote different messages: light touch may convey "*Hello, I am here. Can you respond to me?*" while heavier touch may convey reassurance. Each type of touch elicits a different response from the child. In this way, the provider can set the stage so that touch is expected and calming and becomes part of the process of establishing trust.

Behavioral Features

Interpersonal Distance Interpersonal distance describes the psychological boundary or buffer zone surrounding an individual.[37,38] Children use interpersonal distance as a manifestation of their degree of fear.[39–41] Children who are apprehensive are more alert and responsive to perceived threats in the environment.[42–47] A stranger coming too close or approaching too quickly can lead to an increase in the child's fear. Providers can use interpersonal distance to assess a child's level of fear by observing how close they allow the provider to come without a visible increase in fear.

If the boundary is initially narrow, suggesting a lower level of fear, begin interacting in proximity to the child. If the boundary is wide, with the child displaying a high level of fear when you are at a distance, begin your initial interaction from the edge of the perceived boundary and gradually move closer while observing the child's response. If your interventions are effective, the boundary will shrink as fear decreases, allowing you to move closer to the child (see ENGAGING).

Child–Parent Positioning Child–parent positioning can provide information on the dyad's emotional state. Observe how the child is positioned relative to the parent, along with their respective nonverbal cues. Parent and child are attuned to each other's emotional state, and will often display matching facial expressions, gaze, posture, and gestures (see Matching).

The many facets of the emotional state of the child–parent dyad are illustrated in Renaissance paintings of Madonna and Child. The artists skillfully discern the subtle behavioral features of the dyadic interaction, revealing the underlying emotional states.[48] These depictions represent templates of common scenarios that practitioners who care for children encounter. They can be used to train visual sensitivity, leading to enhanced recognition and interpretation of clinical signs.[49,50] The paintings illustrate features of dyadic matching (Figs. 8-3a and 8-3b). Notice the similarity between the mother and child's facial expression, gaze, arms and hands, gestures, and emotional state.

Parental Cues: The Dyadic Relationship Although structurally referred to as a dyad (from the Latin *duo*—something that consists of two elements or parts), parent and child are functionally one unit and are continuously reading and regulating each other's emotional states.[51–58] This mutual regulation explains why parental responses reflect their child's emotional state and can be used as indicators of how effective your interventions are in engaging the child. Parents will experience the shift in their child's emotional state as you engage the child and establish trust. Parents will visibly brighten and/or focus on the activity that the child has become engaged in. Watch for this positive change in the parents' demeanor.

The parent's emotional state can affect the child.[4,18–20,52–54,59] If the parent is anxious, for example, this may be transmitted to the child, escalating their fear.[59,60] It is therefore important to assess the parent's ability to regulate their

A

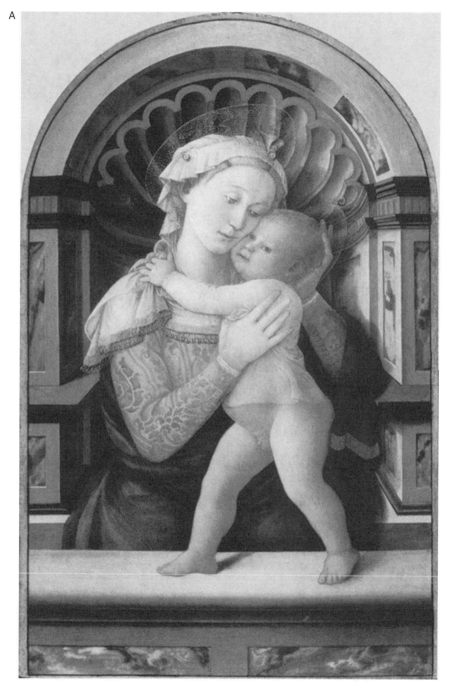

FIGURE 8-3. **(A) Madonna and Child—Filippo Lippi. (Source: AA.VV., Palazzo Medici Riccardi e la Cappella Benozzo Gozzoli, Biblioteca de "Lo Studiolo", Becocci/Scala, Firenze 2000.) (B) Madonna and Child—Johann Nepomuk Ender. (Source: Dorotheum.)**

B

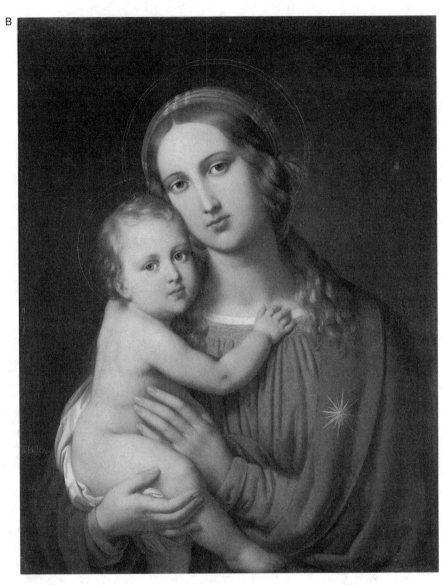

FIGURE 8-3. *(Continued)*

emotional state during medical encounters. Parents who cannot control their emotional responses, and who may be extremely anxious or distraught, will have difficulty helping their child cope. These parents may be given the option to leave the room during the examination or procedure. Parents who have some degree of emotional regulation but are overwhelmed by the current situation can be redirected by being given a specific role or task (e.g., pointing out images in a picture book, reading to the child, playing an interactive game with the child). Parents who have highly developed emotional regulation skills, and who are already actively engaging and focusing the child, can work collaboratively with the provider to manage the child's emotional state during the examination or procedure.[61,62]

Child Engagement A child's level of engagement in an activity or task can be an indicator of the extent of their ability to emotionally regulate. A child who is fully engaged, by themselves or with a parent, in an activity such as watching television, reading a book, or playing a game, demonstrates an ability to focus their attention. These children have a low level of fear and are typically unconcerned by your presence. They can be approached directly and engaged through the activity they are already focusing on (see Arousing Curiosity).

Some children may be engaged in play when they are afraid. They will be acutely aware of your presence and will stop focusing on the activity and become more fearful when you approach them or when you attempt to draw their attention away from the activity. Pay careful attention to where the personal space boundary is with these children, and begin by desensitizing them to your presence (see Desensitization).

Child Responsiveness A child's initial response to the provider, whether they engage or not, is a critical datapoint that determines subsequent engagement strategies (see Monitoring).

Environmental Features

Features from the child's physical environment (e.g., personal objects, toys) can be used to capture attention during the engagement process (see Arousing Curiosity). Additionally, the type and intensity of sensory input (e.g., number of people in the room, ambient light and noise) can be used to determine the extent to which the child's attention is diverted and the methods needed to capture it.

Interpreting the Data

Child development and nonverbal communication principles can be used to analyze and interpret clinical observation data. Pattern recognition, the organization of individual cues into meaningful patterns, is fundamental to the interpretation process, because it serves as the basis for formulating an appropriate set of interventions congruent with the child's emotional state. Salient patterns include those that represent different manifestations of fear at varying ages and developmental levels (i.e., the constellation of cues that indicate low, moderate, or high fear).

Misjudging a child's emotional state may lead to interventions that cause distress. Frightened children, especially young children, have great difficulty controlling their apprehension and cooperating, making common procedures or physical examination difficult to accomplish.[4,24,63–65]

■ ENGAGING

Moving From Fear to Trust

Once the child's emotional state is assessed, a series of integrated engagement methods are employed to capture and anchor the child's attention, facilitating the shift from fear to trust. To form a relationship, the provider and child must be engaged with and paying attention to one another, as engagement and focus are prerequisites for building trust. Engagement methods facilitate focus, allowing the provider to direct the child's attention. The specific engagement methods used, and their sequence, are determined by the child's position on the Fear-to-Trust Axis, their developmental level, and temperament.

Each method acts synergistically with and amplifies the effect of the other methods. We discuss these methods in discrete, sequential steps, although in practice they are often occurring simultaneously. There are five general categories of engagement methods: arousing curiosity, matching, desensitization, distraction, and developmental tasks.

Arousing Curiosity

Arousing curiosity is a nonthreatening method for engaging and capturing the attention of infants and young children through the use of descriptive, declarative, factual statements. Direct questions (e.g., *How are you? What is your name? Is that your teddy bear?*) are not understood by infants and can be threatening to young children, especially if spoken by a provider who is a stranger to the child. When children are afraid and do not trust you, they may avoid responding to open-ended questions; however, they will respond to simple, descriptive statements. Use the individual features that you observe (e.g., the child's clothing or toys) as the basis for these statements. In doing this, you are letting the child know that you are paying attention and that you are aware of them. For children, as with adults, the experience of being noticed is the first step in creating a genuine connection and building trust.

Arousing curiosity is most effective when the provider jointly experiences the curiosity with the child. Instead of simply asking the child what they observe (e.g., "*What are these toys you are holding in your hand?*" "*Which dinosaur do you like best?*"), engage in the observation with them (e.g., "*Look at these gray, scaly dinosaurs and tall palm trees with green, spinning leaves.*"). Recognize the child's individuality by noticing and pointing out aspects unique to them, for example, the color or design of a specific item of clothing (*"You are wearing a beautiful shirt…with red balloons, green circles, and brown tigers."*). Desensitization to your physical presence, gaze, and touch can be integrated into arousing curiosity (see Desensitization). Point to and, if the child shows no signs of increasing fear, touch the described area. *"You have pink shoes,"* as you point to or touch the shoes, *"…and an Elmo sticker on your tummy,"* as you touch the sticker. *"And you have one nose and two ears and one mouth…and mommy has a white shirt."* This may be accompanied by direct eye contact, if the child accepts it at this point in the interaction. Fearful children may not tolerate direct eye contact initially. They will only accept it once trust has been established and the provider is no longer seen as threatening. By engaging in the observation and curiosity with the child, the power differential is mitigated and the child begins to develop a sense of comfort and trust.

In young children, arousing curiosity can be constructed as a narrative. Weave the objects (e.g., the orange tigers on the hospital gowns) into a story, and narrate using parentese: *"You have orange tigers on your shirt. This tiger is very sleepy. It ate a big dinner and now it is soooo sleepy. It's time for it to go to sleep."* The physical examination can be integrated into the story: *"This tiger is sleeping so quietly. Let's see if we can wake it up."* (Palpation of the abdomen.) *"It is sleeping so quietly. Let's see if we can listen to it sleeping."* (Auscultation of heart and lungs.)

Arousing curiosity can be done verbally, as described above, or sensorially. Visual, auditory, sensorimotor, and tactile stimulation (e.g., your touch, shining an otoscope light, light-up toys or other objects, rhythmically and repetitively tapping the stretcher) can be used to arouse curiosity in infants and young children. You have successfully aroused a child's curiosity, and captured their attention, when their gaze tracks what you are describing or pointing to. Gaze tracking is an especially useful indicator that the child is paying attention, as typical listener responses, such as head nodding, eyebrow-raising, and verbal acknowledgments, are absent in preschool-age children.[66]

Matching

During interpersonal interactions, people unconsciously mimic each other's facial expressions, postures, and mannerisms, engendering affinity.[67–69] Matching (i.e., behavioral mimicry, postural congruence, mirroring) refers to similar behaviors occurring at the same time or in sequence.[51,70] Adopting the child's nonverbal cues creates the experience of connectedness and helps build trust.[71] Matching can be done symmetrically (e.g., posture matching posture, gesture matching gesture) or asymmetrically (e.g., voice matching gesture, facial expression matching gesture).[2]

With infants and young children, matching takes place through imitation. In fact, neonates as young as 2 days of age imitate facial expressions and head and finger movements.[72–75] The provider can imitate facial expressions, vocalizations, and gestures, as playful experimentation with hands, feet, and senses is the dominant mode of learning for infants.

Matching takes on a different character in older children. Unlike with imitation, the child is not consciously aware that you are matching them. Observing and matching the child's rhythm and pace can be used to slow down the interaction and capture attention. Positive changes in facial expression and posture, such as relaxation or opening, serve as cues that you are effectively engaging the child. Observe the extent of the child's movement, and notice, as an indication of your effectiveness, how it decreases as their attention is focused.

Desensitization

Originally developed by Joseph Wolpe, systematic desensitization has been used extensively for the treatment of phobias, through graded exposure to the fear-inducing stimulus.[76,77] During medical encounters, children are often apprehensive of strangers and unfamiliar things in the environment (e.g., examination room, stretcher, instruments, monitors, and other equipment). Desensitization may be used to alleviate the child's fear and reduce their negative reaction to the provider and environment.

Desensitization can be direct or indirect and rapid or gradual. Direct desensitization is done with the child, and it can be used to accustom the child to objects that will be used in the physical examination or procedure. Indirect desensitization occurs through the parent, sibling, the child's toy, or other personal objects. Rapid desensitization can be facilitated directly by having the child touch or hold an object that will be part of the physical examination or procedure (e.g., a piece of gauze, a Q-tip, or an otoscope earpiece—"*Can you hold this? Thank you. I have one too, just like you.*") or indirectly, by demonstrating parts of the physical examination on yourself, the child's parents, siblings, or a toy, before approaching the child.

Gradual desensitization involves exposure, in stages, to something (e.g., an object in the examination room) or to someone (e.g., your presence) that is threatening to the child. Gradual desensitization to your presence may be accomplished by coming in and out of the room several times without making eye contact and without speaking to the child, or by entering the room without making eye contact with the child and remaining at a distance as you begin to speak with the parents.

Playing peek-a-boo with the child from outside the room can also be used to desensitize them to your presence. Arousing curiosity sensorially (e.g., entering the room without looking at the child and rhythmically and repetitively tapping on the door, a cabinet, a chair, the stretcher, or a parent's leg, arm, or hand) can capture the child's attention and can also be used to desensitize the child to your presence before you establish physical contact.

Distraction

Distraction, from the Latin *distractio* (to pull apart), represents a diverse group of activities that divert attention from a threatening or fearful situation to a less threatening activity. Distraction can be passive (e.g., watching a video, listening to music) or active (e.g., drawing, reading a book, telling stories, playing with toys, interacting with medical clowns, blowing bubbles, playing videogames, or using a cell phone, computer, tablet, or a virtual reality headset).[18,19,78–81]

Distraction can be used to capture and anchor attention and is most effective when tailored to a child's age and developmental level. Distracting activities that are passive or minimally interactive, and require little cognitive processing, serve only as diversions and do not reliably anchor attention. They often necessitate redirecting and refocusing the child's attention. Distraction typically does not change a child's underlying emotional state. Therefore, by itself, it is insufficient to establish trust. To be effective as an engagement method, distraction must be grounded in clinical observation, as this is the basis for formulating an accurate assessment and appropriate response to the individual child.

Developmental Tasks

Learning is at the core of a child's cognitive and motor development. Children are constantly learning through play and exploration of their environment.[82] The provider can use the child's developmental learning process to capture and anchor their attention by presenting them with a challenging developmental task.[82–84] A developmental task is a learning-based, cognitive and motor activity that the child is actively attempting to master. The provider matches the learning activity to the child's developmental level. Thus, the developmental task facilitates exploration and mastery of skills within the child's zone of proximal development.[85] These provider-guided learning activities mobilize a child's innate curiosity and desire to learn; are inherently engaging, pleasurable, and rewarding (through the joyful experience of discovery and mastery); and anchor a child's attention.[24,82–84,86] This form of guided play is familiar and predictable for children, providing a sense of control.[82,86]

In addition to the myriad commercially available developmental toys, low-tech objects in the examination room (e.g., tongue blades, sterile urine cups, gauze, plastic bags, rolls of tape) can be used as learning tools. The object itself is less important than the task that is demonstrated. The task should be structured, have clear goals, and allow the child to learn at their own pace (e.g., picking up a set of objects and putting them into a specimen cup, one at a time; unscrewing and opening, then closing and screwing on, the lid of a specimen cup; grasping a tongue blade and tapping it against an object; grasping a tongue blade then transferring it from hand to hand; putting two otoscope earpieces together, one inside the other).[83,84,86] The difficulty of the task can be adjusted to fit the child's zone of proximal development, by making it not too difficult (above their developmental skill level) and not too easy (below their developmental level). The process of engaging with a child in their developmental learning communicates to them that you recognize and appreciate the skills they are working on, and it is an integral part of building trust.[82–84,86]

The Deep Dive

Developmental tasks are effective engagement tools for preschool children. As children reach school-age, however, developmental tasks are replaced by what we call the Deep Dive. By this time, children have mastered the basic cognitive and motor developmental tasks and are now interested in more abstract and complex operational tasks.

The Deep Dive is a particular type of vertical conversation used to build an image of an identified area of interest in the patient's mind. Unlike horizontal conversations, which typically move from one topic to another, a vertical conversation identifies a single area of interest and explores it in-depth. The Deep Dive captures and anchors older children's attention in the same way that a developmental task does with preschool-age children.

The Deep Dive begins by scanning for and identifying an opening into the patient's world. As you enter the room, take in the scene. Use individual features that you observe (e.g., the child's clothing, jewelry and other accessories, or hairstyle) as launchpads for beginning the conversation. If there is nothing that grabs your attention, ask the patient what they are interested in. Once you pinpoint an area of interest, begin by asking simple, concrete questions.[i] The questions you pose are designed to help the patient visualize themselves performing an activity (e.g., imagining where they stand relative to the lines

---

[i]For example, if the patient is interested in volleyball, imagine that you know nothing about the sport, but you are curious about how the game is played: "How many people are on a team?" "Are there different positions?" "Where does the server stand?" "How does the server position their feet?" "How do they hold the ball?" "How does someone perform a serve?"

on the volleyball court, inhabiting what it feels like to serve the ball), evoking a detailed mental image. The goal is for the child to become immersed in the image they are creating.

The primary rule for the Deep Dive is having Beginner's Mind. Assume you know nothing about the area of interest. This allows you to ask detailed questions that help the patient build an image. If you bring your preexisting knowledge and assumptions about the topic with you into the interaction, this limits the kinds of questions you can ask and makes it more difficult to help the patient build the image. Place yourself in the role of learner, and let the patient teach you about the topic. Collaborate with the patient. Remain curious and attentive. Imagine that you will be asked, by a colleague, to describe what you learned about the patient's world, when you leave the room.

■ SHAPING THE INTERACTION

There are several contextual factors that substantially impact the provider–child interaction. The provider communicates a set of signals to the child—through encoding, expectancy, and language—that can positively or negatively shape the child's response and the course of the interaction. A child may also be extremely fearful due to a previous negative medical experience, requiring the provider to reframe the experience. Additionally, the environment where the encounter takes place may contain factors that facilitate or hinder the trust building process.

Encoding

Encoding, the expression or sending of cues, often happens automatically, without intention or awareness. What we encode conveys information about our attitudes and emotions, to other people.[21,52,87] We are always communicating nonverbally, and patients are impacted by these communications, even if they are not consciously aware of them.[27,28,53,54,70,87,88] While much nonverbal communication is involuntary, nonverbal behaviors can be deliberately controlled to convey a particular impression. (Note: here, deliberate does not mean fake or inauthentic.)[68,89–91]

Bringing under conscious control and intentionally crafting what you communicate nonverbally is pivotal to shaping the child's response and the course of the encounter. The provider's ability to express caring nonverbally is an essential part of establishing trust. Children's behavior is always in response to something; they are not a priori a certain way (e.g., irritable, resistant, fearful, quiet). What you transmit nonverbally as you first meet the child is what they will respond to. For example, in our own clinical practice we intentionally encode a calm, interested, curious, attentive, and respectful demeanor, which children respond positively to. What we consistently encode in patient interactions is what is commonly referred to as bedside manner.

Expectancy

If we expect certain behavior from another person, we may act in a manner that increases the probability that they will behave as expected.[92-94] This effect, called interpersonal expectancy, has been demonstrated in animal studies and human studies with researchers, school teachers, judges, executives, and healthcare providers.[92,93]

Expectancy can be used by providers to help guide patient interactions. As with encoding, expectancy requires the provider to be consciously aware of what they nonverbally communicate and intentionally craft those communications to promote child engagement. Once the child engages, the provider can rapidly determine, from the child's initial cues and response, how the interaction will go (e.g., *this will go well*) and behave consistently with this perspective (e.g., *I know where we can go, let me show you how to get there*).[95-98] Expectancy works together with engagement methods to facilitate the shift from fear to trust.

This is especially important in fearful and distressed children whose trajectory from fear to trust is not linear. During the process of establishing trust, these children may move two steps forward and then one step backward along the Fear-to-Trust Axis. If the provider's response to these normal vicissitudes is *this is not working* or *this will not go well*, this may be transmitted nonverbally to the child, increasing the probability of a negative outcome.[99-101]

Language

Language is an important factor in managing a child's emotional state. Specific speech patterns and phrasing can create positive or negative expectations that influence a child's emotional state and shape their response.[102,103] While positive expectations facilitate the process of alleviating fear and establishing trust,[104,105] anticipation of negative events (e.g., discomfort, pain) can elicit fear and distress.[102,106-109]

Nocebo effects, from the Latin *nocere* (to cause harm), are negative expectations produced by suggestions of negative outcomes.[102,109-113] During medical encounters with children, the provider's goal is to communicate information that positively influences the child's emotional state, without triggering negative expectations. The process of moving a child from fear to trust involves changing their negative expectations into positive ones.[114]

There are specific parental and provider speech patterns and behaviors associated with increasing fear and distress in children. These include apologizing, criticism, excessive or negative reassurance, giving too much control to the child ("Tell us when you are ready for the shot"), negative expectation, and providing vague information.[18,113,115–119] For example, the phrases *"no shots," "no ouchie,"* or *"no surprises"* are all forms of negative reassurance. Frightened children are not reassured by these type of statements.[113,119–122] These behaviors and speech patterns tend to focus the child's attention on the procedure or examination and the associated fear, distress, or pain, rather than away from these factors. Parental and provider behaviors that can minimize fear and distress include coaching to cope, distraction, encouragement, labeled praise, limited control, positive focus, procedural information, and sensory information.[18,115,116,123]

Reframing Past Negative Medical Experiences

When children present with fear out of proportion to the current situation, this may suggest a previous negative medical experience or that the child has a negative expectation about the medical encounter.[10,19,20] Confirm with the parent if your assessment is accurate, and inquire about what happened to the child (e.g., Was the experience frightening? What was the child's reaction? Was physical immobilization or sedation required? What was done to reduce the child's distress, and how successful was it?).

For young children, approach them as you would a frightened child (see Engaging). For older children, address the negative past experience directly with the child and/or parents and attempt to desensitize and cognitively reframe their past experience by walking them through a series of steps that show them how the present experience will be different.[16,19,20,124–126]

Managing Environment-Related Factors

Medical encounters with children and their parents usually take place in spaces that have been designed to facilitate the provider's performance, while guaranteeing optimal patient safety and operational efficiency. In general, their design is dominated by examination-, procedure- and monitor-related equipment; bright lighting conditions; relatively fixed architecture; and providers entering the room directly and unpredictably. Within this setting, procedural disclosure and preparation often take place in the immediate vicinity of the child, promoting anticipatory fear and anxiety. The overall unpredictability of the encounter, appearance and/or proximity of unfamiliar personnel, presence of frightening materials and information, and limited privacy and space for parents can interfere substantially with a child's sense of control, generating negative expectations and impeding the provider's efforts to positively influence their emotional state.[5,127]

Some children, such as those with Autism Spectrum Disorder, may be unusually sensitive to environmental factors. With these children, targeted improvements in preparation and communication between providers and families, and modifications of clinical environments and patient flow, can improve the quality and success of the medical encounter.[128] Parents report that "autism-friendly" environmental modifications, such as reduced sensory stimulation, warm colors, and absence of fluorescent lighting result in less stressful visits.[128]

In the last decade, there has been growing interest in the effect of a hospital's physical environment on children's emotional well-being.[129] Much of this work is based on Ulrich's Theory of Supportive Design for Healthcare Facilities, which postulates that the hospital environment will reduce stress if it fosters perceptions of control, social support, and positive distraction.[130,131]

A child's sense of control is related to their perception of privacy, autonomy, predictability, and their felt ability to modify aspects of the environment and avoid unexpected events.[131] Having a sense of control reduces feelings of uncertainty and fear. In many medical procedures, children can participate positively and exercise choice within limits set by the provider. Building trust with a child is likely to be enhanced in a familiar and predictable environment.

In unfamiliar and stressful conditions, social support can reduce stress and temper the child's emotions. The physical environment can be designed to make close visual, auditory, and tactile contact between the child and parent possible, without interfering with the medical process. In addition, applying a position-of-comfort approach, in which the child is positioned on the parent's lap or abdomen and gently held and controlled by the parent, reduces distress in both the child and parent and allows for optimal social support and interaction.[132–134]

Medical environments should be designed to foster trust-directed interactions. This implies the absence of negative distractors that may elicit distress and shift the child's attention away from the interaction with the provider. Negative distractors include visible medical materials (e.g., needles, medical instruments), unpleasant ambient noises (e.g., beeping of monitors, loud voices, crying of other children) or smells, unexpected events, and negative expectations expressed by other providers.

Pediatric hospitals have traditionally devoted substantial attention and resources to constructing child-friendly facilities.[135] In an attempt to camouflage the medical atmosphere, the interior design of pediatric procedural rooms is enriched with color, attractive lighting, comic characters, gadgets, toys, and child-directed art. Despite these efforts, there is a lack of research evaluating the impact of this kind of environmental design on children's behavior and emotional state.[136]

Although adding art and other graphic elements to the environment may have some impact on a child's well-being, there are reasons to question the efficacy of this practice. The most important criticism pertains to static design, which limits individualized modifications of the environment according to a child's developmental level, individual characteristics, or emotional needs. A wall or ceiling with comic characters that are popular with one age group or gender may be meaningless, childish, or frightening for another.[137] Though art may be an effective stress-reducer for children, social support is more effective.[138] The most effective distractors create a moderate degree of stimulation and contain evolutionary elements associated with stress reduction, such as smiling faces, live animals, and scenes of nature.[138-141]

After considering the conditions that facilitate optimal medical experiences for children and their families, we designed a procedural environment that embodies ideas of supportive interior design, such as low sensory stimulation, soft and nature-inspired colors and graphics, medical equipment that is hidden or subtly integrated into the environment, and ample space for human interaction. In the procedure room, there are three zones: a welcome and preparation zone, a procedural comfort zone (where providers engage with children and manage their emotional state and physical comfort throughout the course of the procedure), and a medical equipment zone (a physically separate space where the procedural equipment is prepared outside of the child's view and hearing) (Fig. 8-4). The efficacy of this environmental design has been demonstrated through a qualitative peer validation process with children and providers, and in virtual and real-life simulations.[5]

▩ MONITORING

The effectiveness of provider interventions can be assessed by observing changes in the child's level of fear and degree of cooperation. Observe for positive changes in facial expression, gaze, posture, kinesthetics (body movement decreases as the child's attention is absorbed in an activity), interpersonal distance, and parental responses (see Parental Cues).[2,21,142] Effective interventions minimize fear and maximize cooperation.

A child's initial response to the provider can be to engage (positive or negative response) or not engage (no response). Positive response behaviors from the child include: postural relaxation (e.g., opening of arms and body), attentiveness (e.g., looking at a described object or pointing to the object, following the providers' movements and gestures, gazing at the provider), positive facial and vocal expressions, allowance of close interpersonal distance, acceptance of touch, and cooperation. Negative response behaviors—e.g., grimacing, tensing posture, averting gaze, covering body parts, turning or moving away,

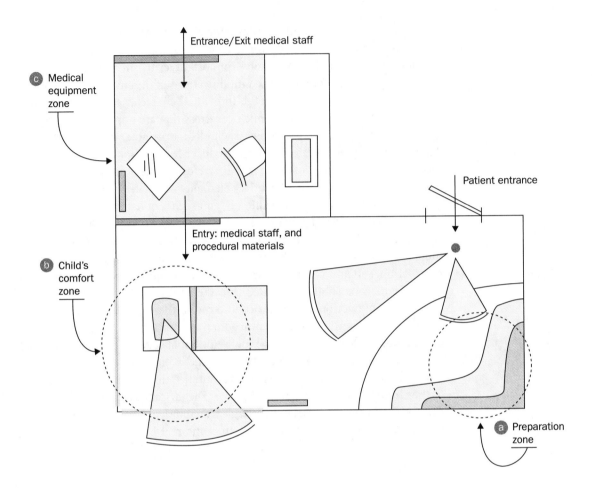

FIGURE 8-4. Environmental configuration.

and decreasing cooperation—convey fear and distress. Any response, whether positive or negative, indicates that the child is engaging; therefore, the provider can use engagement methods to establish trust (see Expectancy).[2-5] No response behaviors occur when the child pays no attention to the provider and behaves as if they are not present.

To establish trust, a child must be capable of engaging. This methodology is not effective with children who will not engage (e.g., forms of autism, certain syndromic patients, and patients with severe developmental delay). Children who have difficulty sustaining engagement (e.g., a child who breaks off engagement after initial connection with the provider, a child whose attention waxes and wanes throughout the interaction) require reassessment as they may be experiencing physical discomfort (e.g., nausea, fever, pain, hunger, lack of sleep from missed daily naptime, poor night's sleep due to illness), limiting their ability to maintain engagement. Addressing their discomfort through pharmacologic means (e.g., antiemetics, antipyretics, analgesics) and/or nonpharmacologic means (e.g., letting the child nap or eat) can help alleviate these symptoms, allowing the child to fully engage (Fig. 8-2).

Bluetooth Pairing: When Trust is Established

A critical part of the monitoring process involves recognizing the features that herald the establishment of trust.[143] We use the term "Bluetooth Pairing" to identify the point at which trust is established and to clearly define the outcome of the methodology. Bluetooth Pairing is indicated by a set of features (positive affect and behavior, mutual attentiveness, and coordination between provider and child) and specific child behaviors (softening of facial expression, relaxing and opening of posture, focusing attention on the provider and the directed activity, and engaging in guided play).[2,144-146] Once established, this trusting relationship becomes the conduit through which the history, physical examination, and treatment flow. It, therefore, determines the quality of the child and family's experience.

■ THE TRUSTING RELATIONSHIP: THE CHILD, THE FAMILY, AND THE PROVIDER

The current crisis of trust in medicine and recent initiatives like the Trust Practice Challenge (an American Board of Internal Medicine initiative to form a compendium of trust-building practices used by providers) highlight the need for a structured understanding of, and education in, patient–provider trust formation.[147-149] This chapter describes a systematic approach to establishing trusting relationships with children in medical encounters, through management of their emotional state. The goals of the methodology are to establish trust and create a positive and rewarding experience for children and their families. The provider also benefits. Through the process of connecting with and contributing to the child and facilitating a positive medical experience, the provider experiences a deep sense of fulfillment. This feeling emanates from the realization of the provider's commitment to making a meaningful impact in patients' lives. These moments remind us why we have dedicated our lives to medicine.

■ FRAMEWORK

This methodology provides a framework and a roadmap for establishing trust with children (Figs. 8-1 and 8-2).

1. Patient Assessment: Start with clinical observation and use it to position the child on the Fear-to-Trust Axis.
2. Engagement Methods—Capturing Attention: Depending on where the child is on the Axis—along with their developmental level, temperament, and prior medical experience—select the appropriate engagement methods and use them to capture the child's attention.
3. Engagement Methods—Anchoring Attention: Once attention is captured, move to a distraction activity, developmental task, or the Deep Dive to anchor attention.
4. Bluetooth Pairing—Establishing Trust with the Child: Continuously monitor the child's responses for the features of Bluetooth Pairing.
5. Bluetooth Pairing—Establishing Trust with Parents: Continuously monitor the parents' responses for positive changes.

ACKNOWLEDGMENTS

The authors acknowledge the Radcliffe Institute for Advanced Study at Harvard University for supporting the development of this work.

REFERENCES

1. Doyle AC. *The adventure of the blanched soldier. The Strand Magazine;* November 1926.
2. Krauss BA, Krauss BS. Managing the frightened child. *Ann Emerg Med.* 2019;74:30-35.
3. Krauss BS, Krauss BA, Green SM. Managing procedural anxiety in children. *N Engl J Med.* 2016;374:e19.
4. Krauss BS, Callgaris S, Green SM, Barbi, E, Current concepts in the management of pain in children in the emergency department. *Lancet.* 2016;387:83-92.
5. Leroy PL, Costa LR, Emmanouil D, van Beukering A, Franck LS. Beyond the drugs: nonpharmacologic strategies to optimize procedural care in children. *Curr Opin Anaesthesiol.* 2016;29(Suppl 1):S1-13.
6. Bijttebier P, Vertommen H. The impact of previous experience on children's reactions to venepunctures. *J Health Psychol.* 1998;3:39-46.
7. Pate JT, Blount RL, Cohen LL, Smith AJ. Childhood medical experiences and temperament as predictors of adult functioning in medical situations. *Child Health Care.* 1996;25:281-298.
8. Weisman SJ, Bernstein B, Schechter NL. Consequences of inadequate analgesia during painful procedures in children. *Arch Pediatr Adolesc Med.* 1998;152:147-149.

9. Dahlquist LM, Gil KM, Armstrong FD, Delawyer DD, Greene P, Wuori D. Preparing children for medical examinations: the importance of previous medical experience. *Health Psychol.* 1986;5:249-259.

10. Duff AJ, Gaskell SL, Jacobs K, Houghton JM. Management of distressing procedures in children and young people: time to adhere to the guidelines. *Arch Dis Childh.* 2012;97:1-4.

11. Chen E, Zeltzer LK, Craske MG, Katz ER. Children's memories for painful cancer treatment procedures: implications for distress. *Child Dev.* 2000;71:933-947.

12. Hermann C, Hohmeister J, Demirakça S, Zohsel K, Flor H. Long-term alteration of pain sensitivity in school-aged children with early pain experiences. *Pain.* 2006;125:278-285.

13. Jones T, DeMore M, Cohen LL, O'Connell C, Jones D. Childhood healthcare experience, healthcare attitudes, and optimism as predictors of adolescents' healthcare behavior. *J Clin Psychol Med Settings.* 2008;15:234-240.

14. Kennedy RM, Luhmann J, Zempsky WT. Clinical implications of unmanaged needle-insertion pain and distress in children. *Pediatrics.* 2008;122(Suppl 3):S130-S133.

15. Taddio A, Chambers CT, Halperin SA, et al. Inadequate pain management during routine childhood immunizations: the nerve of it. *Clin Ther.* 2009;31:S152-S167.

16. Chen E, Zeltzer LK, Craske MG, Katz ER. Alteration of memory in the reduction of children's distress during repeated aversive medical procedures. *J Consult Clin Psychol.* 1999;67:481-490.

17. Cohen LL, Blount RL, Cohen RJ, Ball CM, McClellan CB, Bernard RS. Children's expectations and memories of acute distress: short and long-term efficacy of pain management interventions. *J Pediatr Psychol.* 2001;26:367-374.

18. Cohen LL. Behavioral approaches to anxiety and pain management for pediatric venous access. *Pediatrics.* 2008;122:S134-S139.

19. Duff AJA. Incorporating psychological approaches into routine paediatric venepuncture. *Arch Dis Childh.* 2003;88:931-937.

20. Hearst D. The Runaway Child: managing anticipatory fear, resistance and distress in children undergoing surgery. *Paediatr Anaesth.* 2009;19:1014-1016.

21. Knapp ML, Hall JA, Horgan TG. *Nonverbal Communication in Human Interaction.* 8th ed. Boston, MA: Cengage; 2013.

22. Arnheim R. *Visual Thinking.* Berkeley, CA: University of California Press; 2004.

23. Darwin CR. A biographical sketch of an infant. *Mind.* 1877;2:285-294.

24. Konner M. *The Evolution of Childhood: Relationships, Emotion, Mind.* Cambridge, MA: Belknap Press of Harvard University Press; 2010.

25. Darwin CR. *The Expression of the Emotions in Man and Animals.* London: John Murray; 1872.

26. Charlesworth WR, Kreutzer MA. Facial expressions of infants and children. In: Ekman P, ed. *Darwin and Facial Expression.* New York, NY: Academic Press; 1973.

27. Neumann R, Strack F. Mood contagion: the automatic transfer of mood between persons. *J Pers Soc Psychol.* 2000;79:211-223.

28. Hietanen JK, Surakka , Linnankoski I. Facial electromyographic responses to vocal affect expressions. *Psychophysiology.* 1998;35:530-536.

29. Snow CE. Mothers' speech research: from input to interaction. In: Snow CE, Ferguson CA, eds. *Talking to Children: Language Input and Acquisition.* Cambridge, UK: Cambridge University Press; 1977.

30. DePaulo BM, Coleman LM. Talking to children, foreigners, and retarded adults. *J Pers Soc Psychol.* 1986;51:945-59.

31. DePaulo BM, Coleman LM. Verbal and nonverbal communication of warmth to children, foreigners, and retarded adults. *J Nonverbal Behav.* 1987;11:75-88.

32. Fernald A, Taeschner T, Dunn J, Papousek M, de Boysson-Bardies B, Fukui I. A cross-language study of prosodic modifications in mothers' and fathers' speech to preverbal infants. *J Child Lang.* 1989;16:477-501.

33. Grieser DL, Kuhl PK. Maternal speech to infants in a tonal language: support for universal prosodic features in motherese. *Dev Psychol.* 1988;24:14-20.

34. Ferguson CA. Baby talk in six languages. *Am Anthropol.* 1964;66:103-114.

35. Drescher VM, Gantt WH, Whitehead WE. Heart rate response to touch. *Psychosom Med.* 1980; 42:559-565.

36. Nilsen WJ, Vrana SR. Some touching situations: the relationship between gender and contextual variables in cardiovascular responses to human touch. *Ann Behav Med.* 1998;20:270-276.

37. Hall ET. *The Hidden Dimension.* Garden City, NY: Doubleday; 2000.

38. Little KB. Personal space. *J Exp Soc Psychol.* 1965;1:237-247.

39. Gifford R, Price J. Personal space in nursery school children. *Can J Behav Sci.* 1979;11:318-326.

40. Guardo CJ. Personal space in children. *Child Dev.* 1969;40:143-151.

41. McBride G, King MG, James JW. Social proximity effects on galvanic skin responses in adult humans. *J Psychol.* 1965;61:153-157.

42. Fox E, Mathews A, Calder AJ, Yiend J. Anxiety and sensitivity to gaze direction in emotionally expressive faces. *Emotion.* 2007;7:478-486.

43. Adams RB, Gordon HL, Baird AA, Ambady N, Kleck RE. Effects of gaze on amygdala sensitivity to anger and fear faces. *Science.* 2003;300(5625):1536.

44. Putman P, Hermans E, van Honk J. Anxiety meets fear in perception of dynamic expressive gaze. *Emotion.* 2006;6:94-102.

45. Mogg K, Garner M, Bradley BP. Anxiety and orienting of gaze to angry and fearful faces. *Biol Psychol.* 2007;76:163-169.

46. Mathews A, Fox E, Yiend J, Calder A. The face of fear: effects of eye gaze and emotion on visual attention. *Vis Cogn.* 2003;10:823-835.

47. LeDoux JE. Emotion circuits in the brain. *Annu Rev Neurosci.* 2000;23:155-184.

48. Klinnert MD. The regulation of infant behavior by maternal facial expression. *Infant Behav Dev.* 1984;7:447–465.

49. Dolev JC, Friedlaender LK, Braverman IM. Use of fine art to enhance visual diagnostic skills. *JAMA.* 2001;286:1020-1021.

50. Naghshineh S, Hafler JP, Miller AR, et al. Formal art observation training improves medical students' visual diagnostic skills. *J Gen Intern Med.* 2008;23:991-997.

51. Bernieri FJ, Rosenthal R. Interpersonal coordination: behavior matching and interactional synchrony. In: Feldman RS, Rimé B, eds. *Fundamentals of Nonverbal Behavior.* New York, NY: Cambridge University Press; 1991.

52. Hatfield E, Cacioppo JT, Rapson RL. *Emotional Contagion.* Cambridge: Cambridge University Press; 1994.

53. Dimberg U. Facial reactions to facial expressions. *Psychophysiology.* 1982;19:643-647.

54. Dimberg U, Thunberg M, Elmehed K. Unconscious facial reactions to emotional facial expressions. *Psychol Sci.* 2000;11:86-89.

55. Tronick ED, Als H, Brazelton TB. Mutuality in mother–infant interaction. *J Commun.* 1977;27:74-79.

56. Van Egeren LA, Barratt MS, Roach MA. Mother–infant responsiveness: timing, mutual regulation, and interactional context. *Dev Psychol.* 2001;37:684-697.

57. Cappella JN. Mutual influence in expressive behavior: adult-adult and infant-adult dyadic interaction. *Psychol Bull.* 1981;89:101-132.

58. Stern D. Mother and infant at play: the dyadic interaction involving facial, vocal and gaze behaviors. In: Lewis M, Rosenblum LA, eds. *The Effect of the Infant on its Caregiver.* New York, NY: Wiley; 1974.

59. Bernard R, Cohen L. Parent anxiety and infant pain during pediatric immunizations. *J Clin Psychol Med Settings.* 2006;13:282-287.

60. Lamontagne LL, Hepworth JT, Byington KC, Chang CY. Child and parent emotional responses during hospitalization for orthopaedic surgery. *Am J Matern Child Nurs.* 1997;22:299-303.

61. Kleiber C, Craft-Rosenberg M, Harper DC. Parents as distraction coaches during i.v. insertion: a randomized study. *J Pain Symptom Manage.* 2001;22:851-861.

62. Bauchner H, Vinci R, May A. Teaching parents how to comfort their children during common medical procedures. *Arch Dis Childh.* 1994;70:548-550.

63. White SH. The child's entry into the age of reason. In: Sameroff AJ, Haith MM, eds. *The Five to Seven Year Shift: The Age of Reason and Responsibility.* Chicago, IL: University of Chicago Press; 1996.

64. Kagan J, Herschkowitz N. *A Young Mind in a Growing Brain.* Mahwah, NJ: Lawrence Erlbaum Associates, Inc.; 2005.

65. Flavell JH, Green FL, Flavell ER, Grossman JB. The development of children's knowledge about inner speech. *Child Dev.* 1997;68:39–47.

66. Dittmann AT. The body movement-speech rhythm relationship as a cue to speech encoding. In: Siegman AW, Pope B, eds. *Studies in Dyadic Communication.* New York, NY: Pergamon Press; 1972.

67. LaFrance, M. Nonverbal synchrony and rapport: analysis by the cross-lag panel technique. *Social Psychol Q.* 1979;42:66-70.

68. Lakin JL, Chartrand TL. Using nonconscious behavioral mimicry to create affiliation and rapport. *Psychol Sci.* 2003;14:334-339.

69. LaFrance, M. Posture mirroring and rapport. In: Davis M, ed. *Interaction Rhythms: Periodicity in Communicative Behavior.* New York, NY: Human Sciences Press; 1982.

70. Chartrand TL, Bargh JA. The chameleon effect: the perception-behavior link and social interaction. *J Pers Soc Psychol.* 1999;76:893-910.

71. Chartrand TL, Lakin JL. The antecedents and consequences of human behavioral mimicry. *Annu Rev Psychol.* 2013;64:285-308.

72. Field T, Woodson R, Greenberg R, Cohen D. Discrimination and imitation of facial expressions by neonates. *Science.* 1982;218:179-181.

73. Meltzoff AN, Moore MK. Imitation of facial and manual gestures by human neonates. *Science.* 1977;198:75-78.

74. Meltzoff AN, Moore MK. Newborn infants imitate adult facial gestures. *Child Dev.* 1983;54:702-709.

75. Meltzoff AN, Moore MK. Imitation in newborn infants: exploring the range of gestures imitated and the underlying mechanisms. *Dev Psychol.* 1989;25:954-962.

76. Wolpe J. Psychotherapy by reciprocal inhibition. *Cond Reflex.* 1968;3:234-240.

77. Wolpe J, Lazarus AA. *Behavior Therapy Techniques: A Guide to the Treatment of Neuroses.* Elmsford, NY: Pergamon Press; 1966.

78. Birnie KA, Noel M, Chambers CT, Uman LS, Parker JA. Psychological interventions for needle-related procedural pain and distress in children and adolescents. *Cochrane Database of Syst Rev.* 2018;October 4:10.

79. Gates M, Hartling L, Shulhan-Kilroy J, Macgregor T, et al. Digital technology distraction for acute pain in children: a meta-analysis. *Pediatrics.* 2020;145:1-18.

80. Cohen LL, Cousins LA, Martin SR. Procedural pain distraction. In: McGrath PJ, Stevens BJ, Walker SM, Zempsky WT. *Oxford Textbook of Paediatric Pain.* Oxford, UK; New York, NY: Oxford University Press; 2014.

81. Chan E, Foster S, Sambell R, Leong P. Clinical efficacy of virtual reality for acute procedural pain management: a systematic review and meta-analysis. *PLoS One.* 2018;13:e0200987.

82. Yogman M, Garner A, Hutchinson J, Hirsh-Pasek K, Golinkoff, RM. The power of play: a pediatric role in enhancing development in young children. *Pediatrics.* 2018;142:1-17.

83. Bruner JS, Jolly A, Sylva K, eds. *Play: Its Role in Development and Evolution.* 1st ed. New York, NY: Basic Books; 1976.

84. Piaget J. *Play, Dreams and Imitation in Childhood.* New York, NY: WW Norton & Co.; 1952.

85. Cole M, John-Steiner V, Scribner S, Souberman E, eds. *Mind in Society: The Development of Higher Psychological Processes. L. S. Vygotsky.* Cambridge, MA: Harvard University Press; 1978.

86. Weisberg DS, Hirsh-Pasek K, Golinkoff RM. Guided play: where curricular goals meet a playful pedagogy. *Mind Brain Educ.* 2013;7:104-112.

87. Choi SY, Gray HM, Ambady N. The glimpsed world: unintended communication and unintended perception. In: Hassin RR, Uleman JS, Bargh JA, eds. *The New Unconscious.* Oxford, UK: Oxford University Press; 2005.

88. Dimberg U. Psychophysiological reactions to facial expressions. In: Segerstråle UC, Molnár P, eds. *Nonverbal Communication: Where Nature Meets Culture.* Hillsdale, NY: Lawrence Erlbaum Associates, Inc.; 1997.

89. Goffman, E. *The Presentation of Self in Everyday Life*. New York, NY: Anchor Books; 1959.

90. DePaulo BM. Nonverbal behavior and self-presentation. *Psychol Bull*. 1992;111:203-243.

91. Schlenker BR. Self-presentation. In: Leary MR, Tangney JP, eds. *Handbook of Self and Identity*. New York, NY: The Guilford Press; 2012.

92. Rosenthal R. Covert communication in laboratories, classrooms, and the truly real world. *Curr Dir Psychol Sci*. 2003;12:151-154.

93. Rosenthal R. Covert communication in classrooms, clinics, courtrooms, and cubicles. *Am Psychol*. 2002;57:839-849.

94. Harris MJ, Milich R, Johnston EM, Hoover DW. Effects of expectancies on children's social interactions. *J Exp Psychol*. 1990;26:1-12.

95. Ambady N, Rosenthal R. Thin slices of expressive behavior as predictors of interpersonal consequences: a meta-analysis. *Psychol Bull*. 1992;111:256-274.

96. Ambady N, Rosenthal, R. Half a minute: predicting teacher evaluations from thin slices of nonverbal behavior and physical attractiveness. *J Pers Soc Psychol*. 1993;64:431-441.

97. Ambady N, Bernieri FJ, Richeson JA. Toward a histology of social behavior: judgmental accuracy from thin slices of the behavioral stream. In: Zanna MP, ed. *Adv Exp Soc Psychol*. 2000;32:201-271.

98. Ambady N, Skowronski JJ, eds. *First Impressions*. New York, NY: Guilford Publications; 2008.

99. Word CO, Zanna MP, Cooper J. The nonverbal mediation of self-fulfilling prophecies in interracial interaction. *J Exp Soc Psychol*. 1974; 10:109-120.

100. Learman LA, Avorn J, Everitt DE, Rosenthal R. Pygmalion in the nursing home: the effects of caregiver expectations on patient outcomes. *J Am Geriatr Soc*. 1990;38:797-803.

101. Chen M, Bargh JA. Nonconscious behavioral confirmation processes: the self-fulfilling consequences of automatic stereotype activation. *J Exp Soc Psychol*. 1997;33(5):541-560.

102. Petrie KJ, Rief W. Psychobiological mechanisms of placebo and nocebo effects: pathways to improve treatments and reduce side effects. *Annu Rev Psychol*. 2019;70:599-625.

103. Kirsch I. Response expectancy as a determinant of experience and behavior. *Am Psychol*. 1985;40:1189-1202.

104. Rief W, Shedden-Mora MC, Laferton JA, et al. Preoperative optimization of patient expectations improves long-term outcome in heart surgery patients: results of the randomized controlled PSY-HEART trial. *BMC Med*. 2017;15:4.

105. Kress L, Bristle M, Aue T. Seeing through rose-colored glasses: how optimistic expectancies guide visual attention. *PLoS One*. 2018;13:e0193311.

106. Barsky AJ. The iatrogenic potential of the physician's words. *JAMA*. 2017;318:2425-2426.

107. Perry C, Samuelsson C, Cyna AM. Preanesthetic nurse communication with children and parents—an observational study. *Paediatr Anaesth*. 2015;25:1235-1240.

108. van Laarhoven AIM, Vogelaar ML, Wilder-Smith OH, et al. Induction of nocebo and placebo effects on itch and pain by verbal suggestions. *Pain*. 2011;152:1486-1494.

109. Colloca L, Finniss D. Nocebo effects, patient-clinician communication, and therapeutic outcomes. *JAMA*. 2012;307:567-568.

110. Colloca L, Miller FG. The nocebo effect and its relevance for clinical practice. *Psychosom Med.* 2011;73:598-603.

111. Krauss BS. "This may hurt"—predictions in procedural disclosure may do harm. *Br Med J.* 2015;350:h649.

112. Benedetti F, Lanotte M, Lopiano L, Colloca L. When words are painful: unraveling the mechanisms of the nocebo effect. *Neuroscience.* 2007;147:260-271.

113. Lang EV, Hatsiopoulou O, Koch T, et al. Can words hurt? patient-provider interactions during invasive procedures. *Pain.* 2005;114:303-309.

114. Bartels DJP, van Laarhoven AIM, Stroo M, et al. Minimizing nocebo effects by conditioning with verbal suggestion: a randomized clinical trial in healthy humans. *PLoS One.* 2017;12:e0182959.

115. Racine NM, Riddell RR, Khan M, Calic M, Taddio A, Tablon P. Systematic review: predisposing, precipitating, perpetuating, and present factors predicting anticipatory distress to painful medical procedures in children. *J Pediatr Psychol.* 2016;41:159-181.

116. Campbell L, DiLorenzo M, Atkinson N, Riddell RP. Systematic review: a systematic review of the interrelationships among children's coping responses, children's coping outcomes, and parent cognitive-affective, behavioral, and contextual variables in the needle-related procedures context. *J Pediatr Psychol.* 2017;42:611-621.

117. Blount RL, Corbin SM, Sturges JW, et al. The relationship between adults' behavior and child coping and distress during BMA/LP procedures: a sequential analysis. *Behav Ther.* 1989;20:585-601.

118. Dahlquist LM, Power TG, Carlson L. Physician and parent behavior during invasive pediatric cancer procedures: relationships to child behavioral distress. *J Pediatr Psychol.* 1995;20:477-490.

119. McMurtry CM, McGrath PJ, Chambers CT. Reassurance can hurt: parental behavior and painful medical procedures. *J Pediatr.* 2006;148:560-561.

120. Chorney JM, Tan ET, Kain ZN. Adult-child interactions in the postanesthesia care unit: behavior matters. *Anesthesiology.* 2013;118:834-841.

121. McMurtry CM, Chambers CT, McGrath PJ, Asp E. When "don't worry" communicates fear: children's perceptions of parental reassurance and distraction during a painful medical procedure. *Pain.* 2010;150:52-58.

122. Manimala MR, Blount RL, Cohen LL. The effects of parental reassurance versus distraction on child distress and coping during immunizations. *Child Health Care.* 2000;29:161-177.

123. Mahoney L, Ayers S, Seddon P. The association between parent's and healthcare professional's behavior and children's coping and distress during venepuncture. *J Pediatr Psychol.* 2010;35:985-995.

124. Pickrell JE, Heima M, Weinstein P, et al. Using memory restructuring strategy to enhance dental behaviour. *Int J Paediatr Dent.* 2007;17:439-448.

125. Marche TA, Briere JL, von Baeyer CL. Children's forgetting of pain-related memories. *J Pediatr Psychol.* 2016;41:220-231.

126. von Baeyer CL, Marche TA, Rocha EM, Salmon K. Children's memory for pain: overview and implications for practice. *J Pain.* 2004;5(5):241-249.

127. Lew VK, Lalwani K, Palermo TM. Factors affecting parental satisfaction following pediatric procedural sedation. *J Clin Anesth*. 2010;22:29-34.

128. Davignon MN, Friedlaender E, Cronholm PF, Paciotti B, Levy SE. Parent and provider perspectives on procedural care for children with autism spectrum disorders. *J Dev Behav Pediatr*. 2014;35:207-215.

129. Cartland J, Ruch-Ross HS, Carr L, Hall A, Olsen R, Rosendale E, Ruohonen S. The role of hospital design in reducing anxiety for pediatric patients. *HERD*. 2018;11(3):66-79.

130. Andrade CC, Devin AS. Stress reduction in the hospital room: applying Ulrich's theory of supportive design. *J Environ Psychol*. 2015;41:125-134.

131. Ulrich RS. A theory of supportive design for healthcare facilities. *J Healthc Des*. 1997;9:3-24.

132. Baxter A. Common office procedures and analgesia considerations. *Pediatr Clin North Am*. 2013;60:1163-1183.

133. Lacey CM, Finkelstein M, Thygeson MV. The impact of positioning on fear during immunizations: supine versus sitting up. *J Pediatr Nurs*. 2008;23:195-200.

134. Sparks LA, Setlik J, Luhman J. Parental holding and positioning to decrease IV distress in young children: a randomized controlled trial. *J Pediatr Nurs*. 2007;22:440-447.

135. Komiske B. *Designing the World's Best Children's Hospitals*. Vol. 3. Mulgrave, Victoria, Australia: Images Publishing Group Pty Ltd; 2013.

136. Cohen L, Blount R, Chorney J, Zempsky W, Cousins L. Management of pediatric pain and distress due to medical procedures. In: Roberts M, Steele R, eds. *Handbook of Pediatric Psychology*. 5th ed. 2018.

137. Boyatzis CJ, Varghese R. Children's emotional associations with colors. *J Genet Psychol*. 1994;155:77-85.

138. Eisen SL, Ulrich RS, Shepley MM, Varni JW, Sherman S. The stress-reducing effects of art in pediatric health care: art preferences of healthy children and hospitalized children. *J Child Health Care*. 2008;12:173-190.

139. Sridharan K, Sivaramakrishnan G. Therapeutic clowns in pediatrics: a systematic review and meta-analysis of randomized controlled trials. *Eur J Pediatr*. 2016;175:1353-1360.

140. Vagnoli L, Caprilli S, Vernucci C, Zagni S, Mugnai F, Messeri A. Can presence of a dog reduce pain and distress in children during venipuncture? *Pain Manage Nurs*. 2015;16:89-95.

141. Vos GD, van Os J, Leroy PL, Schieveld JN. Pets or meds: how to tackle misery in a paediatric intensive care unit. *Intensive Care Med*. 2017;33:1492-1493.

142. Birdwhistell RL. *Introduction to Kinesics: An Annotation System for Analysis of Body Motion and Gesture*. Washington, D.C.: Department of State, Foreign Service Institute; 1952.

143. Tickle-Degnen L, Rosenthal R. The nature of rapport and its nonverbal correlates. *Psychol Inq*. 1990;1:285-293.

144. Mehrabian A. Inference of attitudes from the posture, orientation, and distance of a communicator. *J Consult Clin Psychol*. 1968;32:296-308.

145. Mehrabian A. Relationship of attitude to seated posture, orientation, and distance. *J Pers Soc Psychol*. 1968;10:26-30.

146. Mehrabian A. *Nonverbal Communication*. Chicago, IL: Aldine; 1972.

147. Chang S, Lee TH. Beyond evidence-based medicine. *N Engl J Med*. 2018;379:1983-1985.

148. Peabody FW. The care of the patient. *JAMA*. 1927;88:877-882.

149. Lynch TJ, Wolfson DB, Baron RJ. A trust initiative in health care: why and why now? *Acad Med*. 2019;94:463-465.

Interacting Effectively with Individuals with Reduced Facial Expressivity

CHAPTER 9

Amanda R. Hemmesch, Sarah D. Gunnery, and Linda Tickle-Degnen

■ INTRODUCTION

Effective clinical interaction with patients and clients draws upon the same cues and skills necessary for successful interaction in daily life. However, interacting with individuals with health conditions that reduce facial expressivity (such as facial paralysis, autism, cerebral palsy, or Parkinson's disease) requires additional skill and awareness because typical heuristics may lead to mistakes reading emotions when interacting with these individuals. This chapter will introduce important concepts related to person perception that can inform effective clinical interactions with individuals with reduced emotional expressivity, particularly in the face, with a focus on biases that may arise when interacting with individuals with expressive conditions and strategies to address those biases. In the words of biologist Adams A. Wilkins: "*The human face is highly distinctive not only in its set of physical features compared to our animal cousins, but also in being the most expressive face of any creature on Earth, and as such it plays a crucial part in our social existence.*"[1] The clinical encounter is a specialized social interaction that is of great importance to personal and population health. The information in this chapter not only pertains to interactions with clients with reduced facial expressiveness. It is also useful during clinical encounters with clients without expressive disorders because people tend to use the same heuristics when interacting with a variety of other people. Regardless of whether the client has a health condition that affects facial expressivity, clinicians must be cognizant of the critical role the face plays in the effectiveness of clinical decision making and the outcomes of the encounter.

As a normal part of interactions, people make social judgments about others. For example, a clinician might want to determine if a new client seems like a reliable reporter and capable of adhering to recommended treatments. We use information from others, like if they are smiling or not, or if they are talkative or quiet, to form our first impressions of them. Sometimes these first impressions may be correct and other times they may not be. For example, we might assume someone is competent and through our interaction discover that they are successfully managing their chronic health condition, or we might find out that a person who seemed competent is not adhering to treatment or does not understand their condition. Some of the challenges of effective clinical encounters are determining which information to use when forming impressions of clients, and then determining if impressions of clients are correct. Accurate impressions are critical to establishing a working alliance between client and clinician for developing an effective treatment plan that promotes adherence and healthy outcomes.[2]

Research has identified different channels, or different methods, that individuals use to read emotions and form first impressions in clinical encounters and daily life. Verbal cues refer to the content of speech (e.g., someone saying that they are happy). Nonverbal cues include information such as facial expressions, gestures, posture, eye gaze, leaning/social distancing, and dress and grooming, as well as aspects of speech such as tone, prosody (including the rhythms, stresses, and intonations of speech), and pauses. In clinical encounters, clinicians can use verbal and nonverbal cues to attempt to understand their client's emotions or personality (as discussed more in Chapter 5, Perception of Emotion in the Medical Visit, and Chapter 6, Emotion Cues as Clinical Opportunities). In research, these channels can be presented together, in isolation, or in combination to determine how these different channels contribute to the impressions made on others.[3]

Studies based on healthy targets (people who are being judged) and healthy observers (people who are making judgments about others) have shown that first impressions of personality and emotions can be accurate above chance levels even with limited information.[4,5] The ability to form relatively accurate impressions quickly can be adaptive by helping people to avoid potential threats, for example, maintaining distance from someone who seems angry.[6–8] However, research with healthy targets and observers has also demonstrated that heuristics for understanding others can lead to errors or bias. Observers often rely on facial expressions as nonverbal cues during interactions, which is typically adaptive because the face usually provides reliable information about others.[9,10] However, reliance on the face poses problems when interacting with individuals with conditions that affect facial expressivity. For example, people typically assume that someone who smiles at them is friendly (and that someone who does not smile is not friendly). But for someone with facial paralysis who cannot smile, a lack of smile may not necessarily indicate that that person is not friendly; it may just be a symptom of their condition. Someone with facial paralysis may use other methods to try to communicate their friendliness, like by saying "hello" in a cheerful voice. Nevertheless, people may assume that someone with facial paralysis is unfriendly because they did not smile. Research with healthy adults has also shown that people tend to rate more expressive individuals more positively regardless of their actual characteristics, and that this is true for both men and women.[11–14] Again, this positivity bias toward expressivity potentially compromises interactions with individuals with conditions that limit expression, who have fewer channels available to communicate.

People with conditions that reduce expressivity are at risk of being stigmatized because their verbal and/or nonverbal cues may lead people to form inaccurate impressions of them. Stigma refers to a gap between someone's actual identity and how they are perceived by others.[15] When a client is stigmatized, they are typically evaluated negatively, which can contribute to behaviors such as avoidance.[15] It is believed that disease- and disability-related stigma is evolutionarily adaptive because it may help individuals avoid others who are potentially ill or who are unable to contribute to successful group functioning.[16–18] However, individuals who experience stigmatization are at higher risk for depression, anxiety, isolation, and other poor outcomes.[19–21] It is important that clinicians develop the tools and awareness to avoid stigmatizing their clients. Stigma and the related social difficulties could affect the development of a therapeutically beneficial clinician–client relationship, and could cause additional stress to clients who are already managing health conditions, potentially causing additional health issues.[22]

Many acute and chronic conditions can affect verbal and nonverbal expressivity across the lifespan and this puts clients at risk for stigmatization in their lives and in clinical encounters. Research examining conditions that limit expression has found differences in adaptation for individuals with congenital and acquired disorders.[23] In Bogart et al.'s study,[23] adaptation referred to the ability to develop alternative strategies that do not rely on the face for communicating with others, like choosing to laugh audibly in response to jokes instead of smiling, or using clothing and grooming to communicate cues about personality and competence. Individuals with congenital conditions such as cerebral palsy and Moebius syndrome are born with their conditions and therefore have an entire lifetime to develop strategies to adapt well. In contrast, individuals with acquired conditions that may lead to chronic reduction of expression (e.g., Bell's palsy, stroke, Parkinson's disease, depression, dementia, and schizophrenia) develop their conditions later in life, which requires them to learn new skills and strategies for successful functioning. Either way, individuals with expressive conditions may experience a mismatch between their internal emotional state and their emotional behavior. Understanding how individuals with expressive disorders may adapt to compensate for their disorder may help clinicians develop skills that can improve sessions with individuals with congenital or acquired conditions. These strategies may also improve interactions with other clients by making clinicians more aware of the various methods clients may use to communicate.

This chapter will use Parkinson's disease (PD), an acquired condition, as a model for understanding expressive conditions in general. We will include examples from other expressive conditions, such as Moebius syndrome, a rare congenital condition characterized by facial paralysis and the inability to move the eyes from side to side, to illustrate how bias and stigmatization could influence clinical interactions. We will also highlight existing research that suggests methods for achieving more successful interactions with clients with conditions that affect their expressivity. While we use PD as a case for discussing how conditions that affect facial expression can be particularly stigmatizing, emotional expression is compromised by a diverse group of disorders that vary in age of onset, cue channel affected, chronicity, and whether they are diagnostically categorized as physical or psychological health conditions. There are also nonmotor pathways for loss of expression including cognitive and mental health conditions; these nonmotor pathways may result in similar biases and stigma.

■ HEALTHCARE PRACTITIONERS' AND OBSERVERS' BIAS AGAINST REDUCED EXPRESSION

As human beings, we are socialized to read nonverbal cues to recognize emotion in others from an early age. When a person has atypical emotional expression due to a chronic medical condition, healthcare practitioners and other people whom they encounter in their daily lives still use these automatic processes to recognize emotions and other states and traits in the person. When emotion expression is impaired in the face, body, or voice, use of these automatic processes often leads to healthcare practitioners and other observers having negatively biased impressions of the individual due to the mismatch between emotional states and expressive behaviors.

PD is a useful case for examining how people's impressions of those with atypical expression are negatively biased, because PD classically presents itself as a movement disorder that affects the three main channels of nonverbal emotion expression: face, body, and voice. PD is a progressive neurodegenerative disorder that affects a person's ability to move with ease and fluidity.

This causes the person with PD to experience slowness and rigidity in their movement, postural instability, and tremor. Hypomimia, also known as facial masking, is a specific symptom of PD that decreases the ability to communicate with the face due to a decrease in the speed and coordination with which people are able to activate their facial musculature.[24,25] People with PD experience hypomimia to varying degrees. Approximately 70% of individuals with PD have facial masking, and there is preliminary research showing that as facial masking severity increases, both the number and intensity of facial muscle actions decrease.[26,27] There is also evidence that automatic emotion expression (spontaneously smiling when you are happy to see someone) may be more impacted by PD than deliberate expression (smiling to say thank you for a gift).[28]

Though the research investigating exactly how emotion expression is affected by PD is somewhat lacking, there is a substantial body of research that has investigated how practitioners and same-aged peers view people with facial masking. This work has largely found that those with facial masking are perceived as more depressed and less sociable, less socially supportive, and less cognitively capable, even when the severity of the facial masking is quite low.[29,30]

Pentland and colleagues showed silent videos of people with PD and controls with heart disease to physical and occupational therapists[31] and speech therapy students.[32] They found that although targets with PD and those with heart disease did not differ in any characteristics of their actual affect (i.e., depression), targets with PD were rated as more depressed and anxious, less stable and intelligent, and as being poorer social partners, among other negative attributes. This was attributed largely to differences in facial masking.

Similar results were found when investigating perceptions of the voice in people with PD. As compared to a control group with ischemic heart disease, people with PD were rated as more anxious, cold, and withdrawn based solely on vocal qualities. Pitcairn et al. analyzed the vocal characteristics of both groups, and found that it was characteristics of pauses in speech and fundamental frequency that differed between groups.[33]

Biased perceptions of people with facial masking also occur in samples outside of the United States. Both American and Taiwanese doctors, nurses, and rehabilitation practitioners rated people with moderate facial masking more negatively (i.e., more depressed, more cognitively impaired, and less socially skilled) than people with PD who had typical emotion expression in their faces.[30] There are also some interesting interactions between facial masking, culture, and gender. American women with Parkinson's disease were perceived with the most bias by both American and Taiwanese health professionals, presumably due to gender norms whereby women are expected to be more expressive than men are expected to be,[34] and especially in cultures (such as American) that highly value people who draw attention to themselves.

Older adults (e.g., same aged peers) perceive people with PD with similar biases as healthcare professionals. Same aged peers were less likely to want to start a social relationship with women with PD who experienced facial masking than women with PD who had typical facial expression. This effect was not present for men, as men with high and low masking were rated similarly.[32] These findings showed that women experience more negative social outcomes for not showing emotion in their face than men, likely due to women breaking social norms more so than men by not showing expression in their face.[35]

Misinterpreting expressive cues can be especially problematic for people with health conditions like PD because it can lead to a misdiagnosis. For example, Bogart[36] outlined how people with PD who experience hypomimia are often perceived as apathetic, but don't experience the decreased quality of life that is typically seen in people experiencing apathy. Bogart's review supports the idea that people with PD may be misdiagnosed as apathetic because of their expressive facial masking. Research continues to develop with respect to apathy in PD and, as yet, is inconclusive. For example, a recent study found severity of facial masking to be positively associated with severity of apathy,[25] suggesting that there may be a connection between apathy and expressivity in PD.

The effects of facial masking are not limited to people with PD. Care partners who view their partners with PD as having more trouble showing expression in their face report enjoying interacting with their partners less even when controlling for depression in the care partner and the person with PD.[37] Qualitative analyses have shown that facial masking can have detrimental effects on marital relationships[38] and that care partners of people with PD often misperceive facial masking as the person with PD experiencing negative emotions.[39] These findings are correlational and could be interpreted either as care partners being biased in their impressions of their partners based on their lack of facial expressivity or as care partners experiencing the stigma of decreased facial expressivity vicariously through their partners.[22]

There is emerging evidence that the correlation between facial masking and quality of life in people with PD is mediated by the experience of stigma.[40] This gives a potential pathway for clinicians to help maintain their clients' health related quality of life by making a conscious effort in decreasing their own biases around decreased nonverbal expressivity.

Brunswik's lens model[41] can be used as a general diagnostic categorization tool for attempting to untangle the source of one's own clinical impression of a client's nonresponsive, inexpressive behavior during the clinical encounter, independent of the clinical cause of decreased emotional expression. The use of this tool would be to enhance the communication process in order to create an effective clinical encounter that facilitates the clinician's ability to assess the client's presenting problems and their needs accurately before moving on to further symptom testing and intervention.

In the lens model, Brunswik[41] proposed that individuals provide cues, or information, that others use to infer their internal characteristics (e.g., personality, current emotions, or thoughts). This model is illustrated in Fig. 9-1. Cue validity refers to the relationship between a client's internal state and their expressive behavior. Cues may be reliably related to an internal state (like a genuine smile when someone feels happy[42]) or they may be ambiguous, unreliable, or misleading (like when someone smiles when they are nervous[43]). Observers then use the cues they notice to infer something about others' internal characteristics. Ideally, a client would provide reliable cues about what they are thinking or feeling, and a clinician would notice these cues and use them to form an accurate impression of their client. For example, a clinician would notice their client's genuine smile and infer that the person is feeling happy. Cue utilization refers to the relationship between a client's expressive behavior and a clinician's judgments (i.e., what information is a clinician using to form an impression of a client). For example, a clinician may or may not notice a client's smile. Achievement refers to the agreement between the client's internal state and the clinician's impression (i.e., Did the clinician make a correct judgment about the client?). Accuracy is one form of achievement, but achievement in a clinical setting can also refer to establishing an effective working alliance with the client and other stakeholders (e.g., formal and informal caregivers). The lens model also suggests there are many points at which an interaction might be challenging and lead a clinician to form an incorrect impression of a client's emotional state or a more enduring trait. For example, there might not be a reliable relationship between how an individual is feeling and the cues they produce (as is the case in conditions that limit expression), or cues might be missed or misinterpreted.

▨ STRATEGIES FOR ACHIEVING BENEFICIAL OUTCOMES DURING CLINICAL ENCOUNTERS

Emotions in a clinical encounter involve both client and clinician experiences and behavior. The clinician begins forming impressions of the client very quickly and automatically at the beginning of an encounter and forms basic reactions to these impressions. Some of these impressions will be extremely rapid, automatic social impressions about the client's emotional state, their character, and whether or not they appear to be likeable. Other impressions will be estimating the client's ability to participate in the clinical tasks of the encounter to answer the implicit question: *What is the client's likelihood of participating actively and productively in the history-taking and assessment process that can lead to an accurate diagnosis and appropriate therapeutic recommendations?*

Client emotions are fundamental indicators of more than negative or positive emotions in an encounter. Emotional expressivity involves dynamic person-to-person interaction via the several channels of communication outlined above. Expressivity openly displays feelings, intentions, attitudes, and character. According to Boone and Buck,[44] to be emotionally expressive is a signal to others of one's own trustworthiness, and one's willingness to engage in a cooperative relationship. From their viewpoint, expressiveness, particularly of negative and positive emotions, creates likeability because it can signal the open exposure of one's intentions. With this openness, or disclosure of self that makes one vulnerable to another, an observer is able to easily read the expressor's intentions during the formation of a cooperative relationship. The caveat here is that the expressor must be an accurate encoder of their emotions and intentions. Boone and Buck define "expressivity" as an ability to accurately encode one's interior state to be easily "read" by others. If this is the case, the clinician may mistrust that clients with reduced expressivity, that is, those who cannot accurately encode their emotions, are going to participate actively in the exchange of information needed for an effective medical encounter. The lack of dynamic action in any communication channel may create an immediate loss of resources for the exchange of information needed to accomplish clinical tasks. Reduced expressivity also creates the potential for ambiguity and uncertainty to influence clinicians' first impressions and reactions to them. At the same time, as noted above, reduced expressivity creates unfavorable social impressions of character, such as lack of warmth, openness, and caring. To complicate matters, reduced expressivity is also emblematic of poor health: lack of physical, mental, and social vitality, including frailty, sadness, apathy, and interpersonal incapacitation.

All of what can be said about the client's emotions can also be said of the clinician's emotions. Individual variation exists in the expressive tendencies of both client and clinician,[45] and there is situational variation in their emotional expressivity across different tasks and situations outside and inside the clinic.[46,47] The personal traits and states of the people involved in the encounter, in addition to the perception of what types of expression is expected or appropriate for the specific encounter, influence emotion and its expression. A primary difference between the client and the clinician in the medical encounter is the clinician's ethical responsibility and trained expertise to facilitate and influence the course of the encounter to achieve an effective health recommendation. Trustworthiness is mutually developed and earned through the clinician's strategic responses to the expressivity present in the encounter.

How can clinicians enhance their own clinical decision-making process and expressive behavior to decipher and respond to clients whose emotional expressivity is reduced? To answer this question, we expand the unidirectional client-to-clinician flow of behavioral information depicted in Fig. 9-1 to a bidirectional mutuality, shown in Fig. 9-2, that involves cocreated experiences and behavior by the client and clinician. Although this model demonstrates that client and clinician are cocreators of the encounter, our focus is on the clinician's actions as the formally responsible agent in facilitating trustworthiness in the process and outcomes of the encounter.

The clinician can monitor their own decision-making process and their encoding behavior to meet three interrelated achievement goals: (1) an accurate differential diagnosis of the emotional situation in the encounter; (2) an appropriate therapeutic recommendation for the client's presenting problem; and (3) effective triangulation from multiple perspectives, such as from informal caregivers and partners, health specialists, or additional clinician encounters with the client. Table 9-1 presents a rubric of strategies and steps toward meeting these achievement goals. The first two goals are operational during the clinical encounter, and the third is a follow-up to the first two, as

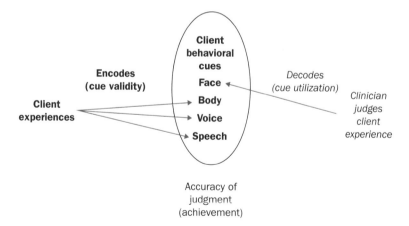

FIGURE 9-1. An unidirectional lens model applied to clinician decision making. In this example, the client encodes (expresses) experience (emotion, thought, personal preferences) via body, voice, and speech while the face does not encode the client's experience due to reduced expressive capacity. The clinician uses only the still face to form an impression of the client's experience. The clinician judges the client's interior experience through the clinician's perceptual "lens" of the client's behavioral cues. The achievement in this model is the clinician's accuracy of their judgment of the client's interior experience. Bold lettering depicts client. *Italic* lettering depicts clinician.

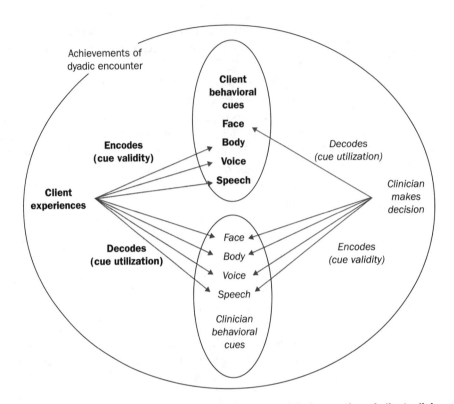

FIGURE 9-2. A bidirectional lens model applied to dynamic interaction of client–clinician dyads during a clinical encounter. In this example, the upper half of the figure depicts that the client encodes their experience into behavioral cues while the clinician uses their own perceptual "lens" of those cues, as shown in Fig. 9-1. The lower half of the figure depicts that the clinician encodes their experience into behavioral cues, in this case, using their face, voice, body, and speech. These clinician cues are then available to the client to form an impression through the client's perceptual "lens" of the clinician's behavior. The achievements in this model are dyadic, transactional outcomes, such as degree of mutual understanding, rapport, or a working alliance. This model can be extended to groups, inclusive of other people in the social ecology of the client's care: such as informal family caregivers or formal *health care* providers on the clinician's team. Bold lettering depicts client. *Italic* lettering depicts clinician.

needed. Although we previously have defined lens model achievement as the accuracy of the clinician's use and interpretation of the client's cues (unilateral model), we now define it from a more dyadic and temporal perspective that aligns with the clinician's medical role and the skills and tasks associated with that role. This chapter focuses on the first achievement goal because it provides the foundation for effective clinical encounters with individuals with expressive conditions.

The first achievement goal is to optimize creating a broad differential diagnosis of the emotional situation. As with all clinical encounters, quickly

■ **TABLE 9-1. Strategies and Steps for Achievement Goals with Clients who have Reduced Expressivity**

Achievement 1: Optimize differential diagnosis of the emotional situation

☐ **Establish the basics of therapeutic rapport by reducing stress, creating trust, and engaging the client in active communication:**
→ Listen and observe attentively.
→ Recognize one's own interpersonal traits, capacities, and preferences, and how one's own interpersonal qualities and behavior feed into dyadic behavior during encounter.
→ Identify positive state and trait capacities of the client for engaging in the encounter
→ Implement strategies to empower the client to mutually engage in decision making, such as encouraging clients to engage in an open-ended conversation about the client's broad concerns of daily living that is pertinent to the presenting problem.

☐ **Maximize accuracy of first impressions**
→ Reduce overgeneralization into the clinic the implicit use of social heuristics that work in one's home and community yet may not correlate with health conditions involving loss of communication channels of expressivity.
→ Turn first impressions into hypotheses and test these hypotheses to rule out and discover potential factors contributing to client's emotional presentation. A series of rating items are arranged below—from general to specific—for starting to describe the factors. Engage the client verbally to help in the ratings listed below:

　　☐ *Chronic Health Condition Severity*: Does the client have a chronic health condition that includes symptoms that can reduce their ability to express emotion?
　　　• Do you think that the client might have a relevant chronic condition?
　　　　○ Probability of likelihood: Zero, Low, Moderate, High, Unsure
　　　• If low, moderate, or high probability, how severe are the symptoms of loss of expression? Which channels of expression are affected?

　　☐ *Acute Health Condition Severity*: Does the client have an acute health condition that includes symptoms that can reduce their ability to express emotion?
　　　• Do you think that the client might have a relevant acute condition?
　　　　○ Probability of likelihood: Zero, Low, Moderate, High, Unsure
　　　• If low, moderate, or high probability, how severe are the symptoms of loss of expression? Which channels of expression are affected?

　　☐ *Positive Emotional Behavior*: To what degree does the client present during the encounter with positive emotional behavior?
　　　• Make a gestalt rating of the frequency and/or intensity of overall positive emotional behavior: Zero, Low, Moderate, High, Unsure
　　　• What behavioral signs relate to your rating?
　　　• What are your subjective impressions of their meaning?

　　☐ *Negative Emotional Behavior*: To what degree does the client present during the encounter with negative emotional behavior?
　　　• Make a gestalt rating of the frequency and or intensity of overall negative emotional behavior: Zero, Low, Moderate, High, Unsure
　　　• What behavioral signs relate to your rating?
　　　• What are your subjective impressions of their meaning?

(continued)

■ **TABLE 9-1. Strategies and Steps for Achievement Goals with Clients who have Reduced Expressivity (*Continued*)**

☐ *State Emotions Contributing to Behavior*: To what degree do you think the client expresses emotions that are state-like, that is due to a particular situation or event that has occurred recently or today?
- Do you think that the client might be experiencing state emotions?
  o Probability of likelihood: Zero, Low, Moderate, High, Unsure
- If low, moderate, or high probability, how confident are you that state emotions are contributing to the client's presentation?
- What are the behavioral signs of the state emotions?

☐ *Trait Emotionality Contributing to Behavior*: To what degree do you think the client expresses emotions that are traitlike, that is, due to enduring personality traits, such as a tendency to negative or positive emotionality or long-lasting characteristics (e.g., neuroticism and/or extraversion)?
- Do you think that the client might be experiencing trait emotionality?
  o Probability of likelihood: Zero, Low, Moderate, High, Unsure
- If low, moderate, or high probability, how confident are you that trait emotionality is contributing to the client's presentation?
- What are the behavioral signs of trait emotionality?

Achievement 2: Create an appropriate message or therapy for the client's presenting problem

☐ **Activate the client's engagement in decision making:**
→ What is the client's view of the problem? How does this align with your view?
→ What is the client's perception of a successful outcome for their problem?
→ What is the client's perception of various therapies that might help the problem to be resolved?
→ What is the client's expressed satisfaction with the encounter, the hoped-for outcome, and the suggested therapies?
→ Ask the client how likely they are to follow up with your suggested next steps, and what they or their family/friends could do to help achieve follow up to suggested therapies and/or activities?

Achievement 3: Are multiple specialist perspectives or encounters needed to reduce ambiguity about the client's presenting problem and possible resolution to it?

☐ **Treat informal caregivers and health partners as part of the team: Determine if family or others accompanying the client can provide more clarity or additional perspectives about the emotional situation.**
☐ **Determine if additional encounters are needed between you and the client.**
→ In-clinic? When? Why is in-clinic visit useful for addressing client needs?
→ Telehealth? When? Why is telehealth useful for addressing client needs?
→ Email? When? Why is email useful for addressing client needs?
☐ **Determine if your regular team members can provide more clarity through informal consultation.**
☐ **Determine if it would be helpful to refer client to other medical or therapy specialists:**
→ Biological/physical process ambiguity: Refer to appropriate medical pathologists and therapists whose specialization area is physical rehabilitation in the fields of speech and language pathology, physical therapy, and occupational therapy.
→ Psychological process ambiguity: Refer to appropriate psychiatrists, psychotherapists, and psychiatric specialists in the fields of social work, nursing, and occupational therapy.
→ Social process ambiguity: Refer to appropriate case and social workers, and occupational therapists who specialize in social participation.

creating a rapport bond is an important first step for establishing an effective working alliance with the client.[2,47] Establishing rapport creates a climate favorable to activating the client's available channels of communication, including cues emanating from facial and bodily movement, vocal prosody, and speech content. The activation of the client's repertoire of cues optimizes the information available for accurate detection of the client's emotional experience and presenting health concerns (cue utilization and validity). Rapport begins with a recognition of how clinician and client behavior are mutually intertwined in a temporal flow, as shown in Fig. 9-2. The clinician creates a climate facilitative of rapport by listening and observing attentively; recognizing the quality of the flow of communication; and modeling a respectful and caring positive regard. Simple tips for setting the tone for a productive working alliance with clients with expressive conditions include the following:

- Brief introductions and exchange of pleasantries upon entry (e.g., "What's up with this weather?"), if it is appropriate to do so. It would not be appropriate to be cheery and light if a client was obviously in distress. A more concerned response would be appropriate (e.g., "How are you feeling today?").
- Elimination of external distractions and making sure the client is hearing and seeing clinician behavior. This involves silencing cell phones, and positioning of chairs for optimizing the sensory processes (e.g., vision, hearing) underlying communication.
- Self-adapting the speed of clinician verbal and nonverbal behavior to the speed of the cognitive processing and behavior production capacities of the client. For example, clients who are anxious or have neurological conditions may have reduced processing of another's behavior and production of their own responses.[48] The client may otherwise be cognitively capable of self-reporting emotional experience and health problems.
- Empowering the client to actively participate in the encounter.[49,50] Examples include providing information about what to expect from the encounter, such as what questions will be asked, what tests should be conducted, and what are the expected outcomes of the encounter. It is often helpful to start question-asking with simple yes/no questions that help frame the content of the encounter (e.g., "Do you have any particular issues or problems you want to talk with me about today?"), followed by open-ended questions with probes to understand details of the client's experience and perceptions. Typical probes include: "tell me more about that" and "why do you think you've been experiencing this issue?"

With practice and experience, this first achievement goal can be reached quickly and effectively. A major complicating factor is the clinician having enough time to spend with a client who may be functioning at a slower communication pace than the clinician. Use of extra follow-up emails and telehealth can augment the initial clinical encounter. Several encounters may be necessary, if possible, to achieve a successful rapport.

Across clinical populations, the autobiographical and qualitative literature of patient experiences is replete with calls for clinicians to listen to them with patience and caring concern, to lighten their day with social niceties, such as light humor, and to recognize the personal rejection and distress clinicians can cause by not engaging in an authentic, trusting relationship with the client. Saxton,[51] growing up with spina bifida, found that providers "*never asked me what I wanted for myself...*" and she guided others like her to say to providers: "*Before you do anything else, just listen to me.*" Craig,[52] on the other hand, described how her husband's nurse began her home visits: "*...by listening. And anything Ed wanted to tell her was relevant. She let him tell her, in his own way and in his own time, about everything that was happening to his body. And in that way, she came to know his soul.*" Watt,[53] who experienced chronic pain, described his favorite nurse: "*I believed she would make things better. It was never anything she said. It was something in her face.*" Crepeau and Garren[54] reported the experience of a hand therapist and her client with severe elbow injury and medical complications from a traffic accident. The therapist first had a negative impression of him: "*... I don't remember what it was about him... but I thought, oh, I don't even think I want to have this guy on my schedule... I just thought he was a jerk....*" Slowly over several encounters the therapist strategically started using humor in their sessions: "*we started this bantering rapport, not putting each other down, but just giving little digs to make each other laugh.*" And both therapist and client reported thoroughly enjoying one another and their sessions together. The client never missed a session.

To meet the achievement goal of optimizing a broad differential diagnosis of the emotional situation with a client with reduced expressivity, it is important to maximize the accuracy of the clinician's impression of the client. This requires the clinician to self-monitor how effectively their communication is progressing, and to strategize how to optimize accuracy and reduce bias in the impressions being formed of the client. First impressions form rapidly and automatically, based on highly overlearned sociocultural norms that are subject to self-confirmation in everyday social life. We observe what we expect to observe, unless we consciously apply constraints on these "natural" social cognitive processes. Consequently, the clinician must exercise strategic constraints on biases. One means to do so is by invoking scientific reasoning to test and counter one's own biases, assumptions, and expectations (see Table 9-1 for a strategic approach to this).[55,56] This requires calling to consciousness and observing these processes that drive our inferences, then forming them into testable hypotheses: not as a formal research study, but as a lived practice in one's clinical work.

Our research work and support-group education with people with PD and caregivers have helped us to develop recommendations for implementing straightforward and relatively quick strategies for countering biases that reduce accurate impressions of clients with reduced expressivity. Two case vignettes are used to help describe how these strategies work. These vignettes are based on informal discussions among people with Parkinson's disease and caregivers with one of the authors (LTD), and are created here with no actual names, formal documentation, or quotes:

Case #1—Inaccurate diagnosis of depression (false-positive decision result)

Mr. Smith had PD for quite some time and was a leader of a local support group. He described a clinical encounter with a doctor. In preparation for the doctor's appointment that day, Mr. Smith needed extra time to complete his morning routine due to his slowed and rigid parkinsonian movement. After grooming, dressing, eating, and taking his medications, he and his wife rushed to make the appointment on time. While driving they argued about something that made them both angry: something that in retrospect seemed minor. However, the incident exacerbated Mr. Smith's bradykinesia (slowness) and facial rigidity, a common effect of negative social interactions in Parkinson's. Upon arrival, Mr. Smith found that it was impossible to convince the doctor that he was not depressed through his words. The outcome of the visit was a new prescription for depression, which was not Mr. Smith's primary reason for visiting the doctor. Mr. Smith explained, during the support group, that his face had frozen into a grimace during the argument with his wife and his expression could not be changed during the encounter. He also described that his Parkinsonism presentation typically resulted in glaring, unblinking eyes when he was "frozen" and that this was interpreted as anger by others.

Mr. Smith reported that he experienced no depression symptoms; however, his face was frozen into a fixed grimace that appeared to the doctor an expression of sadness, consequently resulting in prescription of an unneeded medication. Mr. Smith had no apparent problem expressing his emotional experience verbally. However, his facial expression did not match what he was telling the doctor. I had no access to Mr. Smith's wife to determine if she was aligned with Mr. Smith's perception of depression or with the doctor's impression. It can be helpful for spouses, friends or formal patient advocates to fill in communication gaps or correct a clinician's misinterpretations when client self-advocacy is not working in clinical encounters.[57,58] In any case, it is important not to assume that one person's perspective is any more valid than another person's in the complex matters of healthy living and healthcare. Rather, seeking and listening to various and even apparently conflicting perspectives offer opportunities for the clinician to achieve a better understanding of the central problems and issues that require immediate attention and resolution, and which issues might require attention at a later time.

Case #2—Inaccurate diagnosis of absence of pathological pain (false-negative decision result)

Mrs. Jones was a caregiver for her father with PD. She reported that her father, Mr. Ames, had difficulty flexing and rotating his arm, which are actions needed for many basic daily activities, such as washing one's hair, dressing, reaching for an object on an upper shelf, and driving safely. A rehabilitation therapist was "ranging" his shoulder joint (to achieve greater range of motion in the arm) by cradling his arm and progressively and slowly moving it into a more externally rotated and flexed position. Mr. Ames told the therapist, in a slow, monotone, and quiet voice, along with an inexpressive face, that he felt pain. He repeated his spoken experience of pain throughout the ranging. The therapist thought Mr. Ames was not reporting his experience accurately. Unfortunately, the ranging tore Mr. Ames rotator cuff, an outcome quite debilitating for someone like Mr. Ames. His chronic shoulder pain was exacerbated, and it would take a long time to heal, if at all, from the incident. Mrs. Jones was very angry about the situation and had not been present when the tear occurred.

In this case, the low emotional expressiveness of Mr. Ames' speech was unconvincing to the therapist who may have responded to the mismatched messages of Mr. Ames' speech content and expressionless nonverbal behavior. In both Case #1 and Case #2, the health providers were more convinced by their impression of the client's nonverbal behavior presentation than by the client's spoken words. Typically, unless dementia is present, people with Parkinson's are capable of reporting their own needs, symptoms, and other internal experiences.[59] In any case, the communication process is complicated by mismatched messages among various channels of expression. Added to this ambiguity are comorbidities of aging, the possibility of dementia, and of depression and anxiety, as well as a wide range of retention or loss of expression among the multiple channels of communication.

What can be done as a clinician in order to achieve accurate differential diagnosis of emotion in such complex and ambiguous communication scenarios? Table 9-1, Achievement 1, describes strategic steps to improve the clinician's impressions of a client. In both Case #1 and Case #2 above, the clinicians overgeneralized into the clinic their well-learned social experience that had been developed outside of the clinic. Social interaction occurs within a social ecology, in which social cues can be used effectively and accurately, or ineffectively and inaccurately, to negotiate daily life.[7] The meaning of specific social cues—such as an expression in the face, voice, or body—in one context of the social milieu can mean one thing (e.g., depression), yet be overgeneralized, or inaccurately extended, into a different social context, with the same cue having the same meaning to the observer, but it no longer accurately indicates the experience or motives of the target (e.g., presence of a movement problem).[60] Errors in forming impressions can result. These errors can become imprinted into social stereotypes or short-cut heuristic impressions that are impervious to falsification. As we have described, stigma may result when the overgeneralization creates a negative social identity in the observed individual.

The first step to deal with overgeneralization of social cue meaning is for the clinician to become aware of this as an issue. The art of being a clinician must also be the science of being a clinician. They are inseparable. The clinician attempts to activate their training in creating a differential diagnosis and scientific (evidence-based) reasoning with a mind-set toward testing and falsifying one's own confidently formed, intuitive, and automatic first impressions. If a person looks like they are unmotivated, unfriendly, vacant, cognitively incapable, or a poor candidate for engaging in an effective working alliance with the clinician, it is incumbent on the clinician to attempt to falsify these predictions and focus on correct attributions. This chapter does not focus on the more welcomed clinic patient—motivated, friendly, present, bright with a positive working alliance, but rather assuming a more challenging patient encounter requiring the provider to have a broader differential diagnosis. Patient traits such as calmness, stoicism, toughness, and masked outrage might co-occur with reduced emotional expressiveness and have positive social meaning in certain contexts, such as an empowered response to difficult situations, and False-Negatives (Case #2, no pain) must be filtered out in favor of True-Positive and Negative impressions. The examination of accuracy in decision making found overconfidence in experts, inclusive of medical experts, to be a major concern related to inaccurate decisions.[56] The message is that clinicians must retain a skeptical perspective about their own skills and translate their inferences into testable hypotheses while providing opportunities to clients that expand their cue encoding repertoire.

Listed in Table 9-1 are a series of questions generated to provide options for expanding and testing one's own inferences. The questions are answered by the clinician, and can be used also to elicit confirmation or disconfirmation of the clinician with ratings of likelihood and confidence that the impression is accurate. These questions are guides to the clinician's investigation of the medical chart, and interview of the client, caregivers, and specialists. The questions in the table can be used also with the client to provide their verbal perspective on the clinician's emerging viewpoints. The table contains questions designed to assess the degree to which the client's contributions to emotional presentation include chronic and acute health conditions and the experience of positive and negative emotions, as well as whether these experiences of emotion appear to be statelike (temporary or situational) and traitlike (enduring and generalized across situations).

In Case #1, Mr. Smith had the chronic disease of PD, and his facial expression loss was of a moderate to higher level, so that while he tended to be upbeat and have positive emotions, he had had a situational (state) emotion of anger or distress going into his encounter with his doctor, and the doctor registered his facial expression as indicative of depression, a trait problem of enough enduring magnitude as to need medication. In Case #2, as in all cases, there is always a level of uncertainty and ambiguity. It is important for clinicians to directly acknowledge that multiple perspectives are needed to address the broad differential diagnosis of considerations. Mr. Ames was described by his daughter in a manner that suggested Mr. Ames to have more severe sequelae of PD than Mr. Smith, having reduced expressivity in both face and voice, and a rotator cuff injury either due to PD or an acute traumatic event. Mr. Ames was self-reporting via words his negative response to his therapist's ranging of his arm, but was not showing it in his nonverbal behavior, so the therapist assumed that Mr. Ames was not self-reporting his experience accurately. Had these clinicians followed a different reasoning pathway about the potential effects of loss of expression on their diagnostic impressions, they may have prevented their inaccurate impressions.

One simple and effective strategy to decipher whether a client's reduced expressivity is indicative of emotion, or due to other factors, is to directly ask them about their mood, perhaps with a self-report measure such as the Positive Affect–Negative Affect Scales.[61] Probing further, a clinician could have them describe a recent negative (problem-oriented, frustrating) event followed by a positive (satisfying) recent event or activity.[62] Takahashi and colleagues[62] found people with Parkinson's generally show reduced expressivity during their description of negative events and activated expressivity during positive event description. These simple questions are mild mood manipulations (negative versus positive). When people, regardless of health status, are experiencing negative moods such as sadness, their expressions generally involve less activity in facial muscles and posture—there is a drawing in and down in physical vitality. On the other hand, a positive mood manipulation involved in describing a positive event tends to activate movement in the face and body—a drawing out and up—even among those with PD. The combination of these two types of questions may broaden the range of client cues or show that the client cannot broaden their repertoire of expressivity. By attempting to elicit more cues through two different forms of questions, the clinician can observe the client's capacity to produce a fuller repertoire of cues, and also notice if there is a change or no change in client expressivity.

It is important to observe the various channels of communication and determine which channel, if any, seems more active or inactive. These types of simple socioemotional questioning strategies can help to test one's inferences. Since in general clinicians often conduct problem-oriented histories, they may already be doing a mild negative mood manipulation and can use this to note the client's demeanor. We suggest trying, at an appropriate time in the interview when light-heartedness is not seen as callousness, a simple question about positive events or activities to determine if a person is actually experiencing positive emotions in their lives and can express this via both words and nonverbal channels.

We have discussed in detail the first achievement goal, because this is the most pressing problem for the clinician to accurately diagnose the situation of a client with reduced expressivity. The second achievement goal is a deepening of the working alliance, with suggested best practices for doing so (see Table 9-1). The third achievement goal is an expansion of the lens model to a larger stakeholder network than the dyad represented in Fig. 9-2. It represents the clinician's effectiveness in accessing the larger social ecology of the client's health provision activities. Consultation from specialists, including informal caregivers who know the client well, and medical specialists who have expertise in different areas of the biopsychosocial continuum of health, creates a wider picture of convergence or divergence of various perspectives. This expanded social ecology offers more clues about the client's emotional expressivity profile and further reduces any ambiguities in their presenting health problems.

■ TRAINING IMPLICATIONS BEYOND THE CLINICAL ENCOUNTER

We have used the example of loss of expression with PD to illustrate how to address this clinical population's reduced expressivity. It is an extreme case, in that several channels of expressivity can be compromised in this neurodegenerative disorder, and the presenting symptoms of the disease can be quite unpredictable and a complex syndrome of motor and nonmotor symptoms.

Table 9-1 can be revised and refined as needed for other clinical populations in which the client's interior experience is uncertain or ambiguous to the clinician. There will be differences in the nuances and substance of how to address reduced expression in others. In general, people vary in their degree of emotional expressivity, and this is moderated by personality, gender, age cohort, and culture of origin. Expressivity is a continuum rather than dichotomous (e.g., present/absent). The clinician's understanding of a client's emotional experience is not necessarily the end-state of the differential diagnosis process—it may be a step toward understanding what the investigatory next steps are to be. Our point is to provide the lens model as a device for generating strategies for decision making to improve accurate clinical impressions and provide person-centered health provision.

The rubric for strategizing during person-centered encounters with a single client can form part of a more formalized systematic training with clinicians. For example, the last author (LTD) incorporates this approach for teaching students and providers working in neurology and neurorehabilitation. This rubric approach is particularly useful for educating providers about how to conduct person-centered evidence-based practice, particularly with clients and families who are living with incurable chronic and disabling diseases. The lens model suggests two further types of educational interventions to improve clinical communication with individuals with expressive disorders, those focused on clinicians/observers or those focused on clients.

Clinician-Focused Interventions

The most relevant interventions to improve clinical communication with clients with expressive conditions focus on building clinicians' skills, which may improve interactions with other clients as well. The lens model proposes that clinicians could be trained to improve their ability to determine which expressive channels are and are not impaired in their clients. By focusing on functioning cues, clinicians may be able to avoid biased and stigmatizing impressions of their clients and improve their capacity to understand and respect clients' emotional, cognitive, and daily activity experience of living with their socially debilitating health conditions.

Bogart and Tickle-Degnen[63] tested two types of training designed to reduce observers' bias and improve the accuracy of impressions of extraversion in individuals with facial paralysis. Extraversion is associated with a tendency to feel and express positive emotion and to be drawn to activities and situations in which sociability is enacted and valued. They compared education (instructing observers to focus on voice and body when forming impressions), education and feedback (education plus learning how some targets rated themselves), and a control group that received no education or feedback. Results suggested that both education and a combination of education and feedback reduced bias in observers' first impressions, but neither intervention significantly improved accuracy. Even a reduction in bias against clients with reduced expressivity may improve clinical encounters.

Client-Focused Interventions

Interventions designed for clients often aim to improve clients' ability to provide cues to observers. Some interventions focus on basic biological processes that may be involved in reduced cue validity, and we defer to medical and pharmacological experts with respect to this type of intervention. Rather we focus on behavioral interventions. Previous research has found that individuals who use nonimpaired channels of communication to compensate for impaired channels are perceived more positively than those who do not use alternative forms of expression.[64–68] For example, a focus group study found that people with Moebius syndrome, a type of congenital and bilateral facial paralysis, used tone of voice, gestures, touch, clothing, and verbal disclosure as methods for communicating that did not rely on facial expressions.[65] Any client who is capable of learning new skills could practice using more alternative communication channels to provide more cues about their internal states and traits.

Beyond medications for improving biopsychosocial functioning, clinicians may also recommend rehabilitation to help clients improve communication. For example, facial rehabilitation[69] and Lee Silverman Voice Treatment have been shown to improve facial expression in PD,[70] and may be helpful particularly for individuals who have potentially recoverable motor conditions, such as stroke and Bell's palsy. However, this is often very intensive and time consuming, and the gains may not persist after therapy is completed.

Clinicians may also recommend other types of activities to improve expressivity. If a client has reduced expressivity due to cognitive loss or depression, a different form of treatment based on the nonmotor mechanisms of these conditions is required. "Enjoyment" interventions (e.g., focused on music or dance) might be suitable for many forms of loss of expression because positive affect is an activator for expressiveness.[62] Elefant et al.[71] found improvements (relative to baseline) in facial expressiveness for individuals with PD after a 20-week group singing intervention, and a review found that some singing interventions can also improve speech.[72] Similarly, dance programs for individuals with PD suggest some benefit for motor symptoms as well as for elevating mood and motivating individuals to exercise and stay socially engaged.[73] However, the potential benefits of expressivity interventions might be temporary during the activity itself and not have lasting effects. A focus on person-centeredness requires a viewpoint that the quality of the clinical interaction can generate better clinical communication, including expressiveness, and that the effectiveness of communication exchange can be strategically influenced by the clinician's self-reflection and behavior.

■ CONCLUSION

This chapter has demonstrated that individuals with reduced expressivity due to acute or chronic medical conditions may experience bias and stigma within and outside clinical settings. The existing literature examining PD provides a useful model for understanding how reduced expressivity may lead clinicians to form inaccurate impressions of clients. Effective clinical communication requires both clients and clinicians to consider the encoding and decoding of verbal and nonverbal cues. The lens model can help clinicians develop effective strategies for encounters with individuals with expressive conditions, including directly asking about emotional states and providing opportunities for clients to report on both positive and negative experiences to gather more expressive information to test clinician's hypotheses about clients' states and traits.

REFERENCES

1. Wilkins AS. *Making Faces: The Evolutionary Origins of the Human Face*. Cambridge, MA; London, England: Belknap Press of Harvard University Press; 2017: ix.

2. Fuertes JN, Toporovsky A, Reyes M, Osborne JB. The physician-patient working alliance: theory, research, and future possibilities. *Patient Educ Couns*. 2017;100(4):610-615.

3. Slepian ML, Bogart KR, Ambady N. Thin-slice judgments in the clinical context. *Annu Rev Clin Psychol*. 2014;10:131-153.

4. Ambady N, Bernieri FJ, Richeson JA. Toward a histology of social behavior: Judgmental accuracy from thin slices of the behavioral stream. *Adv Exp Soc Psychol*. 2000;32,201-271.

5. Ambady N, Rosenthal R. Thin slices of expressive behavior as predictors of interpersonal consequences: a meta-analysis. *Psychol Bull*. 1992;111(2):256.

6. Berry DS, Finch Wero JL. Accuracy in face perception: a view from ecological psychology. *J Pers*. 1993;61(4):497-520.

7. McArthur LZ, Baron RM. Toward an ecological theory of social perception. *Psychol Rev*. 1983;90(3):215.

8. Zebrowitz, LA. *Social Perception*. Buckingham, UK: Open University Press; 1990.

9. Darwin C. *The Expression of the Emotions in Man and Animals*. Oxford, UK: Oxford University Press; 1998.

10. DePaulo BM. Nonverbal behavior and self-presentation. *Psychol Bull*. 1992;111(2):203.

11. Matsumoto D, Kudoh T. Cultural similarities and differences in the semantic dimensions of body postures. *J Nonverbal Behav.* 1987;11(3):166-179.

12. Montepare JM, Zebrowitz-McArthur L. Impressions of people created by age-related qualities of their gaits. *J Pers Soc Psychol.* 1988;55(4):547.

13. Riggio RE, Friedman HS. Impression formation: the role of expressive behavior. *J Pers Soc Psychol.* 1986;50(2):421.

14. Shrout PE, Fiske DW. Nonverbal behaviors and social evaluation 1. *J Pers.* 1981;49(2):115-128.

15. Goffman E. *Stigma: Notes on the Management of Spoiled Identity.* New York, NY: Simon & Schuster; 1963.

16. Kurzban R, Leary MR. Evolutionary origins of stigmatization: the functions of social exclusion. *Psychol Bull.* 2001;127(2):187.

17. Neuberg SL, Smith DM, Asher T. Why people stigmatize: toward a biocultural framework. In: Heatherton TF, Kleck RE, Hebl MR, Hull JG, eds. *The Social Psychology of Stigma.* New York, NY: The Guilford Press; 2000:31-61.

18. Phelan JC, Link BG, Dovidio JF. Stigma and prejudice: one animal or two? *Soc Sci Med.* 2008;67(3):358-367.

19. Hebl MR, Tickle J, Heatherton TF. Awkward moments in interactions between nonstigmatized and stigmatized individuals. In: Heatherton TF, Kleck RE, Hebl MR, Hull JG, eds. *The Social Psychology of Stigma.* New York, NY: The Guilford Press; 2000:275-306.

20. Katz I. *Stigma: A Social-Psychological Perspective.* Hillsdale, NJ: Lawrence Erlbaum Associates, Inc.; 1981;2(3):4.

21. Yang LH, Kleinman A, Link BG, Phelan JC, Lee S, Good B. Culture and stigma: adding moral experience to stigma theory. *Soc Sci Med.* 2007;64(7):1524-1535.

22. Pescosolido BA. The stigma complex. *Annu Rev Sociol.* 2015;41:87-116.

23. Bogart KR, Tickle-Degnen L, Ambady N. Compensatory expressive behavior for facial paralysis: adaptation to congenital or acquired disability. *Rehabil Psychol.* 2012;57(1):43-51.

24. Bologna M, Fabbrini G, Marsili L, Defazio G, Thompson PD, Berardelli A. Facial bradykinesia. *J Neurol Neurosurg Psychiatry.* 2013;84(6):681-685.

25. Ricciardi L, De Angelis A, Marsili L, et al. Hypomimia in Parkinson's disease: an axial sign responsive to levodopa. *Eur J Neurol.* 2020;27(12):2422-2429.

26. Gunnery SD, Naumova EN, Saint-Hilaire M, Tickle-Degnen L. Mapping spontaneous facial expression in people with Parkinson's disease: a multiple case study design. *Cogent Psychol.* 2017;4(1):1376425.

27. Pitcairn TK, Clemie S, Gray JM, Pentland B. Non-verbal cues in the self-presentation of Parkinsonian patients. *Br J Clin Psychol.* 1990;29(2):177-184.

28. Schwartz R, Pell MD. When emotion and expression diverge: the social costs of Parkinson's disease. *J Clin Exp Neuropsychol.* 2017;39(3):211-230.

29. Hemmesch AR, Tickle-Degnen L, Zebrowitz LA. The influence of facial masking and sex on older adults' impressions of individuals with Parkinson's disease. *Psychol Aging.* 2009;24(3):542.

30. Tickle-Degnen L, Zebrowitz LA, Ma HI. Culture, gender and health care stigma: practitioners' response to facial masking experienced by people with Parkinson's disease. *Soc Sci Med.* 2011;73(1):95-102.

31. Pentland B, Pitcairn TK, Gray JM, Riddle W.Jr The effects of reduced expression in Parkinson's disease on impression formation by health professionals. *Clin Rehabil.* 1987;1(4):307-312.

32. Pentland B, Gray JM, Riddle WJ, Pitcairn TK. The effects of reduced non-verbal communication in Parkinson's disease. *Br J Disord Commun.* 1988;23(1):31-34.

33. Pitcairn TK, Clemie S, Gray JM, Pentland B. Impressions of parkinsonian patients from their recorded voices. *Int J Lang Commun Disord.* 1990;25(1):85-92.

34. Briton NJ, Hall JA. Beliefs about female and male nonverbal communication. *Sex Roles.* 1995;32(1-2):79-90.

35. Hall JA. Nonverbal behavior, status, and gender: how do we understand their relations? *Psychol Women Q.* 2006;30(4):384-391.

36. Bogart KR. Is apathy a valid and meaningful symptom or syndrome in Parkinson's disease? A critical review. *Health Psychol.* 2011;30(4):386.

37. Gunnery SD, Habermann B, Saint-Hilaire M, Thomas CA, Tickle-Degnen L. The relationship between the experience of hypomimia and social wellbeing in people with Parkinson's disease and their care partners. *J Parkinson Dis.* 2016;6(3):625-630.

38. Chiong-Rivero H, Ryan GW, Flippen C, et al. Patients' and caregivers' experiences of the impact of Parkinson's disease on health status. *Patient Relat Outcome Meas.* 2011;2:57-70.

39. Wootton A, Starkey NJ, Barber CC. Unmoving and unmoved: experiences and consequences of impaired non-verbal expressivity in Parkinson's patients and their spouses. *Disabil Rehabil.* 2019;41(21):2516-2527.

40. Ma HI, Gunnery SD, Stevenson MT, Saint-Hilaire M, Thomas CA, Tickle-Degnen L. Experienced facial masking indirectly compromises quality of life through stigmatization of women and men with Parkinson's disease. *Stigma Health.* 2019;4(4):462.

41. Brunswik E. Representative design and probabilistic theory in a functional psychology. *Psychol Rev.* 1955;62(3):193-217.

42. Gunnery SD, Ruben MA. Perceptions of Duchenne and non-Duchenne smiles: a meta-analysis. *Cogn Emot.* 2016;30(3):501-515.

43. Lyons KD, Tickle-Degnen L, Henry A, Cohn E. Impressions of personality in Parkinson's disease: can rehabilitation practitioners see beyond the symptoms? *Rehabil Psychol.* 2004;49(4):328.

44. Boone T, Buck R. Emotional expressivity and trustworthiness: the role of nonverbal behavior in the evolution of cooperation. *J Nonverbal Behav.* 2003;27:163-182.

45. Kring AM, Smith DA, Neale JM. Individual differences in dispositional expressiveness: development and validation of the Emotional Expressivity Scale. *J Pers Soc Psychol.* 1994;66(5):934-949.

46. Bernieri FJ, Gillis JS, Davis JM, Grahe JE. Dyad rapport and the accuracy of its judgment across situations: a lens model analysis. *J Pers Soc Psychol.* 1996;71(1):110-129.

47. Tickle-Degnen L, Gavett E. Changes in nonverbal behavior during the development of therapeutic relationships. In: Philippot P, Feldman RS, Coats EJ, eds. *Nonverbal Behavior in Clinical Settings*. New York, NY: Oxford University Press; 2003:75-110.

48. Beauchamp MH, Anderson V. SOCIAL: an integrative framework for the development of social skills. *Psychol Bull*. 2010;136(1):39-64.

49. Johnson MO. The shifting landscape of health care: toward a model of health care empowerment. *Am J Public Health*. 2011;101(2):265-270.

50. Street RL, Haidet P. How well do doctors know their patients? Factors affecting physician understanding of patients' health beliefs. *J Gen Intern Med*. 2011;26(1):21-27.

51. Saxton M. The something that happened before I was born. In: Brightman A, ed. *Ordinary Moments: The Disabled Experience*. Syracuse, NY: Human Policy Press; 1985:127-140.

52. Craig J. *Between Hello and Goodbye*. Los Angeles, CA: Tarcher; 1991.

53. Watt B. *Patient: A True Story of a Rare Illness*. New York, NY: Grove Press; 1996.

54. Crepeau EB, Garren KR. I looked to her as a guide: the therapeutic relationship in hand therapy. *Disabil Rehabil*. 2011;33(10):872-881.

55. Djulbegovic B, Guyatt GH. Progress in evidence-based medicine: a quarter century on. *Lancet*. 2017;390(10092):415-423.

56. Kahneman D, Klein G. Conditions for intuitive expertise: a failure to disagree. *Am Psychol*. 2009;64(6):515-526.

57. Ball J. Managing Parkinson's disease symptoms while hospitalized for non-PD related conditions. *J Parkinson Dis*. 2013;3(Suppl.1):212.

58. Lyons KD, Tickle-Degnen L. Dramaturgical challenges of Parkinson's disease. *OTJR*. 2003;23:27-34.

59. Mikos AE, Springer US, Nisenzon AN, Kellison IL, Fernandez HH, Okun MS, Bowers D. Awareness of expressivity deficits in non-demented Parkinson disease. *Clinical Neuropsychol*. 2009;23(5):805-817.

60. Zebrowitz LA. Overgeneralization effects in perceiving nonverbal behavior: evolutionary and ecological origins. *J Nonverbal Behav*. 2003;27(2):133-138.

61. Watson D, Clark LA, Tellegen A. Development and validation of brief measures of positive and negative affect: the PANAS scales. *J Pers Soc Psychol*. 1988;54(6):1063-1070.

62. Takahashi K, Tickle-Degnen L, Coster WJ, Latham NK. Expressive behavior in Parkinson's disease as a function of interview context. *Am J Occup Ther*. 2010;64(3):484-495.

63. Bogart KR, Tickle-Degnen L. Looking beyond the face: a training to improve perceivers' impressions of people with facial paralysis. *Patient Educ Couns*. 2015;98(2):251-256.

64. Bogart KR, Tickle-Degnen L, Ambady N. Communicating without the face: holistic perception of emotions of people with facial paralysis. *Basic Appl Social Psych*. 2014;36(4):309-320.

65. Bogart KR, Tickle-Degnen L, Joffe MS. Social interaction experiences of adults with Moebius syndrome: a focus group. *J Health Psychol*. 2012;17(8):1212-1222.

66. Cole J, Spaulding H. *The Invisible Smile: Living Without Facial Expression*. Oxford, UK: Oxford University Press; 2008.

67. Meyerson MD. Resiliency and success in adults with Moebius syndrome. *Cleft Palate Craniofac J.* 2001;38(3):231-235.

68. Wang SM, Tickle-Degnen L. Emotional cues from expressive behavior of women and men with Parkinson's disease. *PloS One.* 2018;13(7):e0199886.

69. Ricciardi L, Baggio P, Ricciardi D, et al. Rehabilitation of hypomimia in Parkinson's disease: a feasibility study of two different approaches. *Neurol Sci.* 2016;37(3):431-436.

70. Dumer AI, Oster H, McCabe D, Rabin LA, Spielman JL, Ramig LO, Borod JC. Effects of the Lee Silverman Voice Treatment (LSVT˚ LOUD) on hypomimia in Parkinson's disease. *J Int Neuropsych Soc.* 2014;20(3):302-312.

71. Elefant C, Lotan M, Baker FA, Skeie GO. Effects of music therapy on facial expression of individuals with Parkinson's disease: a pilot study. *Musicae Scientiae.* 2012;16(3):392-400.

72. Barnish J, Atkinson RA, Barran SM, Barnish MS. Potential benefit of singing for people with Parkinson's disease: a systematic review. *J Parkinson Dis.* 2016;6(3):473-484.

73. Bek J, Arakaki AI, Lawrence A, Sullivan M, Ganapathy G, Poliakoff E. Dance and Parkinson's: a review and exploration of the role of cognitive representations of action. *Neurosci Biobehav Rev.* 2020;109:16-28.

A Trauma-Informed Approach to Emotion Communication in the Clinical Encounter

Ben Kaplan, Greeshma Somashekar, Missy Brown, Bria Adimora Godley, Asif Khan, Enioluwafe Ojo, and Amy Weil

■ INTRODUCTION

Karina holds her face in her hands and rocks back and forth, cursing under her breath. You are seeing her for an annual physical before she leaves home to attend college in a neighboring state. As her primary care physician, you've known Karina for 3 years and have never been concerned about her health or development. Today, despite her layers of clothing and makeup, she appears emaciated. Your older sister struggled with an eating disorder when you were growing up, so you tend to notice when someone has lost weight quickly.

After a brief conversation with Karina about her summer, you ask, "Have you had any issues with dizziness or feeling more tired than usual?" "Have you noticed a change in your appetite or eating habits?" "Any recent stressors in your life?" Karina's consistent answer to all of these questions is a simple "no." She doesn't make eye contact. When you bring up the change in her weight, she slams her hand on the counter and says, "That's it. I'm done talking to you. You obviously don't get it. Don't pretend like you care. Nobody gives a damn."

She stares at you, and you stare back. You wait. You try to create space. She stares at her feet. You wait a little longer. Eventually, you say, "Help me understand." This is when she begins rocking back and forth again. You get halfway through her physical, but when you ask if you can proceed with an abdominal exam, Karina abruptly sits up and runs out of the exam room. Everything happens too fast for you to react or respond.

You're left with a half-completed college physical form, a delayed clinic schedule, your own unsettled feelings and an uneasy sense of apprehension about Karina's well-being.

Challenging emotional scenarios like this one—based on a real clinical encounter from one of this chapter's co-authors (with the name changed)—are common in clinical practice. Healthcare is inherently emotional, and directly impacts the physical and psychological well-being of patients and clinicians alike. Of course, patients and clinicians experience positive emotions of joy, relief, and satisfaction when engaged in collaborative, mutually healing care. But experiences of illness may unearth deep-rooted feelings of sadness, anger, guilt, shame, denial, loneliness, fear, inadequacy, confusion, and more in patients and clinicians. Clinicians may inadvertently trigger these emotions within a clinical encounter, causing unintended harm to the patient. Conversely, clinicians caring for ill patients are vulnerable to stress, vicarious trauma, compassion fatigue, the opening of personal wounds, and a negative sense of self due to perceived failures–all of which contribute to the growing prevalence of perceived moral injury and burnout among healthcare workers.[1] These emotions are further complicated by each individual's experience in a labyrinthic healthcare system plagued by increasing administrative burden, rising costs, widening disparities in access and outcomes, and a long history of structural racism, homophobia, transphobia, and other forms of structural violence. Despite this, emotion remains a relatively untouched topic in medical education.

The above vignette reflects the many interconnected factors that influence how we handle emotions in a clinical encounter. In this scenario, you and Karina are independent actors who bring your individual personalities, experiences, perspectives, and traumas to the described interaction. What could be done differently in this situation to promote shared understanding and foster healing? What can we do—and more importantly how can we be—as clinicians to meet our patients where they are? How can we adapt dynamically to emotional situations in which patient and clinician trauma may limit open communication and collaboration?

While many strategies have been introduced to improve clinical communication, we often use these techniques without a clear acknowledgment of trauma's role in the patient–physician encounter—particularly with respect to emotion. Trauma may impair one's ability to perceive, process, and communicate emotion, and requires an explicitly trauma-informed approach to navigating emotionally charged patient encounters. Techniques to acknowledge, cope with, and ameliorate trauma can improve emotional communication.[2] In future interactions with Karina, you may consider offering a shared deep-breathing exercise to promote a sense of safety and mutuality, or acknowledging her apparent discomfort with an empathic statement. You may make a point of offering her as many choices as possible throughout your conversation, from which chair she sits in to the topics you discuss. If you are to continue developing a healthy, supportive therapeutic alliance with Karina, you may also consider exploring the ways in which her emaciated appearance triggers you in some way.

These and other strategies are part of a trauma-informed approach to emotion communication in clinical practice, the subject of this chapter. In what follows, we describe trauma, its mechanism of affecting health, and the key principles of a trauma-informed approach to emotion communication, as well as illustrative examples of how to apply these principles in practice. This framework is followed by a discussion of mindfulness and resilience-based strategies to address primary and vicarious/secondary trauma among healthcare professionals, as well as guidance on designing and maintaining trauma-informed systems in healthcare.

▨ WHAT IS TRAUMA?

Defining Trauma

The Substance Abuse and Mental Health Services Administration (SAMHSA) defines trauma as resulting from "an event, series of events, or set of circumstances that is experienced by an individual as physically or emotionally harmful or life threatening and that has lasting adverse effects on the individual's functioning and mental, physical, social, emotional, or spiritual well-being."[3] Some events are widely if not universally acknowledged as "traumatic events": for example, a near-fatal car crash, or the sudden death of a loved one. However, the wording of SAMHSA's definition emphasizes that trauma lies not in an event itself, but rather in a person's *experience of* that event. A person may be traumatized by an event that others see as relatively innocuous, or conversely may experience little to no traumatization in response to an event that others would deem catastrophic; often, this response can be influenced by prior experiences. Its subjective, often unpredictable, profoundly personal nature makes trauma particularly difficult—but all the more critical—to discuss with our patients and colleagues.

From "Shell Shock" to Posttraumatic Stress Disorder: The Rise of Trauma in Popular Discourse

Trauma first came to national attention in 1980, when the American Psychiatric Association included Posttraumatic Stress Disorder (commonly known as "PTSD") in the third edition of the Diagnostic and Statistical Manual of Mental Disorders (DSM-III).[4] This diagnosis was initially developed based on observations of Vietnam War veterans, building on a long history of terms like "shell shock," "war neurosis," "soldier's heart," and other descriptors of the unusual but remarkably consistent emotional and behavioral symptoms seen in many soldiers upon their return from combat.[4] The manifestations of PTSD are diverse and often debilitating, and may generally be divided into four categories: "intrusion" symptoms (including re-experiencing the traumatic event through flashbacks or nightmares), "avoidance" symptoms (including avoiding trauma-related thoughts, feelings, or environmental triggers), "cognitive/mood" symptoms (including negative thoughts or feelings, feelings of isolation, or inability to recall key features of the trauma), and "arousal/reactivity" symptoms (including irritability, aggression, or hypervigilance). Based on the DSM-V criteria, a formal diagnosis of PTSD requires the following[5,6]:

1. Direct or indirect exposure to death, threatened death, actual or threatened serious injury, or actual or threatened sexual violence
2. One or more intrusion symptoms
3. One or more avoidance symptoms
4. Two or more cognitive/mood symptoms
5. One or more arousal/reactivity symptoms
6. Duration of symptoms lasting more than one month
7. Symptoms causing distress or functional impairment
8. Symptoms not due to medication, substance use, or other illness

However, it is essential to note that *any of these symptoms may occur in individuals who have experienced trauma, even if all of the diagnostic criteria of PTSD are not met.* We include these symptoms here as a framework for considering the many possible responses to trauma.

Intimate Partner Violence: Understanding the Role of Power and Control

Trauma and PTSD have since been further understood in the context of intimate partner violence (IPV), a pattern of physical and/or emotional abuse or coercion "perpetrated by someone who is, was, or wishes to be involved in an intimate or romantic relationship with an adult or adolescent victim."[1] Although IPV can happen to any person, irrespective of gender identity, sexual orientation, race, age, socioeconomic status, 85% of cases are perpetrated by men against women. Internationally, the term "Gender-Based Violence" is used to acknowledge violence at the personal, community, and state levels perpetrated by men upon women in more gender-stratified communities (communities with more gender inequality).[7] Domestic Abuse Intervention Programs developed the "Duluth Model" to summarize the abuses of power and control that often occur in IPV, including physical and emotional intimidation; coercion and threats; economic abuse; male privilege; use of children to induce guilt and relay messages; minimizing, denying, and blaming; using isolation; and emotional abuse.[8,9]

Identifying, communicating about, and addressing IPV is an extremely important and nuanced topic that goes beyond the scope of this chapter; please see Appendix A for further information and additional resources. With this said, the Duluth Model invites a broader conversation about the role of power and control in many traumatic experiences. Trauma almost always involves an acute perceived loss of power or control, resulting in a cascade of physical and emotional responses that often has lasting effects. Long after a traumatic experience has transpired, a trauma survivor may continue to experience severe distress in future interactions, particularly with authority figures.[10] Trauma inflicted by a person who was previously seen as trustworthy—such as an intimate partner, or a parent—may result in long-term challenges with emotional attachment, trust, and interpersonal security. This in turn may impair the formation of healthy relationships, including those with clinicians.[11]

Triggers, ACEs, and the Window of Tolerance: A Neurodevelopmental Framework for Understanding the Acute and Chronic Effects of Trauma

Trauma may affect a person's emotional and physical health throughout their lifetime, starting as early as childhood. Psychoanalyst John Bowlby's (1907–1990) Theory of Attachment posits that adaptive social and emotional development hinges on a healthy "dyadic" relationship in which infants and young children are completely dependent on a caregiver, often a parent, and most commonly their mother.[12] This safe dyadic foundation may be disrupted by a wide variety of childhood traumas. Felitti et al.'s Adverse Childhood Experiences (ACE) Study found that over 60% of study participants (adult attendees of a primary care clinic in San Diego) recalled at least one traumatic childhood experience, or ACE.[13] Furthermore, exposure to more categories of ACEs—including psychological, physical, or sexual abuse, but also witnessing IPV, and other traumatic family experiences such as a parent in prison or suffering with addiction—demonstrated a linear association with a higher risk of many adverse long-term health outcomes, including obesity, infection, and heart, lung, and liver disease.[13] A similar relationship was also observed between ACEs and future alcohol and drug use, depression, and suicide attempts, which was largely attributed to the development of these behaviors as "maladaptive" survival strategies for coping with traumatic experiences.[13]

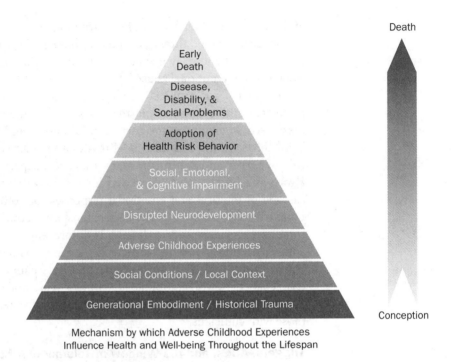

Mechanism by which Adverse Childhood Experiences
Influence Health and Well-being Throughout the Lifespan

**FIGURE 10-1. Adverse Childhood Event (ACE) Pyramid.
Source: Reproduced from Ref. 14.**

The "ACE Pyramid" depicted in Fig. 10-1 summarizes a proposed pathway by which ACEs, mediated by "high-risk" or maladaptive coping behaviors, lead to earlier and more sicknesses, and ultimately foreshortened lifespans (Fig. 10-1).[14] Of note, the ACE Study's retrospective design likely underestimated the prevalence of ACEs due to recall bias.[15] Additionally, the study was conducted in a mostly White, middle-class population. It has since been replicated in more diverse populations, with additional ACEs including economic hardship and discrimination identified as disproportionately affecting low-income and racial/ethnic minority households.[16] Figure 10-1 addresses the role of generational/historical trauma and socioeconomic context in shaping a person's exposure to ACEs, placing these variables at the base of the "ACE pyramid" (Fig. 10-1).[14]

Since the ACE study, researchers have further elucidated the neurobiological pathways by which trauma may be encoded in the mind and body, disrupting Neurobiological processes in both children and adults. The following paragraphs explore in greater depth the physiologic and pathophysiologic responses to trauma, in order to provide a framework for identifying the presence of trauma and intervening when necessary.

As we move through the world every day, our brains constantly receive and synthesize sensory information from our surroundings. A typical physiologic response to this information involves intermittent activation or arousal, mediated by the sympathetic nervous system, followed by a gradual settling or relaxation, mediated by the parasympathetic nervous system (predominantly the dorsal, or "back," vagus nerve).[17] A traumatic experience disrupts this physiologic equilibrium, eliciting a sudden "fight-or-flight" response to perceived danger without a return to baseline relaxation. The prefrontal cortex, which controls focus, attention, and rational thinking, is impaired. The amygdala, a central structure in the brain's fear circuitry, sends a distress signal to the hypothalamus, which in turn activates a biochemical cascade via the hypothalamus–pituitary–adrenal (HPA) axis.[18] As part of this cascade, the adrenal gland produces cortisol, a hormone that activates the sympathetic nervous system and swiftly mobilizes the body's energy stores.[19–21]

Chronic overactivation of this fear circuitry may affect the development and regulation of other brain systems, including those that control learning, memory, and mood.[20,22] Over time, without a secure, safe foundation, repeat trauma may reduce a person's "window of tolerance": that is, the range of external stimuli within which they feel calm and in control, smoothly alternating between gradual sympathetic activation and parasympathetic relaxation.[23] As a result, they may be more likely to experience sympathetic hyperactivation in response to seemingly innocuous stimuli, including sensory *triggers* that elicit memories and emotions associated with a specific traumatic experience.[10] Some triggers, like revisiting the location of a prior trauma, are easier to identify and avoid; others, like experiencing similar weather conditions, are less predictable, but often just as distressing. A person may also be triggered by an interpersonal or even spatial dynamic that reflects the loss of power or control they felt during a past traumatic experience. For instance, a person who has experienced IPV in the past may experience severe distress when spoken to in a raised voice or touched without consent. A person who was previously involved in a school shooting may have a similar reaction to somebody inadvertently blocking the door during a conversation. Without a clear understanding of trauma, such a response may seem like an "over-reaction"—but this is not the case. Rather, this is a conditioned, automatic physiological and emotional response to assure safety against perceived danger.

Trauma survivors may also experience a higher degree of sympathetic arousal at baseline, marked by "fight" symptoms (e.g., anger, combativeness) and "flight" symptoms (e.g., anxiety, mistrust, and hypervigilance see Table 10-1).[24] At extremely high levels of arousal, the dorsal vagal nerve triggers a reactionary hypoarousal, or "freeze," marked by "collapse" symptoms (e.g., depression or hopelessness) and "dissociation" symptoms (described in greater depth below).[20,22,25] Symptoms from any or all of these categories may be observed in individuals who have experienced acute or prolonged trauma. Some behavioral scientists have proposed that deliberate self-harm (e.g., cutting), substance use, and other maladaptive coping mechanisms among trauma survivors may represent attempts to control this often unpredictable biochemical dysregulation.[23]

Some people with a history of trauma may also experience dissociation, an unconscious protective mechanism mediated by the dorsal vagal nerve. During a "dissociative episode," a person temporarily disconnects from their own emotions, thoughts, memories, body, and/or present circumstances to avoid experiencing the pain and stress of trauma. Dissociation may occur in the moment of a traumatic event itself, or in response to a posttraumatic trigger that may or may not be recognized by observers. A person experiencing dissociation may appear "shut down" or unresponsive to communication, almost as though in a trance. They may appear frozen, or they may behave erratically and appear extremely distressed. After "coming to" or emerging from this dissociative state, they may have little to no recollection of what just occurred.[26] Those who have experienced particularly severe traumatic stress may even manifest several discrete personalities which may emerge or re-emerge in response to triggers, a phenomenon termed "Dissociative Identity Disorder" (formerly known as Multiple Personality Disorder).[26]

Altogether, neurobiological derangements from trauma can have lasting effects on the body. Over time, repeated stress stimuli may result in a phenomenon called *allostatic load*, in which a person's homeostatic "set point" is increased to accommodate higher levels of cortisol, as well as proinflammatory molecules called *cytokines*.[27] Chronically elevated levels of these molecules may contribute to higher rates of heart disease, cancer, autoimmune disease, and other illnesses among those who have experienced ACEs or other traumatic events.[27] Further, multiple studies have suggested that trauma and chronic stress may exert *epigenetic effects*, causing changes to DNA that are passed to future generations outside of typical genetic mechanisms.[28] For example, chronic stress may lead to shortening of *telomeres*, the repetitive nucleotide sequences that protect DNA from deterioration. This triggers cells to die prematurely, potentially resulting in higher rates of disease, accelerated aging, and lower overall health among those who have experienced trauma—as well as their descendants.[29]

Such a detailed discussion of neurobiology may seem out of place in a chapter about emotional communication strategies. However, it is especially crucial to understand trauma's neurodevelopmental underpinnings in this context, for two main reasons. First, we emphasize that while trauma is a deeply personal and subjective experience, it has repeatedly demonstrated a consistent, objective neurodevelopmental imprint, which translates into adverse emotional and physical health outcomes. Simply put, trauma is real, and its presence within emotional interactions merits rigorous consideration. Second, we feel that this insight into trauma's neurobiological underpinnings offers hope. As we describe in the following sections, relationship-building, mindfulness-based somatic practices and other strategies may help activate the ventral (or "front") vagus nerve, reversing many of the neurobiological processes described above and expanding the "window of tolerance." By forming trusting, respectful, informed relationships with those who have experienced trauma, we may begin to harness resilience and foster healing—for our patients, our colleagues, and ourselves.

Race-Based Traumatic Stress: Acknowledging the Emotional Trauma of Structural Violence

Before embarking on a discussion of trauma-informed strategies for emotional communication, the authors would like to highlight the often severe emotional trauma of structural violence, which is less often discussed than the trauma sustained from primary events like IPV, child abuse, or combat. Coined by sociologist Johan Gultang, structural violence describes a subtler form of violence in which social, political, cultural, and economic constructions prevent individuals and communities from meeting societal and basic needs.[30] Pertinent examples include ageism, nationalism, racism, sexism, and ableism; many of which have demonstrated significant contribution to disease prevalence and outcomes.[31,32] Much like trauma sustained from primary events, the trauma of structural violence can also stem from a loss of power and control, resulting in a similar biochemical cascade that may ultimately shape how a patient or clinician expresses or perceives emotion in a clinical context.[33]

> *Consider a 44-year-old Black woman who presents to a clinic with elevated blood pressure, fatigue, and upper back pain. Her clinician, a white male, begins collecting a medical history. During the interview, the patient appears defensive and speaks in a guarded tone. Last week, the police in a nearby city murdered an unarmed 17-year-old Black boy, sparking a widely publicized debate about extra-judicial killings of Black men and outrage from community members. She has two sons, 25 and 15 years old.*

Race-based traumatic stress refers to the emotional stress and pain one experiences as a result of discrimination due to racial or ethnic identification.[34] It is a form of toxic stress that occurs in response to structural violence, specifically experiences of racism, including media attention of violence toward minority groups, daily "microaggressions," and lower access to basic resources and societal privilege. Starting from a young age (as noted in the "expanded ACEs" study referenced earlier[16]), cumulative race-based traumatic stress may elicit a similar physiologic response to that seen in ACEs, IPV, and other acute traumatic events. Over time, this may result in a heightened sensitivity to danger, sense of a foreshortened future, depression, and maladaptive coping mechanisms, as well as physical symptoms including upper back pain and fatigue, and conditions such as hypertension.[35] Black women are among the highest-risk groups for the cumulative toxic stress of structural violence, including race-based traumatic stress.[36] Based on a number of high-quality studies, the "weathering hypothesis" proposes that toxic stress-mediated telomere shortening causes accelerated "biological aging" (i.e., earlier deterioration of overall health) in Black women.[29]

While this patient's hypertension, fatigue, and back pain should be evaluated with the same diagnostic rigor as one would for any other patient, it is also essential to be mindful of the ways in which the experience of structural violence may affect her overall physical and emotional health, as well as her emotional perception and behavior within this clinical encounter. Last week's shooting may have triggered her chronic race-based traumatic stress, or possibly a specific traumatic memory of her own, resulting in sympathetic hyperactivation. This stress may be compounded by the vulnerability of being in an unfamiliar clinical setting, as well as mistrust of the healthcare system based on centuries of abusive, coercive, and nonconsensual research and clinical practices against Black people.[1-5] The race and/or gender of the clinician may also be triggering for her. Her low tone and closed-off body language may be misinterpreted as an expression of hostility when they may represent an adaptive response to prolonged, potentially *intersectional trauma:* that is, trauma endured from a combination of personal and/or structural experiences.[37] However, without inquiring sensitively, the clinician will never know which factors are true for her. Use of trauma-informed emotional communication skills will greatly aid the clinician in serving this patient.

While not discussed in depth in this chapter, a similar dynamic may affect those experiencing other forms of structural violence, like ageism, ableism, transphobia, homophobia, misogyny, and weightism. All of these may overlap with each other and with the traumatic experiences described above, underscoring the importance of an intersectional approach to understanding and managing trauma. Ultimately, we must work to approach all clinical interactions—particularly those with a heightened level of emotional intensity—with the understanding that any person, regardless of their presentation, may be a survivor of acute or chronic trauma, while acknowledging that some groups of people are more likely to have experienced the trauma of structural violence based simply on their identity, appearance, or socioeconomic circumstances.

▦ WHAT IS TRAUMA-INFORMED CARE?

SAMHSA defines and advocates for a trauma-informed approach to healthcare—also referred to as trauma-informed care (TIC)—in their 2014 report, "SAMHSA's Concept of Trauma and Guidance for a Trauma-Informed Approach."[38] This report, developed in consultation with subject-matter experts as well as trauma survivors, establishes the need for a "multipronged, multiagency public health approach" to recognizing and treating trauma.[38] Beyond strategies for individual patient care, SAMHSA advocates for "an organizational or community context that is trauma-informed, that is, based on the knowledge and understanding of trauma and its far-reaching implications."[38] They further assert that such an approach is essential to promoting positive outcomes and minimizing harm both for patients and for healthcare staff. They specifically highlight the importance of this approach within a clinical context, citing the impact of many patients' trauma histories on their health, and the potential of health interventions to aid in healing from trauma.[38]

SAMHSA provides four critical "assumptions" common to a TIC approach, referred to as the "four Rs": the *realization* of trauma's widespread impact on clients, families, and staff; the *recognition* of trauma's signs and symptoms; an appropriate institutional and interpersonal *response* to this information; and an active effort to *resist re-traumatization*.[38] Regarding the first two Rs, "realization" and "recognition," we emphasize that a person's trauma is very often invisible to others. To this end, a number of professional societies recommend regular screening for ACEs, IPV, and other forms of trauma, often using standardized questionnaires; see Appendix A for a more in-depth discussion of screening for IPV. In addition to the signs and symptoms listed in Table 10-1, certain patterns of clinical care may raise concern for the presence of trauma. These are summarized in Table 10-2.

Regarding the second two Rs, "response" and "resist re-traumatization," SAMHSA offers six "key principles" that may be used to guide trauma-informed behaviors and policies. These principles include *safety*; *trustworthiness and transparency*; *peer support*; *collaboration and mutuality*; *empowerment, voice, and choice*; and *cultural, historical, and gender issues*.[38] Understanding that trauma deeply shapes and is shaped by emotional interactions, we can use SAMHSA's six

■ **TABLE 10-1. Symptoms of Sympathetic "Hyperarousal" and Parasympathetic "Hypoarousal"**

Sympathetic "hyperarousal"	**Parasympathetic** "hypoarousal"/"freeze"
"Fight" symptoms: Rage, anger, irritation, frustration, combativeness	**"Collapse" symptoms:** depression, hopelessness, shame, fatigue, preparation for death
"Flight" symptoms: Panic, fear, anxiety, worry, concern, hypervigilance, mistrust	**Dissociation symptoms:** numbness, emotional "shut-down," memory loss

Source: Adapted from Ref. 25.

■ **TABLE 10-2. Care Patterns Concerning for Presence of Trauma**

- Poor control of chronic medical conditions, including nonadherence to prescribed treatment
- Repeat visits to ED or clinic
- Patient is reluctant to undergo physically invasive exams, including genital or oral exam
- Inconsistent primary care, including late/sporadic prenatal care in women experiencing IPV
- In cases of IPV, partner (if present in clinical encounter) could appear anywhere on the spectrum from controlling/overly involved to indifferent

"key principles" to derive strategies for maintaining a trauma-informed approach to emotion communication in a clinical setting. We have briefly defined these "key principles," along with corresponding communication strategies and sample phrases, in Table 10-3. The following section will describe many of these strategies in greater detail, using illustrative clinical scenarios.

■ TRAUMA-INFORMED STRATEGIES FOR GUIDING EMOTION COMMUNICATION IN A CLINICAL ENCOUNTER

During her first shift as a resident in the Emergency Department (ED), Stephanie overhears sniffling coming from Room Four. She looks at the ED tracking board and sees that the patient is a 19-year-old woman, Alexa. The chief complaint reads, "vaginal issues." Upon entering Alexa's room, in which she is separated from another patient by just a thin curtain, Stephanie hears Alexa tell the nurse that she has just been sexually assaulted by her boyfriend, who came home intoxicated after a night of drinking. Alexa turns towards Stephanie, her eyes red and puffy. Stephanie pauses.

■ **TABLE 10-3. Summary of Communication Strategies and Sample Phrases by Principle of Trauma-Informed Care**

Principle	Communication strategies	Sample phrases
Safety: Ensure and convey physical and emotional safety for patients, staff, and clinicians.	Observe the Four Cs: **Calm:** Minimize extra stimuli; speak in a calm, even tone; maintain nonthreatening body language; clear path to exits. **Contain:** Offer private room; ensure confidentiality; only discuss what patient is comfortable discussing; respect patients' personal space and minimize unnecessary physical touch (unless patient consents to use of therapeutic touch). **Care:** Share verbal messages of support and acknowledgment; use signage, pins, brochures, and other visual cues to convey support for a diverse array of identity groups (e.g., a "Black Lives Matter" sign, or gender-inclusive "pronoun pins" for staff). **Cope:** Offer a centering exercise, e.g., mindful deep breathing; work with patient to develop a safety/well-being plan.	"This [ER / hospital / clinic] is one of the safest places you can be right now, even if it can look a bit chaotic at times." "We don't have to discuss any details you're not comfortable sharing." "I'm sorry ____ has happened,.. ____ is not your fault. My team and I are here to help you." "I hear you." "Shall we take some slow, deep breaths together? "In the event that something bad were to happen to you, or you were in danger, do you have a plan for who you would contact and a safe place to go?"
Trustworthiness and Transparency: Maximize transparency in as many clinical and administrative processes as possible, with the goal of building and maintaining trust with patients, family members, and staff.	**Trustworthiness:** State and ensure confidentiality; welcome supportive friends/family if applicable. **Transparency:** Clearly disclose any state- or institution-specific limits to confidentiality; clarify professional role; explain steps and procedures in advance.	"Everything you tell me today is confidential." *[Clearly state any exceptions related to patient safety such as mandated reporting]* (after assessing for safety) "Is there anyone here with you today? Would you like them to join us?"

(continued)

■ **TABLE 10-3. Summary of Communication Strategies and Sample Phrases by Principle of Trauma-Informed Care** (*Continued*)

Principle	Communication strategies	Sample phrases
Peer Support and Mutual Self-help: Value the lived experiences and perspectives of people with trauma histories; encourage these patients to connect with others who share similar experiences, to harness resilience and promote healing.	Provide information on local peer support groups and other organizations that support those who have experienced trauma; discuss and normalize the traumatic response; provide printed educational materials at the patient's educational level and in their preferred language.	"People respond to trauma in different ways. Many people may experience flashbacks, nightmares, sleep changes, feelings of decreased interest, isolation, and other short- or long-term symptoms. These are an expected part of the response to trauma. We can talk more about them whenever you'd like." "Would you like some printed information on trauma that you can read later on? If that feels less safe you can also keep this safety card in your phone case" "[Name of organization] is a great local organization that connects people who have experienced trauma through group meetings and other resources. Would you like their contact information? You can reach out to them whenever you choose."
Collaboration and Mutuality: Promote shared decision-making and mutual collaboration with patients, employees, and students who have a history of trauma.	**For individuals:** Use body language to convey attentiveness (sit at eye level, maintain eye contact, lean slightly forward); minimize distractions in clinical space; offer shared "centering exercise"; verbally emphasize the importance of shared decision making. **For institutions:** Actively solicit anonymous feedback from patients, employees, and trainees regarding necessary changes, as well as confidential reporting of bias or mistreatment.	"Before we talk more, would you like to do a quick mindfulness exercise to help us center our thoughts together? This is totally optional." "There are a number of different steps we could take next." "I want us to work together to come up with a plan that works best for you." "How does this plan sound to you?"

Empowerment, Voice, and Choice: Ensure that patients retain choice and control during decision making, while promoting patient empowerment with an emphasis on skill building.	**Empowerment:** Clarify patient's goals; acknowledge resilience and bravery; offer self-administration of sensitive exams; offer positive coping strategies. **Voice:** Pause frequently to allow patient to speak; use empathic statements. **Choice:** Provide options for care; obtain consent and assent as appropriate for each component of the visit and physical exam.	"What are your priorities for today's visit? I want to make sure we address what's important to you." "You are in control of everything we do and talk about here today." "Please tell me if anything I do or say makes you uncomfortable." "That sounds very frustrating / painful." "You are very brave for sharing your story with me. Thank you." "Is there anything I can do to help make this experience more comfortable for you?" "A physical exam would help me better understand what treatment you need, if any. Is it OK if I [describe specific maneuvers and rationale] today?"
Combatting Structural Violence: Institutions and individuals recognize and mitigate the traumatic effects of structural violence on patients, employees, and students, using behaviors, policies, protocols, and processes that are responsive to their racial, ethnic, cultural, and gender needs.	**For individuals:** Sensitively inquire about experiences of structural violence in patients with higher risk of these experiences (e.g., patients of racial/ethnic minority identities); inquire about and respect religious/cultural preferences regarding care to the extent possible. **For institutions:** Hire and support a diverse clinical staff that represents the many identities and experiences of their patient population; provide mandatory training on diversity, equity, and inclusion (DEI), bias/mistreatment, and trauma-informed care for all employees and students; provide welcoming signage and signals such as pronoun pins; offer interpreters at all steps of the clinical process, including scheduling and checkout.	"Experiencing [racism / sexism / homophobia / xenophobia, etc.] can be very stressful, and even traumatic. Do you feel like any of these have been affecting you?" Even though I can't know everything about your experiences of [racism / sexism / homophobia / xenophobia, etc.], I want you to know that I am sorry that you have gone through [racism / sexism / homophobia / xenophobia, etc.], and want to be your ally to help in any way that I can. "Do you have any religious or cultural beliefs that might affect your care today? I want to make sure I am accommodating your specific needs as best I can."

Source: Adapted from "Fostering Resilience and Recovery: A Change Package for Advancing Trauma-Informed Primary Care," National Council for Behavioral Health, 2020, and Ref. 38.

Patients with a history of trauma require a "safe, trusting, available, and predictable healthcare environment that does not re-traumatize."[39] In that moment of pause, how can Stephanie use the principle of *safety* to guide her interaction with Alexa?

As the nurse finishes taking Alexa's vitals, Stephanie introduces herself calmly and quietly. "Hi Alexa, my name is Dr. Velasquez, and I am the doctor who will be taking care of you today. Room 23 is open—would it be OK if we went there to talk briefly?" Alexa nods affirmatively and walks with Stephanie to room 23, a private room with no other patients. After they both enter the room, Stephanie says, "Please feel free to sit wherever you'd prefer." Alexa sits in a chair near the door. Stephanie asks, "Is it OK if I close the door so we can speak confidentially?" Alexa again nods. Stephanie closes the door, and sits down on a chair in the opposite corner.

Stephanie continues to monitor her own body language, leaning slightly forward and making clear eye contact with Alexa while maintaining a calm, neutral facial expression. She speaks in a soft, even tone of voice. "Everything you tell me is strictly confidential. In this state, doctors are not required to get Law Enforcement involved in these situations, but we can discuss that as an option if that's something you'd like to do. Before we start, I'd like to clarify that you're in control of everything that happens here. I'm here to listen to you and help you, and I'm going to be here for you the entire time you're in the emergency department. I will talk you through and explain anything we do, and will get your permission before proceeding. If you ever have any questions or feel uncomfortable, please let me or your nurse know. Remember, we are here for you."

Stephanie pauses, leaving space for Alexa to process the words. After counting to ten in her head, Stephanie asks, "What are you most concerned about? I want to make sure we address your priorities." She notices that Alexa is looking down at her hands and at the door more than she's looking at her. After another ten seconds, Stephanie says, "The hospital is the safest place you could be right now. Security is here to prevent unauthorized personnel from entering." Alexa nods and tearfully begins telling Stephanie what happened.

Upon recognizing that Alexa had come to the ED following a traumatic event, Stephanie asks to move their conversation to a private room. Limiting the presence of external stimuli helps ensure the safety and well-being of patients who may be experiencing hypervigilance or other manifestations of sympathetic hyperarousal following a traumatic event.[24] Patients may feel safer discussing frightening or upsetting topics in a private room, away from nonparticipatory healthcare staff.[24] Stephanie also monitors her body language and tone to be as nonthreatening as possible. She is also careful not to block the door, understanding that Alexa may be highly sensitive to perceived danger at this time. She mentions the hospital's security guards to explicitly reassure Alexa of her physical safety, including from her assailant.

When considering other strategies for conveying emotional and physical safety in a clinical encounter, we recommend following Kimberg and Wheeler's "Four Cs" of TIC, introduced in the table above: *Calm, Contain, Care,* and *Cope*.[11] Minimizing extra stimuli, speaking in a calm, even tone, maintaining nonthreatening body language, and leaving a clear, unobstructed path to the nearest exit can all help promote a sense of *calm* in the interaction, conveying to the patient that they are in a safe space. Offering a private room whenever possible, ensuring confidentiality, and limiting the detail of the trauma history when appropriate can help *contain* the traumatic event and limit the risk of re-traumatization. After a patient describes a traumatic experience, sharing a message of support and acknowledgment—for example, "I am here for you," or, "You are brave for sharing your story"—can remind them that you are an ally who *cares* about their health and well-being. Offering to participate in a centering exercise, like mindful deep breathing, can promote positive *coping* skills while creating a sense of shared safe space.

Stephanie's emphasis on *trustworthiness and transparency* is closely connected to the sense of safety she promotes. She conveys *trustworthiness* by stating the confidentiality of their conversation; this may be enhanced by welcoming a supportive friend or family member into the encounter whenever possible, as well as offering support from a hospital or local Rape Crisis Service if available. In the interest of *transparency*, it is also important to inform patients of the limits of confidentiality with respect to their medical records, including any opt-in or opt-out policies regarding confidentiality, as well as your jurisdiction's specific laws regarding mandated reporting to law enforcement.[10] Stephanie further promotes transparency by clarifying her professional role and explaining what Alexa can expect while in the ED. Where applicable, it may also be helpful to provide written materials that the patient can review in private, including information about local resources.

Stephanie uses several strategies to promote a sense of *empowerment, voice, and choice* in her interaction with Alexa. Stephanie *empowers* Alexa by telling her, "You're in control of everything that happens here." You may empower your patients by acknowledging their resilience and bravery as they share their experiences with you and offering self-administration of sensitive exam maneuvers, including self-swabbing and self-guided speculum insertion.[24] Stephanie prioritizes Alexa's *voice* by telling her, "I'm here to listen to you and help you," and frequently pausing to allow her to speak. We also recommend acknowledging and validating patients' emotions with empathetic statements such as, "I hear you" or, "That sounds very frustrating." Stephanie offers Alexa as many *choices* as possible, inquiring regarding her priorities and allowing her to direct the flow of their interaction. Even seemingly small choices, like where to sit in the room or the gender of the staff involved in their care, can help a patient to feel more in control of an otherwise stressful situation.[24] In addition to a formal informed consent process, it is crucial to obtain assent from patients before completing each aspect of the physical exam, as touch (especially nonconsensual touch) may be triggering or re-traumatizing for patients with a history of trauma.[40] Similarly, be sure to ask patients' permission before allowing any new people to enter the room, or involving law enforcement.[24]

Stephanie uses both verbal and nonverbal cues to promote a sense of *collaboration and mutuality* in her conversation with Alexa. Sitting at eye level with Alexa, leaning forward, and making eye contact help convey attentiveness and respect for what Alexa has to say. In fact, merely sitting during an encounter with a patient is associated with greater patient-reported satisfaction, a sense of being understood, and even a longer perceived duration of the encounter.[41] Additionally, minimizing distractions (including moving patients to a private room, as discussed above) can improve the sense of connection and focus between patient and clinician.[42] Later in their conversation, Stephanie may also consider offering Alexa some positive coping strategies, including deep breathing and mindfulness-based exercises that help activate the parasympathetic nervous system and promote relaxation. Leading Alexa through one or more of these exercises may contribute to a sense of shared space and effort between herself and Alexa, while helping Alexa to build a positive practice for mitigating the stress of her traumatic experience.

While Stephanie does not specifically address *peer support and mutual self-help* in this early portion of her conversation with Alexa, she could accomplish this later on by providing Alexa with information regarding a local organization that supports those who have experienced trauma.[24] Some patients may benefit from a referral to a trauma support group, where they may build trusting, healing relationships with other trauma survivors. Others may benefit from educational materials designed by people who have experienced trauma themselves. Learning about the many potential physical and emotional reactions to traumatic experiences—especially from the perspective of other trauma survivors—can normalize these symptoms, paving the way for the development of healthy coping strategies.[43]

In the above clinical scenario, Alexa presents to the emergency department shortly following a traumatic event. However, as discussed in the preceding sections, ACEs and other more remote traumatic events may still play an active role in a present-day clinical encounter.[44] Consider the following scenario (adapted, with names changed, from a real case):

Dr. Wallace's next patient is Terrance "Terry" Williamson, a 61-year-old White man who has seen her for primary care for over a decade. According to the medical assistant, Terry's primary concern today is difficulty with urination, which is a new issue for him. While reviewing his chart, Dr. Wallace recalls Terry's history of child abuse, which he disclosed at a previous visit. She remembers having an intensely emotional conversation with Terry about his traumatic childhood experiences, including being prostituted by his parents, who struggled with untreated substance and alcohol use disorders.

Over the past 15 years, Dr. Wallace has developed a close and trusting therapeutic partnership with Terry. On several occasions, Terry has told Dr. Wallace that he tends to be more "on guard" around other clinicians but is more willing to share details of his life, past and present, with her. Dr. Wallace has seen Terry through his alcohol use disorder, as well as six months of incarceration. She recalls the moment in which Terry came out to her as gay after a decades-long marriage to a woman. She thinks about how much more empowered and happy Terry has seemed over the past several years, how much joy and satisfaction he feels in his volunteer work at the local community garden. She knocks on the clinic room door. "Come in." She opens the door. "Good to see you again, Terry!" "Hey doc."

Terry is seated on the exam table, his eyes downcast, hands clasped together. Dr. Wallace moves to avoid blocking the door. Terry is quieter today than he has been recently, not his usual gregarious self. "May I sit?" Asks Dr. Wallace, gesturing towards the chair farthest from the door. Terry nods affirmatively. Dr. Wallace sits and says, quietly, "I'm here for you, Terry. What can I do to help you feel safe and comfortable today?"

Terry looks up. "That's the thing, doc. I don't know if you can help." Terry goes on to describe several months of frequent urination, as well as difficulty maintaining an erection. Dr. Wallace talks through the possible causes of Terry's symptoms and potential treatment options. When she brings up a referral to a specialist, Terry's eyes widen. "I don't want to see anyone but you, doc."

Dr. Wallace does her best to reassure Terry that she can facilitate a careful referral to a specialist she trusts, but Terry maintains that he's not interested. "You know I'm a private person. I don't need anyone else knowing my business."

Dr. Wallace pauses for a moment, allowing time for Terry to elaborate. He doesn't. After a period of silence, she offers to print out a list of specialists in the area, along with their photos and brief biographies. After returning from the printer, she points out four specialists, two male, and two female, who specialize in the urologic care of LGBTQ+ individuals. Terry takes out a pen, circles these clinicians' photos, and agrees to look into a few options before his follow-up appointment in 2 weeks.

Dr. Wallace uses many of the strategies described in the prior scenario to convey safety, offer choice, and empower Terry to lead the conversation and voice his concerns. In a significant departure from the prior scenario, which took place in the Emergency Department, this encounter underscores the role of *clinician continuity* (i.e., the ability for a patient to be seen by a consistent clinician or small set of clinicians) in TIC. Through a year-long relationship of providing affirming, compassionate care, Dr. Wallace has built a trusting therapeutic alliance with Terry, who is now able to openly and honestly convey his concerns. Conversely, Dr. Wallace has become attuned to how Terry's history of trauma has impacted his physical and mental health in the past, allowing her to intuit that his current symptoms may be triggering his past trauma. Indeed, TIC is often a long, dialogical process of laying emotional groundwork and building trust.

However, the closeness of this therapeutic alliance may also present its own challenges. As described earlier in this chapter, individuals who have experienced trauma—especially ACEs—often struggle to develop secure relationships. Once a patient and clinician have developed a safe therapeutic alliance, as Dr. Wallace and Terry have done, it may be difficult for the patient to feel safe or comfortable working with other healthcare professionals. Empowering patients to see other clinicians when necessary—in Terry's case, a urologist, whose specialized training will ensure an optimal clinical outcome—is an often challenging but crucial part of developing a functional therapeutic alliance. It helps to draw upon a close professional network of trusted colleagues and peers, whose care and trustworthiness you may vouch for yourself. Some patients may appreciate printed information on local clinicians, including headshots and brief biographies, which help to humanize these clinicians and promote a sense of trustworthiness.

This case also highlights the importance of an intersectional approach to TIC. Dr. Wallace is aware that Terry has experienced at least two major ACEs: being prostituted, a form of sexual abuse, as well as witnessing substance abuse in both of his parents. In addition to the above challenges with forming new therapeutic alliances, Dr. Wallace intuits that Terry may be particularly uncomfortable regarding his urologic care due to his history of sexual abuse.

This makes her efforts to promote a sense of trustworthiness among these new clinicians all the more important. Dr. Wallace is also aware that Terry has also relatively recently come out as gay, and may have endured prolonged traumatic stress related to this aspect of his identity, both before and since coming out. Referring Terry to a trusted urologist colleague who specializes in the care of LGBTQ+ people—or, if desired, one who self-identifies as a member of the LGBTQ+ community—may add another layer of comfort, familiarity, and safety.[43]

The above scenarios focus on patients with recent or remote histories of interpersonal trauma, specifically sexual assault and/or abuse. As important as it is to maintain a trauma-informed approach to communication surrounding interpersonal trauma, experiences of structural trauma also merit careful consideration. The following scenario focuses on Brian, a fourth-year medical student, and one of his patients, Jo.

Brian, a fourth-year medical student, goes to the Emergency Department to admit Jo, one of the hospital's "frequent fliers." Jo is a 17-year-old Black person who identifies as non-binary, and uses they/them/theirs pronouns. They have been to the ED 12 times in the past eight months for diabetic ketoacidosis (DKA). Every time Jo is admitted, they are treated for DKA, advised to take their insulin as prescribed, and discharged. Psychiatry has been consulted multiple times due to the concern that Jo may be exhibiting passively suicidal behavior by failing to take their insulin.

Before Brian can ask about Jo's symptoms, Jo launches into an indictment of the staff at the hospital. Jo says that the ED physician has refused to give them pain medication and that the nurses were rough with them. "Dr. Oakley keeps calling me a 'she,'" Jo says. "And they keep yelling at me for not taking my insulin, but I got fired from my job, and now I can't afford it." Jo says they feel afraid, mistreated, and alone. Brian sits down on a chair several feet from Jo's ED bed, and listens in silence as Jo tells their story. When Jo is done, Brian remains silent for several seconds, before replying in a calm, even tone. "I'm Brian. My pronouns are he, him, and his. I'm the doctor who will be taking care of you here in the emergency department. What's your name, and what are your preferred pronouns?"

Jo looks down at their hands, and then up again. "I'm Jo. They, them, theirs." Brian replies, "Hello, Jo. Thank you for telling me your story. I believe you. I'm so sorry that has happened. You don't deserve to be treated that way." After explaining the confidentiality of their interaction, Brian asks Jo what matters most to them regarding their care. Jo replies, "Could you get me some pain meds? Not opioids—my brother was addicted to them for a while. But the doctor won't even let me have Tylenol."

Brian employs many previously discussed strategies in his direct communication with Jo: introducing himself and his role; speaking calmly; sitting at eye level with Jo without obstructing the door; asking Jo about their priorities with respect to their care; acknowledging and validating their anger. However, Jo's story reveals an intersection of interpersonal and structural violence that occurred within what should be a safe, welcoming clinical space—all before Brian even entered the room.

Jo has already been labeled by clinicians as a *"frequent flier,"* a dismissive, often derogatory term used to imply that patients who frequently return to the hospital may be "gaming the system" for benefits beyond medical treatment.[45] Furthermore, Jo has been repeatedly chastised for not taking their insulin, in apparent ignorance of their inability to afford this medication. Clinicians are more likely to assume that their Black and Latinx patients are "noncompliant," among other negative stereotypes, when compared to their White patients.[46] Jo also reports undertreatment of their pain despite no obvious contraindications, which is unfortunately consistent with research demonstrating that healthcare professionals both underperceive and undertreat pain in their Black patients relative to their White patients.[47] Additionally, Jo has repeatedly been *misgendered* (i.e., referred to by pronouns corresponding to a gender identity that is not their own; in this case, "she, her, hers" rather than "they, them, theirs"), which may enhance *gender dysphoria* and is associated with several adverse mental health outcomes, most concerningly an astronomical rate of suicide, among transgender and gender nonconforming individuals.[48]

SAMHSA advocates for engaging "cultural, historical, and gender issues" in the provision of TIC. We want to reframe this principle to *recognize and mitigate the traumatic effects of structural violence* within a clinical encounter. Recognizing that Jo's repeated misgendering may be contributing to their stress within this encounter, Brian states his pronouns and asks Jo for theirs, in addition to their name. Outside of his direct interaction with Jo, how can Brian further respond to this encounter in a way that accounts for Jo's experiences of structural violence?

Brian finds Jo's ED physician, a White man in his 60's named Dr. Oakley, and asks if Jo has a contraindication to receiving pain medication. "Oh, her?" Dr. Oakley asks, looking over at Jo's bed. "She's in here all the time. Always wants narcotics. She can have Tylenol if she wants—does she not have an order in?"

Brian replies, "No, they don't have an order in for pain," emphasizing Jo's correct pronouns. "OK," replies Dr. Oakley. "I can change that for her." He adds Tylenol to Jo's order set. After a moment, Brian says, "Just to clarify, Jo uses they/them pronouns."

Even when Jo is not in the room, Brian uses ancillary communication skills to advocate for their needs by asking Dr. Oakley to treat Jo's pain and reminding him of the correct pronouns. Such recently coined "upstander" advocacy[49] directly counters a "hidden curriculum" that perpetuates bias and mistreatment against transgender and gender nonconforming patients, as well as racial/ethnic minority, low-income, and other marginalized patients. Without this intervention, Jo may be forced to advocate for theirself more insistently, speaking at a louder volume or in a more dissatisfied tone. As their stress is compounded by worsening pain, continued misgendering, and other microaggressions, the feeling of being repeatedly ignored may trigger memories of loss, abandonment, or disempowerment from prior structural and/or interpersonal traumas.

Additionally, Jo's increasing expressions of distress may be misinterpreted and pathologized by clinical staff less familiar with trauma.[43] Borderline personality disorder (BPD) is characterized by "unstable interpersonal relationships, fear of abandonment, difficulties in emotion regulation, feelings of emptiness, chronic dysphoria or depression, as well as impulsivity and heightened risk-taking behaviors."[50] Overlap between these symptoms and the symptoms of trauma discussed above likely contributes to the strong association observed between BPD and a history of trauma.[51] Unfortunately, the stigma surrounding BPD may further challenge the formation of meaningful therapeutic alliances for these patients.[52] The resultant cycle of distress and dismissal contributes to subpar clinical outcomes, underscoring the importance of listening to, validating, and responding to the emotions of our patients who have experienced trauma.

This encounter may also present an important opportunity to connect Jo with a primary care clinician, as well as a trauma-informed case manager who can help ensure that Jo has access to food, housing, transportation, and other fundamental resources. Empowering Jo to foster a therapeutic alliance with a healthcare professional could help to mitigate the stress they have experienced in their challenging, potentially traumatizing interactions with the healthcare system thus far. Keeping in mind Jo's experiences of structural violence, it is particularly important to offer the option of a *race-concordant* healthcare professional who is experienced in the care of LGBTQ+ (especially transgender and gender nonconforming) individuals. Considering all healthcare professionals hope to provide excellent, compassionate care for each of their patients, it is important to cultivate a sensitivity to our patients' potential experiences of structural violence. With this said, multiple studies have demonstrated that while patients of racial/ethnic minority identities consistently report lower satisfaction, communication quality, and participatory decision-making with their clinicians than do White patients, this disparity is significantly improved when these patients are cared for by physicians of the same racial/ethnic identity (i.e., patient–physician race concordance).[53,54] (See Chapter 12, Culture and Emotions in the Medical Encounter, for further discussion of diversity.) Limited racial/ethnic diversity among healthcare professionals in many practices and health systems—due to employment discrimination,[55] wage discrepancy,[56] and other manifestations of racism among institutional leadership—is just one of many ways in which institutional bias contributes to the continued re-traumatization of minority patients.

Identifying and mitigating instances of structural violence may be more challenging for some than the communication strategies described previously. However, this effort is one of our most important opportunities as trauma-informed healthcare professionals to validate our patients' distress, advocate for their needs, and promote their health and well-being. It can also be helpful to utilize signs, brochures, and other visual cues that convey a sense of safety and belonging to patients of historically and presently marginalized identity groups. For instance, multiple studies have suggested that "pronoun pins" (i.e., pins worn by faculty, staff, and students, displaying their respective preferred gender pronouns) and LGBTQ-centric brochures and signage often indicate a welcoming environment to LGBTQ+ individuals.[57-59] Similarly, prominently displaying a "Black Lives Matter" sign in your clinic or office can help convey a commitment to antiracism and promote a sense of safety and belonging among BIPOC (black, indigenous, and people of color) patients. These visual cues do not replace individual and systemic efforts to mitigate structural violence; rather, they remind patients, staff, and students of an institution's continued commitment to these efforts.

■ TRAUMA-INFORMED SYSTEMS: SUPPORTING PATIENTS AND PROFESSIONALS FROM THE GROUND UP

Trauma-Informed Systems: Definition and Justification

The case of Jo and Brian underscores the importance of designing *trauma-informed systems*. In addition to providing compassionate, trauma-informed patient care, healthcare professionals and students are in a critical position to advocate for institutional policies and structures that minimize direct or covert trauma to our patients. Consider the following scenario:

Hafsa is a middle-aged Arabic-speaking refugee woman with multiple visits to the Emergency Department over the past year, due to recurrent urinary tract infections and uncontrolled diabetes. When the student "hotspotting" team, along with a professional medical interpreter, entered Hafsa's public housing apartment for their first home visit, she and her 12-year-old daughter greeted them with nervous smiles. The team introduced themselves and assured Hafsa of the confidentiality of their visit. Hafsa became tearful when she learned that an interpreter accompanied the student team. She was dreading having to rely on her daughter to interpret for her. She explained how horrible she feels as a mother having to rely on her daughter to communicate at the grocery store, the bank, or even the emergency department. The team asked her if she was ever offered interpreters in any of those places. She avoided the question, but the rest of the visit went well as the team focused on building rapport.

As the group delved into her health needs over the next few weeks, Hafsa shared a large folder filled with after-visit summaries from the ED, unfiled "charity care" applications, and unfilled prescriptions. When the team politely asked Hafsa what was preventing her from taking the prescribed antibiotics or connecting with a primary care doctor, it was evident that there were other barriers beyond the cost of her care. As Hafsa began to trust the team, she shared that she had stopped going to her primary care doctor after a phone interpreter told her she would die soon if she did not start taking insulin. She also expressed discomfort with often being assigned a male clinician in the past without being given an option. Based on her cultural and religious practices as a Muslim, she preferred to be seen by female clinicians if available, especially for intimate care such as OBGYN and physical therapy. Afraid, traumatized, and unable to afford costly medications, she had stopped engaging with healthcare altogether.

After six home visits that focused primarily on rebuilding trust through non-judgmental listening, Hafsa felt empowered to identify the social, financial, and health barriers that prevented her from feeling healthy in all domains of her life. She soon re-established primary care with a better understanding of her disease process, and drastically improved management of her diabetes. She is now optimistic about her ability to manage her health and expressed interest in leading support groups to assist others in her community to improve their health. With Hafsa's permission, the team spoke with her primary medical clinic about the importance of using in-person interpreters whenever possible, without mentioning Hafsa specifically.

Hafsa's care demonstrates aspects of all six major components of TIC. The student team, which may be less intimidating to many patients than medical professionals, met Hafsa in her home, a space in which she feels physically and psychologically *safe*. The student team fostered *trustworthiness* with Hafsa by ensuring confidentiality and building rapport over several visits. They *empowered* Hafsa by listening attentively and validating her concerns. The in-person professional interpreter offered excellent *peer support* and helped mitigate the stress Hafsa had experienced due to a language barrier. Hafsa was also able to express her desire to establish care with a female primary care clinician according to her cultural and religious practices, allowing the student team an opportunity to ensure this for her in the future. Additionally, noting how Hafsa's trauma appeared to be mitigated by the presence of an in-person interpreter, the team advocated for a meaningful *systems-level change* (a change to a policy, community standard, or other structure that impacts many people employed and/or served by an organization) by asking her clinic to use in-person interpreters whenever possible.

The National Child Traumatic Stress Network (NCTSN) defines a trauma-informed system as follows[60]:

> A trauma-informed child and family service system is one in which all parties involved recognize and respond to the impact of traumatic stress on those who have contact with the system including children, caregivers, and service providers. Programs and agencies within such a system infuse and sustain trauma awareness, knowledge, and skills into their organizational cultures, practices, and policies. They act in collaboration with all those who are involved with the child, using the best available science, to maximize physical and psychological safety, facilitate the recovery of the child and family, and support their ability to thrive. A service system with a trauma-informed perspective is one in which agencies, programs, and service providers:

1. Routinely screen for trauma exposure and related symptoms.
2. Use evidence-based, culturally responsive assessment and treatment for traumatic stress and associated mental health symptoms.
3. Make resources available to children, families, and providers on trauma exposure, impact, and treatment.
4. Engage in efforts to strengthen the resilience and protective factors of children and families impacted by and vulnerable to trauma.
5. Address parent and caregiver trauma and its impact on the family system.
6. Emphasize continuity of care and collaboration across child-service systems.
7. Maintain an environment of care for staff that addresses, minimizes, and treats secondary traumatic stress, and that increases staff wellness.

While the NCTSN gears their recommendations toward pediatric care, the utility of such a system in the care of adults is clear. In addition to the individual behavioral strategies described in the preceding sections, trauma-informed systems employ larger-scale strategies and policies to minimize re-traumatization and promote safety, autonomy, and healing in patients and professionals.

For example, to address item #6 above, consider a protocol for identifying and reaching out to patients with high no-show rates or extended gaps in care and establishing these patients with a dedicated case manager. Rather than merely dismissing these patients as "noncompliant," this system could help to mitigate the root causes of this pattern, including financial stress, limited transportation, mistrust of clinicians due to personal or historical trauma, and other barriers to care. Considering Hafsa's case above, it is also important that all patients have access to an interpreter who speaks their primary language, so that they may express their needs as accurately and comfortably as possible. Regarding item #1, while healthcare professionals should regularly and sensitively screen for trauma exposure and related symptoms in their patients, health systems should also employ accessible, anonymous feedback channels whereby patients and employees may safely report bias, mistreatment, and other adverse experiences within the healthcare environment.

Keeping in mind Hafsa's case, as well as the earlier case of Jo and Brian, a crucial aspect of item #2 is the recruitment and support of a workforce that represents the diverse identities and experiences of the population it serves. This effort may be bolstered by mandatory institution-wide educational interventions, including Diversity, Equity and Inclusion (DEI)[61,62] and Safe Zone[63] trainings. While these programs are by no means sufficient to address the full depth and breadth of structural violence, they may help create a professional and educational community that is more sensitive to the potential of their words and actions to perpetuate or mitigate its effects.

Vicarious Trauma and Compassion Fatigue: Using Trauma-informed Systems to Promote Wellness and Prevent Burnout Among Medical Professionals

While the preceding sections have focused on trauma and its manifestations in patients, item #7 invites the use of trauma-informed systems to help mitigate *vicarious trauma* among medical professionals. While attentive, empathic, and emotional listening is a necessary component of TIC, repeatedly witnessing patients' recollection of traumatic experiences may introduce vicarious (also known as secondary) trauma. Described by the American Counseling Association as "the emotional residue of exposure from patient stories, which creates tension and preoccupation for the listener," vicarious trauma often has many similar effects to primary trauma.[64] Further, witnessing another person's trauma may be triggering to individuals with their own histories of trauma.[64]

Without proper emotional regulation and institutional support, repeated secondary trauma may lead to *compassion fatigue* and *burnout*, two closely related psychological stress responses. Compassion fatigue describes a combination of exhaustion, anger, irritability, "maladaptive" coping behaviors (e.g., alcohol/drug use), reduced capacity for sympathy and empathy, and impaired decision making that results from continued exposure to individuals who have experienced trauma.[65] Burnout describes feelings of detachment, cynicism, ineffectiveness, fatigue, and reduced satisfaction with one's professional work due to repeated stress in the professional setting.[66] Both of these contribute to performance impairment and adverse health outcomes, including rising suicide rates, among medical professionals and students (see Chapter 16, Striving and Thriving: Challenges and Opportunities for Clinician Emotional Wellness for more details).[1,65–67]

To illustrate this phenomenon, let's return to the discussion of Alexa, the patient who presents to the ED following a sexual assault, and Stephanie, the resident physician who is caring for her.

> *As Alexa describes the assault, Stephanie feels herself tensing up and notices her heart racing; her memory flashes to one night in college when a male friend climbed into her dorm bed with her and tried to coerce her into having sex against her will. She can see the memory clearly even though it happened almost 10 years ago; she still remembers the color of the jersey he was wearing, and her roommate's alarm clock that read 3:23 am in a glowing green font. Stephanie makes a conscious effort to relax her shoulders and slacken her face, taking a deep breath to calm her nervous system so as not to make Alexa even more distraught.*

Healthcare professionals are not immune to trauma; in fact, 68% of the healthcare workforce have experienced at least one episode of violence, abuse, or neglect at some point in their lives.[1] This scenario depicts the intersection of vicarious and primary trauma, as hearing Alexa's story triggers Stephanie to have a flashback of her own prior sexual assault. Stephanie vividly reexperiences visual details from this traumatic experience, distracted (albeit briefly) from her conversation with Alexa. By recognizing this trigger and engaging in a grounding exercise, Stephanie not only minimizes her own traumatic stress, but also reflects a sense of calm back onto Alexa.[68] If she is to remain emotionally available to her patients in their most challenging moments, it is crucial that Stephanie herself receives adequate support from a healthcare system that is sensitive to her own experiences of primary and vicarious trauma.

Addressing vicarious trauma and preventing burnout require a multi-pronged approach, combining individual- and systems-level interventions. Students and employees should be supported in making personal "wellness plans" incorporating individual and group mindfulness and body-based self-care practices, including physical exercise, yoga, meditation, reflective writing, and outdoor time, as well as opportunities to connect with peers and build community. These may all help to mitigate sympathetic hyperactivation and stimulate parasympathetic activation.[1] Health professional schools and health systems may help destigmatize mental health and promote self-care by offering free, anonymous counseling for students and employees and a cross-cover system (i.e., a system by which one clinician provides care for another's patients, with reciprocity at a later date) that allows for "mental health days" when necessary. Other specific scenarios call for their own interventions: for instance, excused absences and increased availability of school-sponsored, race-concordant mental health services for Black medical students and employees in light of increased publicization of police brutality against Black people.

As healthcare professionals, regardless of our specific clinical roles or personal experiences, we are all complex, multifaceted individuals who have met at the common goal of caring for others. We must work together to create a system that aids us in caring for others, while caring for ourselves as well.

■ THE PATH FORWARD: EFFECTING AND ADVOCATING FOR NECESSARY CHANGE

Trauma may be spoken or unspoken; recognized or unrecognized; acute or chronic; interpersonal or structural. Often, it is an intersection of many or all of these qualities. It may belong to the patient, to the clinician, or both. Trauma shapes a person's expression and perception of emotion; so, too, may an emotional exchange trigger the emergence of a prior traumatic experience or inflict new trauma itself. Trauma has well-documented biological effects, contributing to adverse health outcomes across several domains. Still, it remains an underrecognized and underaddressed presence within many clinical encounters. Without a thorough understanding of trauma and its effects on our patients, our colleagues, and in many cases ourselves, we miss crucial opportunities to aid in the healing process—and, at worst, risk unintentionally contributing to trauma through our own words and actions.

With this in mind, we urgently advocate for the widespread adaptation of a trauma-informed approach to emotion communication in a clinical setting, encompassing both interpersonal and systems-level interventions. Acknowledging and responding to trauma in an emotional interaction requires closely monitoring one's body language, tone of voice, word choice, and many other factors described throughout this chapter and in Table 10-3. It also involves actively maintaining an awareness of structural trauma, advocating for our patients' safety and well-being, and mitigating the impact of structural violence via institutional change. Just as we must monitor and adjust our own behavior, we must work to ensure that our colleagues, practices, and broader institutions also take responsibility for minimizing traumatization and re-traumatization of their patients and employees.

We hope that Table 10-3 will serve as an action plan for developing an individualized trauma-informed practice. Those looking to start a conversation about TIC in their respective institutions may consider distributing this table to institutional leadership and colleagues and holding a practice meeting to discuss them in an open, respectful environment. We are aware that Trauma-Informed Medical Education (TIME) competencies are being developed by a national group. Once validated, we urge the implementation of structured undergraduate and graduate medical education and faculty development in this critical area.[69]

Institutional leaders can contribute to these efforts by supporting employees and students in developing trauma-informed practices and policies, while adopting interventions to protect their health and well-being. Healthcare professionals and students are far from immune to trauma; on the contrary, caring for others can be a significant source of vicarious/secondary trauma, in addition to triggering past primary traumatic experiences. There is an urgent need for institutionally sponsored mental health resources for healthcare professionals and students, clearly defined pathways for reporting incidents of bias, mistreatment, and abuse, and protected space for these individuals to attend to self-care. The role of trauma-informed strategies in burnout prevention represents an important area of future research. However, the authors feel strongly that a lack of formal evaluation should not delay the implementation of these changes any further.

The authors acknowledge that an in-depth discussion of trauma and TIC is likely new to many readers. The changes we describe in this chapter—particularly on an institutional scale—will not happen overnight. This is all the more reason that we must start implementing these changes now: for our patients, and for each other. All of our well-being depends on it.

REFERENCES

1. Barnhill J, Fisher J, Kimel-Scott K, et al. *Trauma-Informed Care: Helping the Healthcare Team Thrive, in Trauma-Informed Healthcare Approaches.* Cham, Switzerland: Springer; 2019:197-213.

2. Dunkley BT, Wong SM, Jetly R, et al. Post-traumatic stress disorder and chronic hyper-connectivity in emotional processing. *Neuroimage Clin*. 2018;20:197-204.

3. Substance Abuse and Mental Health Services Administration (SAMHSA). Trauma and Violence. 2020. https://www.samhsa.gov/trauma-violence. Accessed October 9, 2020.

4. Crocq MA, Crocq L. From shell shock and war neurosis to posttraumatic stress disorder: a history of psychotraumatology. *Dialogues Clin Neurosci*. 2000;2(1):47-55.

5. National Center for PTSD, U.S. Department of Veterans Affairs. DSM-5 Criteria for PTSD. 2019. https://www.brainline.org/article/dsm-5-criteria-ptsd. Accessed October 20, 2020.

6. American Psychiatric Association. *Diagnostic and Statistical Manual of Mental Disorders*, 5th ed. Washington, D.C.; 2013.

7. Sanjel S. Gender-based violence: a crucial challenge for public health. *Kathmandu Univ Med J (KUMJ)*. 2013;11(42):179-184.

8. Rakovec-Felser Z. Domestic violence and abuse in intimate relationship from public health perspective. *Health Psychol Res*. 2014;2(3):1821.

9. Domestic Abuse Intervention Programs. "Wheels." 2017. https://www.theduluthmodel.org/wheels/. Accessed October 20, 2020.

10. Center for Substance Abuse Treatment (US). Understanding the impact of trauma. In: *Trauma-Informed Care in Behavioral Health Services*. Rockville, MD: Substance Abuse and Mental Health Services Administration (US), Treatment Improvement Protocol (TIP) Series, No. 57; 2014, Report No. (SMA) 14-4816.

11. Kimberg L, Wheeler MB. Trauma and trauma-informed care. In: King TE, Wheeler MB, eds. *The Medical Management of Vulnerable and Underserved Patients: Principles, Practice and Populations*. Upper Saddle River, NJ: McGraw-Hill Professional; 2016.

12. Flaherty SC, Sadler LS. A review of attachment theory in the context of adolescent parenting. *J Pediatr Health Care*. 2011;25(2):114-121.

13. Felitti VJ, Anda RF, Nordenberg D, et al. Relationship of childhood abuse and household dysfunction to many of the leading causes of death in adults: the Adverse Childhood Experiences (ACE) Study. *Am J Prev Med*. 1998;14(4):245-258.

14. Centers for Disease Control and Prevention. The ACE Pyramid. 2020. https://www.cdc.gov/violenceprevention/aces/about.html. Accessed October 24, 2020.

15. Winham SJ, Motsinger-Reif AA. The effect of retrospective sampling on estimates of prediction error for multifactor dimensionality reduction. *Ann Hum Genet*. 2011;75(1):46-61.

16. Wade RJ, Shea JA, Rubin D, Wood J. Adverse childhood experiences of low-income urban youth. *Pediatrics*. 2014;134(1):e13-e20.

17. Gill L. Understanding and Working with the Window of Tolerance. Adapted from Levine, Ogden and Siegel. 2017. https://www.attachment-and-trauma-treatment-centre-for-healing.com/blogs/understanding-and-working-with-the-window-. Accessed October 10, 2020.

18. Sherin JE, Nemeroff CB. Post-traumatic stress disorder: the neurobiological impact of psychological trauma. *Dialogues Clin Neurosci*. 2011;13(3):263-278.

19. Schore AN. Relational trauma, brain development, and dissociation. In: Ford JD, Courtois CA, eds. *Treating Complex Traumatic Stress Disorders in Children and Adolescents: Scientific Foundations and Therapeutic Models*. New York, NY: Guilford Press; 2013:3-23.

20. Shin LM, Liberzon I. The neurocircuitry of fear, stress, and anxiety disorders. *Neuropsychopharmacology.* 2010;35(1):169-191.

21. Harvard Health Publishing. Understanding the Stress Response: Chronic Activation of This Survival Mechanism Impairs Health. 2011. https://www.health.harvard.edu/staying-healthy/understanding-the-stress-response. Accessed October 10, 2020.

22. Teicher MH, Andersen SL, Polcari A, Anderson CM, Navalta CP. Developmental neurobiology of childhood stress and trauma. *Psychiatr Clin North Am.* 2002;25(2),397-426.

23. Corrigan FM, Fisher JJ, Nutt DJ. Autonomic dysregulation and the Window of Tolerance model of the effects of complex emotional trauma. *J Psychopharmacol.* 2011;25(1):17-25.

24. Fischer KR, Bakes KM, Corbin TJ, et al. Trauma-informed care for violently injured patients in the emergency department. *Ann Emerg Med.* 2019;73(2):193-202.

25. Walker, RJ. Polyvagal Chart. Adapted from Cheryl Sanders, Anthony "Twig" Wheeler, and Stephen Porges. 2017. https://www.rubyjowalker.com/PVchart6.pdf. Accessed October 10, 2020.

26. Şar V. The many faces of dissociation: opportunities for innovative research in psychiatry. *Clin Psychopharmacol Neurosci.* 2014;12(3):171-179.

27. Lee DY, Kim E, Choi MH. Technical and clinical aspects of cortisol as a biochemical marker of chronic stress. *BMB Rep.* 2015;48(4):209-216.

28. Yehuda R, Lehrner A. Intergenerational transmission of trauma effects: putative role of epigenetic mechanisms. *World Psychiatry.* 2018;17(3):243-257.

29. Simons RL, Lei MK, Beach SRH, et al. Economic hardship and biological weathering: the epigenetics of aging in a U.S. sample of black women. *Soc Sci Med.* 2016;150:192-200.

30. Farmer PE, Nizeye B, Stulac S, Keshavjee S. Structural violence and clinical medicine. *PLoS Med.* 2006;3(10):e449.

31. Chang E-S, Kannoth S, Levy S, Wang S-Y, Lee JE, Levy BR. Global reach of ageism on older persons' health: a systematic review. *PLoS One.* 2020;15(1):e0220857.

32. Jones CP. Levels of racism: a theoretic framework and a gardener's tale. *Am J Public Health.* 2000;90(8):1212-1215.

33. Menakem, R. *My Grandmother's Hands: Racialized Trauma and the Pathway to Healing Our Hearts and Bodies.* Las Vegas, NV: Central Recovery Press; 2017.

34. Carter RT. Racism and psychological and emotional injury: recognizing and assessing race-based traumatic stress. *Couns Psychol.* 2007;35(1):13-105.

35. Sawyer PJ, Major B, Casad BJ, Townsend SS, Mendes WB. Discrimination and the stress response: psychological and physiological consequences of anticipating prejudice in interethnic interactions. *Am J Public Health.* 2012;102(5):1020-1026.

36. Geronimus AT, Hicken MT, Pearson JA, Seashols SJ, Brown KL, Cruz TD. Do US black women experience stress-related accelerated biological aging? a novel theory and first population-based test of black-white differences in telomere length. *Hum Nat.* 2010;21(1):19-38.

37. Wallace T. Impact of Trauma, Violence and Stress on Health. http://file.lacounty.gov/SDSInter/bos/supdocs/113136.pdf. Accessed October 24, 2020.

38. Substance Abuse and Mental Health Services Administration. SAMHSA's Concept of Trauma and Guidance for a Trauma-Informed Approach. HHS Publication No. (SMA)

14-4884. Rockville, MD: Substance Abuse and Mental Health Services Administration; 2014.

39. Roberts SJ, Chandler GE, Kalmakis K. A model for trauma-informed primary care. *J Am Assoc Nurse Pract.* 2019;31(2):139-144.

40. Elisseou S, Puranam S, Nandi M. A novel, trauma-informed physical examination curriculum for first-year medical students. *J Teach Learn Resour(MedEdPORTAL).* 2019;15:10799.

41. Swayden KJ, Anderson KK, Connelly LM, Moran JS, McMahon JK, Arnold PM. Effect of sitting vs. standing on perception of provider time at bedside: a pilot study. *Patient Educ Couns.* 2012;86(2):166-171.

42. Marr M. Attending to the Story. Closler. October 13, 2020. https://closler.org/clinical-reasoning/attending-to-the-story. Accessed October 15, 2020.

43. Verbal communication with Amy Weil, MD, on October 25, 2020.

44. Earls MF. Trauma-informed primary care: prevention, recognition, and promoting resilience. *N C Med J.* 2018;79(2):108-112.

45. Goldman B. Derogatory slang in the hospital setting. *AMA J Ethics.* 2015;17(2):167-171.

46. Hall WJ, Chapman MV, Lee KM, et al. Implicit racial/ethnic bias among health care professionals and its influence on health care outcomes: a systematic review. *Am J Public Health.* 2015;105(12):e60-e76.

47. Hoffman KM, Trawalter S, Axt JR, Oliver MN. Racial bias in pain assessment and treatment recommendations, and false beliefs about biological differences between blacks and whites. *Proc Natl Acad Sci USA.* 2016;113(16):4296-4301.

48. Russell ST, Pollitt AM, Li G, Grossman AH. Chosen name use is linked to reduced depressive symptoms, suicidal ideation, and suicidal behavior among transgender youth. *J Adolesc Health.* 2018;63(4):503-505.

49. Minow ML. Upstanders, Whistle-Blowers, and Rescuers (Koningsberger Lecture series, Faculty of Law, Utrecht) (Dec. 15, 2014).

50. Brüne M. Borderline Personality Disorder: Why "fast and furious"? *Evol Med public Heal.* 2016;2016(1):52-66.

51. Porter C, Palmier-Claus J, Branitsky A, Mansell W, Warwick H, Varese F. Childhood adversity and borderline personality disorder: a meta-analysis. *Acta Psychiatr Scand.* 2020;141(1):6-20.

52. Aviram RB, Brodsky BS, Stanley B. Borderline personality disorder, stigma, and treatment implications. *Harv Rev Psychiatry.* 2006;14(5):249-256.

53. Shen MJ, Peterson EB, Costas-Muñiz R, et al. The effects of race and racial concordance on patient-physician communication: a systematic review of the literature. *J Racial Ethn Health Disparities.* 2018;5(1):117-140.

54. Laveist TA, Nuru-Jeter A. Is doctor-patient race concordance associated with greater satisfaction with care? *J Health Soc Behav.* 2002;43(3):296-306.

55. Serafini K, Coyer C, Brown Speights J, et al. Racism as experienced by physicians of color in the health care setting. *Fam Med.* 2020;52(4):282-287.

56. Ly DP, Seabury SA, Jena AB. Differences in incomes of physicians in the United States by race and sex: observational study. *BMJ.* 2016;353:i2923.

57. Croghan CF, Moone RP, Olson AM. Working With LGBT baby boomers and older adults: factors that signal a welcoming service environment. *J Gerontol Soc Work*. 2015;58(6):637-651.

58. Quinn GP, Alpert AB, Sutter M, Schabath MB. What oncologists should know about treating sexual and gender minority patients with cancer. *JCO Oncol Pract*. 2020; 16(6):309-316.

59. Wilkerson JM, Rybicki S, Barber CA, Smolenski DJ. Creating a culturally competent clinical environment for LGBT patients. *J Gay Lesbian Soc Serv*. 2011;23(3):376-394.

60. The National Child Traumatic Stress Network. What is a Trauma-Informed Child and Family Service System? https://www.nctsn.org/sites/default/files/resources//what_is_a_trauma_informed_child_family_service_system.pdf. Accessed October 10, 2020.

61. O'Connor MR, Barrington WE, Buchanan DT, et al. Short-term outcomes of a diversity, equity, and inclusion Institute for Nursing Faculty. *J Nurs Educ*. 2019;58(11):633-640.

62. Winters, M-F. Equity and Inclusion: The Roots of Organizational Well-Being. Stanford Social Innovation Review. October 2020.

63. The Safe Zone Project. 2020. https://thesafezoneproject.com/curriculum/. Accessed October 26, 2020.

64. American Counseling Association. "Fact Sheet #9: Vicarious Trauma." https://www.counseling.org/docs/trauma-disaster/fact-sheet-9---vicarious-trauma.pdf. Accessed October 15, 2020.

65. Cocker F, Joss N. Compassion fatigue among healthcare, emergency and community service workers: a systematic review. *Int J Environ Res Public Health*. 2016;13(6).

66. Maslach C, Leiter MP. Understanding the burnout experience: recent research and its implications for psychiatry. *World Psychiatry*. 2016;15(2):103-111.

67. Linzer M, Levine R, Meltzer D, Poplau S, Warde C, West CP. 10 bold steps to prevent burnout in general internal medicine. *J Gen Intern Med*. 2014;29(1):18-20.

68. Isobel S, Angus-Leppan G. Neuro-reciprocity and vicarious trauma in psychiatrists. *Australas Psychiatry*. 2018;26(4):388-390.

69. Brown T, Berman S, McDaniel K, et al. Trauma-Informed Medical Education (TIME): advancing curricular content and educational context. *Acad Med*. July 2020.

70. Chen P-H, Jacobs A, Rovi SLD. Intimate partner violence: IPV in the LGBT community. *FP Essent*. 2013;412:28-35.

71. Smith SG, Chen J, Basile KC, et al. The National Intimate Partner and Sexual Violence Survey (NISVS): 2015 Data Brief—Updated Release. Atlanta, GA: National Center for Injury Prevention and Control, Centers for Disease Control and Prevention; 2018.

72. Sohal H, Eldridge S, Feder G. The sensitivity and specificity of four questions (HARK) to identify intimate partner violence: a diagnostic accuracy study in general practice. *BMC Fam Pract*. 2007;8:49.

■ APPENDIX A: IDENTIFYING AND MITIGATING INTIMATE PARTNER VIOLENCE (IPV)

There are a number of features that can be used to raise concern for IPV, many of which relate to the power dynamics discussed above. These features are summarized in Table A-1.

However, even if these features are not present, it's still important to maintain a high index of suspicion for IPV, given its prevalence across a wide range of demographics, especially women and LGBTQ+ individuals.[70] Results of the National Intimate Partner and Sexual Violence Survey (NISVS), published in 2017, indicated that roughly one in three women and nearly one in six men had experienced at least one experience of contact sexual violence (defined as "rape, being made to penetrate, sexual coercion, and/or unwanted sexual contact") at some point in their lives, with roughly one in four women and one in nine men reporting contact sexual violence, physical violence, and/or stalking by an intimate partner.[71]

■ TABLE A-1. Features Concerning for a History of IPV

Associated diagnoses, signs, and symptoms	Features of the clinical encounter
• Recurrent sinus/dental problems and "defensive injuries" (e.g., injury to arms sustained while covering the face) concerning for physical abuse • Depression, anxiety, psychosis, substance use disorder • Chronic pain, especially pelvic • Unwanted pregnancy (reproductive coercion), irregular vaginal bleeding, sexual dysfunction, recurrent UTIs particularly concerning for sexual abuse	• Reluctance to undergo genital exam, pap smear, oral exam, or other physically invasive exams • Inconsistent primary care, including late/sporadic prenatal care • Poor control of chronic medical conditions • If present, partner may appear anywhere on the spectrum from controlling and overly involved to indifferent

■ TABLE A-2. HARK Questionnaire

- Humiliation: Within the last year, have you been humiliated or emotionally abused in other ways by your partner or your ex-partner?
- Afraid: Within the last year, have you been afraid of your partner or ex-partner?
- Rape: Within the last year, have you been raped or forced to have any kind of sexual activity by your partner or ex-partner?
- Kick: Within the last year, have you been kicked, hit, slapped, or otherwise physically hurt by your partner or ex-partner?

Source: Adapted from Ref. 75.

For this reason, many medical organizations recommend screening for IPV at an initial visit and annually, using the HARK survey and other validated questionnaires to ask patients about their level of safety at home and (if applicable) within their romantic relationship (see Table A-2).[72] Screening, inquiring, and communicating with patients about IPV can be very challenging, especially if a partner is present at the visit. If you are suspicious of IPV, it is critical to speak with the patient without their partner present and postpone inquiry if this is not possible.[43] Statements like, "This is a question I ask all of my patients" can help normalize screening and inquiries that may come up during the clinical encounter, and make the patient feel more comfortable.

Emotion and Gender

Valerie Carrard, Anely Bekbergenova, and Marianne Schmid Mast

■ INTRODUCTION

Women and men differ in how they feel, express, and manage emotions,[1] and these gender differences also affect clinical practice. Female physicians expressing concern, being considerate, and talking about feelings with patients do not get the same credit for their patient-centered communication as do male physicians.[2] Female patients expressing fear are less likely to obtain the necessary treatment for anxiety disorder because they are perceived as "hysterical."[3] A priori assumptions, often unconscious, such as implicit stereotypes affect how we treat women and men and such stereotypes also affect social interactions in the medical domain. While missing an emotional cue in an interaction at work (e.g., not noticing that my colleague is sad) might not hamper work performance much, missing emotional cues in patients might have detrimental effects (e.g., missing cues of sadness or despair resulting in a patient's suicide).

The present chapter applies a gender lens on the discussion about how medical caretakers and patients feel and express emotions, how they read emotions in others, and how they manage their own emotions. Gender is a social and individual construct. It has to be noted, however, that almost all the literature on the topic assumes that participants are cisgender; that is, they self-identify with the gender assigned to them at birth. In most studies, participants self-declare their gender but are given only two choices without the possibility to indicate alternative, nonbinary genders or their sexual orientation, neither of which we are able to address in this chapter. Only very recently has the research community started to look at different conceptions of gender and sexual orientation.[4,5]

When talking about gender differences, we do not mean that all women are like this and all men are like that. We talk about gender differences if in a study the authors report statistically significant differences between women and men. This always means that there is still substantial heterogeneity in the population and that when we encounter one single individual and we only know their gender, we do not know where in the distribution this person stands. This attention to gender heterogeneity is highly relevant for the medical practice and means that if I, as a clinician, have a hypothesis about a person and their emotions based on knowing whether they are a man or a woman (e.g., knowing that research shows that women express sadness more easily than men), I need to put this hypothesis to test in the actual interaction with the patient (maybe this man does not show me his sadness because men tend to hide sadness more than women do or maybe this man is simply not sad).

We review research related to the general population, to patients, or to different healthcare providers such as medical doctors, advanced practice providers, physical and occupational therapists, physician assistants, medical assistants, or genetic counselors. However, most research on emotions in healthcare looking at gender differences compares male and female physicians. Studies comparing male and female nurses or other allied health professionals are also considered in the present chapter, but they are scarcer.

■ GENDER EMOTION STEREOTYPES IN THE HEALTHCARE CONTEXT

According to Social Role Theory, the traditional division of labor between women and men makes us see women as compassionate, kind, caring, and concerned about creating and maintaining interpersonal relationships[6] and men as dominant, self-assured, independent, and competitive.[6] These differences then become culturally established norms that define how women and men ought to behave in our society, including when, where, and by whom emotions should be expressed.[7] Fischer[8] proposes that emotions are stereotypically attributed to one or the other gender according to a powerful–powerless continuum. Dominance and power are stereotypically considered to be male attributes.[9] Thus, emotions such as sadness, anxiety, and fear are considered to be typically female emotions, because they are generally expressed in situations that one is powerless to change.[8] On the other hand, anger, pride, and contempt are typically attributed to men because they reflect an attempt to gain power and control over a situation or reflect the privilege afforded to men in having such feelings.[8]

As we will see in the following pages, these gender stereotypes are prescriptive of the way a man or a woman should feel and express emotions. Moreover, these gender emotion stereotypes affect whether and to what extent a felt emotion is displayed. It is indeed important to distinguish between felt emotions and expressed emotions because expressed emotions are affected by what are called display rules, meaning that before showing an emotion one feels, the gender stereotypical expectations are applied and might filter to what extent or whether the emotion will be expressed at all. Health professionals might train themselves, for instance, to look for what is not communicated and maybe ask men specifically about the emotional aspects, knowing that men are less likely to talk about emotions than women.[10] For instance, a male patient may feel pain but not mention it to his doctor, because according to the gender emotion stereotype, he is supposed to be strong and endure pain.

Additionally, gender emotion stereotypes affect how we perceive emotions in others. To illustrate, with equal scores on a depression scale, women are more likely to be diagnosed with depression than men are.[11] Knowing the gender emotion stereotypes can help healthcare providers explore potentially unexpressed feelings and to be aware of implicit expectations shaping their perception and medical assessment. However, if there are differences in how women and men experience emotions, then the stereotypes reflect true differences—therefore, should we then still call them stereotypes? Indeed, women and men differ in the emotions experienced and sometimes these differences map onto the gender emotion stereotypes and sometimes they do not. But even when there are actual differences in felt emotions, stereotypical expectations make us perceive the differences in an exaggerated way. A stereotype thus polarizes our view of women being sad and men being angry, for example.

Stereotypes also influence the way healthcare professionals are perceived. Nowadays, physicians are encouraged to show communal characteristics such as being empathic, caring, and compassionate, which are stereotypically defined as feminine qualities. However, even though the number of female physicians increased in the past decade, being a doctor is still considered a technical, prestigious, and agentic profession, characteristics typically associated with men.[12] This leads to a dilemma in gender roles: Women are not stereotypically associated with the physician profession, whereas men are less associated with the behavioral characteristics now deemed desirable for this same profession. There is a similar dilemma in the nursing profession: It is historically linked to the female social role, where stereotypically feminine qualities are prevalent,[13] and there is a higher rate of women in the profession.[14] However, men are increasingly entering the nursing profession[15] and the discrepancy between the characteristics of the profession and the stereotypical male social role can create cognitive dissonance in the eyes of patients treated by male nurses[16] and can hinder the creation of trusting relationships.[17] This problematic can similarly arise for men entering any medical profession primarily undertaken by women such as respiratory therapists, physicians' assistants, physical therapists, speech-language pathologists, occupational therapists, dieticians, dental assistants, or home-health aides.[18]

■ GENDER DIFFERENCES IN FEELING, EXPRESSION, AND PERCEPTION OF PATIENTS' AND PROVIDERS' EMOTIONS

Sadness in Patients and Providers

Women report experiencing more intense and long-lasting feelings of sadness than men[19] and they also express more sadness than men,[20] including crying, although this difference might be moderated by culture[21] and is inconsistent during infancy.[22] It has been argued that sadness relates to situations in which one feels powerless and given the relatively low power position of women in our society, sadness is stereotypically seen as a female emotion.[23]

It is thus difficult to gauge whether women are sadder than men or whether they allow themselves to feel sadder and/or feel more at liberty to report feelings of sadness. Therefore, the well-documented predominance of women presenting symptoms of clinical depression[24] might partly be due to women being more attuned to their feelings of sadness and/or being more inclined to report sadness compared to men. The gender norms about sadness might indeed explain why women over-report (i.e., higher risk of false-positive for women) and men under-report (i.e., higher risk of false-negative for men) depressive symptoms, making the accurate diagnosis of depression tricky.[11,25,26] Consequently, clinicians should keep in mind that, due to gender stereotypes, male patients might have more difficulty in expressing their sadness and disclosing depressive symptoms; clinicians might have to probe them about sadness to obtain an accurate account of how sad they actually feel.

The expression of sadness triggers different reactions when expressed by women compared to men. Research shows that men who express sadness suffer from social exclusion, whereas women who express sadness do not.[27] The fact that sadness is stereotypically expected more from women than from men can explain why one can feel particularly touched or uncomfortable in front of a crying man. As a clinician, it is important to be aware that gender stereotypes can trigger negative reactions to men's displays of sadness. Healthcare providers can counteract this by asking themselves whether they would be equally negatively affected when in front of a crying woman and acknowledging the sad feeling in the male patient by naming it (e.g., I can see that you are sad or this seemed to make you sad).

The expression of sadness has been shown to be detrimental to leadership regardless of gender as both male and female leaders are evaluated more negatively if they express sadness compared to neutral emotion.[28] These findings have direct application for clinicians, who find themselves in leadership roles with their trainees, colleagues, and patients. Given the evidence suggesting that expression of sadness may lead to reduced perception of competence,[29] clinicians might want to modulate their display of sadness while still remaining authentic. A reduced display of sadness is also advised because research shows that in breaking bad news situations, expressing hope is important for the patient.[30] So, having a provider who expresses a mixture of moderate sadness combined with hope is most likely the best combination for patients confronted with bad news. Studies in the healthcare context show that, overall, female healthcare providers (physicians, medical students, interns, and nurses) and related staff (medical interpreters and psychosocial professionals) are more likely to report sadness, depression,[31] and crying.[32] Reflecting the gender norms that condone sadness in women but not in men, female healthcare providers are more likely to report sadness when dealing with difficult patient–provider discussions and are more likely to report experiencing grief in response to a patient's death. However, there is evidence that male and female physicians' experience of sadness does not differ in intensity. As a result, there is a need for medical education practices to focus on emotion management and to normalize the experience of sadness for female and for male healthcare providers especially because medical students and interns report a lack of support in learning how to cope with stress and sadness.[32]

Fearful Patients, Fearful Provider

Just as for sadness, fear is stereotypically related to a lack of power and attributed more easily to women. Many self-report studies confirm that adult women report a greater number of fears and they experience fears more intensely than men.[33] It is socially acceptable for women to show fear, whereas for men it is not, or at least to a lesser degree.[34] A meta-analysis showed that women express significantly more fear both behaviorally and physiologically (i.e., heart rate) when presented with fear-inducing audiovisual images.[35] Also, women's preponderance for anxiety disorders is well-documented.[36]

In clinical practice, female patients have been shown to express more intense fear of treatments related to coronary arteriography[37] or dental care.[38] In line with the gender emotion stereotype, women might be more prone to express their concerns about those treatments, whereas male patients might be equally fearful but not speak up, because they do not want to appear weak. Clinicians should thus be particularly attentive to male patients expressing their concerns when discussing treatment options. Men might not voice them so openly; they may need to be asked directly about their potential fears concerning a treatment. On the bright side, it has been shown that even if women are expected to express fear more frequently than men, the way women and men are perceived when expressing fear does not substantially differ.[39] So male patients have something to be gained when they voice their fears or concerns because they will not be perceived more negatively if they do. The healthcare provider can offer help for the male patient to express fears in a face-saving way by for instance assuring him that most patients report feeling anxious about the treatment at hand and asking whether it is the case for him as well.

The literature regarding gender differences among healthcare providers in terms of expressions of fear is mostly related to the fear of one's own death. Studies report mixed findings with some showing gender differences[40] and others not.[41] Some studies report that healthcare providers who are more exposed to the death of their patients, like surgeons, manage their fear of death better than healthcare providers with less exposure to patient death, such as psychiatrists.[41] Fear of death might be reduced via specific training or mentoring, and should be part of clinical training because, similar to coping with sadness, medical students report the need for support in the management of the fear of their own death.[42]

Related to fear is the expression and feeling of anxiety that has been shown to differ between male and female medical students. Female students report significantly higher rates of anxiety[43] and female medical trainees report feeling more fear of repercussions (e.g., losing license, malpractice accusations) after committing medical errors.[44] Research suggests that this can be explained by female medical students perceiving themselves as being less competent and having less self-confidence than male students, despite comparable levels of actual performance.[45] Reassurance of female students with respect to their career choice, potential to succeed and provision of successful female role models in their domain can help alleviate their fear.[46] Hospitals and clinics as well as medical schools can be mindful of how they portray the different clinical professions and can provide testimonies of successful female healthcare providers which can inspire female students.

Detrimental Effect of Anger when Expressed by Female Patients and Female Providers

Stereotypically, anger is seen as a masculine emotion as it relates to the stereotype of men being in control, strong, and prone to aggressive behavior.[23] However, reviews show that there is no real difference in the frequency or intensity of felt anger between men and women.[47] Still, due to social norms, women have the tendency to control and downplay their anger.[47] Conversely, men generally show more aggressive behavior.[47]

Moreover, anger is contextual and men typically express more anger when there is a threat toward their power and status, whereas women express more anger when their interpersonal relationships are at stake.[47] Thus, it seems that women and men tend to express more anger in a context that is stereotypically attributed to their gender (power and status for men and interpersonal relations for women). In clinical practice, providers might have to be mindful that female patients might react with anger when the prescribed treatment means that they cannot be in close contact with their loved ones whereas male patients might react with anger when the prescribed treatment means that they cannot go to work. Moreover, men are less willing to seek help for a health issue[48] and might express more anger when doing so because for them it implies loss of control.[49]

With respect to the healthcare providers, gender does not seem to influence the extent to which physicians feel anger or describe themselves as generally angry.[50] However, female physicians, unlike male physicians, report an increased capacity to control their anger with age.[50] The way anger is perceived also coincides with gender stereotypes. Anger is an indicator of higher status and men who express anger benefit from a higher status referral and are attributed more independence in their job compared to women who express anger.[51] Correspondingly, women who express anger are perceived as less competent and are allocated lower status, whereas the expression of anger does not negatively influence how men are perceived.[52] For clinical practice, this can mean that because displays of anger are expected less from women, clinicians might perceive angry female patients as "difficult patients." Research also shows that women who are angry are devalued only when there is no apparent reason for their anger.[52] So, a healthcare provider who puts effort into figuring out where the anger of a female patient comes from will be able to take that patient more seriously. This underscores that perspective taking is an important skill for clinicians to possess.

The same stereotype that labels angry women as incompetent also affects clinicians. Female physicians are perceived as less competent when they display anger[53] and as more competent when they express a neutral emotional reaction rather than anger.[28] As anger is stereotypically expected of a person with high status, the negative judgment of female physicians who express anger might be the consequence of an incongruence between what is expected of a stereotypical woman (not expressing anger) and of a stereotypical doctor (high status). As a consequence, using patient-centered communication and refraining from showing anger might be particularly important for female healthcare providers.

Prosocial Emotions Are Beneficial

Prosocial emotions are emotions that facilitate affiliative social behaviors. Research indicates that compared to boys, girls are socialized to feel more responsible for others' well-being and are thus expected to be more prosocial.[54] Research confirms that women are more likely to be compassionate, to share, help, and show kindness.[21] Inversely, women are less likely than men to harm others and feel more guilt when they do.[55] Additionally, women typically score higher on self-reported perspective taking (taking the psychological point of view of others) and empathic concern (sympathy and concern for unfortunate others) as measured with the Interpersonal Reactivity Inventory (IRI).[56] They also experience generally more affective responsiveness to others' emotions (emotional contagion) than men.[57]

As in the general population, gender differences regarding prosocial emotions can be observed in the healthcare context. On average, female physicians display more prosocial behaviors such as smiles, nods, active partnership behaviors, and positive talk than male physicians.[58] Patients evaluate these kind of behaviors differently when expressed by male or female physicians. Analogue patients reported more satisfaction when they received the expected nonverbal behaviors based on gender, i.e., when female physicians displayed more prosocial nonverbal behaviors (e.g., gazing, forward leaning, soft voice) and when male physicians showed more "antisocial" nonverbal behaviors (e.g., large interpersonal distance, loud voice).[2] Thus, physicians' behaviors are evaluated in accordance with gender norms and patients are more satisfied when physicians show gender-expected behaviors.

Clinicians' ability to take the patients' perspectives is a core component of the recommended patient-centered care. Numerous studies showed gender difference using the self-reported "perspective taking" and "empathic concern" scales of the IRI or the Jefferson Scale of Physician Empathy (JSPE).[59] The JSPE is a self-report questionnaire measuring physicians' "perspective taking" (sample item: "Physicians' understanding of the emotional status of their patients, as well as that of their families, is one important component of the physician–patient relationship"), "compassionate care" (sample reversed item: "Attention to patients' emotions is not important in history taking"), and "ability to stand in patients' shoes" (sample reversed item: "Because people are different, it is difficult to see things from patients' perspectives").[60] Results of both the IRI and JSPE show that female physicians and female medical students score higher in all measured dimensions,[61] but especially in the construct of "perspective taking."[62] Moreover, longitudinal studies show that medical students' JSPE scores drop from the first to the last year of their studies, but female medical students have overall higher scores compared to male students and their drop is less steep than that of male students.[63] Similar trends were observed in nursing care, where perspective taking has also been described as essential.[64] A study measuring the Empathizing and Systemizing Quotient (EQ-SQ) questionnaire[65] revealed that male nursing students scored significantly higher in the empathizing (sample item: "I really enjoy taking care of other people") compared to other male students (e.g., social sciences, engineering, and business students), but lower than compared to other female nursing students.[66]

On top of self-reported questionnaire assessments, standardized patients also rate female medical students as showing more emotional support ("The student supports my emotions") and better perspective taking ("This student understands my perspective") than male students.[67] Communication behavior studies based on observer coding further confirm that female physicians engage in more inquiry about feelings, exploration of emotional concerns, and statements of concern than male physicians.[58] It is important to note that, like self-reported questionnaires, external observer ratings might still be influenced by gender stereotypes and trigger gender-congruent ratings. Nevertheless, one study suggests that patients' perception of their physician's prosocial abilities is more driven by the actual physician's verbal behavior than by gender stereotypes.[68] The results show that, even when participants reading consultation transcripts are misinformed about the gender of the physician, actual female physicians' transcripts are perceived as putting themselves more in the patient's shoes, treating the patient more as an equal partner, better understanding the patient's point of view, and being more responsive to the patient as compared to transcripts stemming from male physicians.

Overall, taking the perspective of the patients and being responsive to their emotions seem to be a strong suit of female healthcare providers. However, the stereotype of women being more prosocial might hinder the positive effect of these female qualities on patient outcomes. A study has indeed shown that high levels of patient-centeredness are related to better patient outcomes for both female and male physicians, but moderate levels of patient-centeredness (including emotional responsiveness) are related to better patient outcomes for male physicians only.[69] This indicates that male physicians do not need to display high levels of emotional responsiveness to have a positive impact on patients, because it is a behavior less expected from them. On the other side, emotional responsiveness is expected from female physicians, because they are women and they would have to display especially high emotional responsiveness to benefit from more positive patient outcomes.[2,70] Given that men typically display less emotional responsiveness than women,[71] but that female physicians need to display an especially higher level of emotional responsiveness to benefit from positive patient outcomes, both male and female clinicians can benefit from having medical curricula reinforce this skill.

Gender Differences in Overall Emotionality

Research suggests that men have an overall tendency to downplay their emotions more than women do.[72] Men have been labeled as "internalizers" who show less emotional expression despite physiological arousal, whereas women rather are "externalizers," expressing emotions in the absence of physiological arousal[72] or "generalizers," showing concordance between physiological arousal and their emotion expression.[73]

Emotionality is stereotypically attributed to women and studies confirm that on average women feel emotions more frequently and intensely[21] and are more nonverbally expressive[1] than men are. This general difference in emotionality has critical implications in clinical settings. It implies that male patients are less likely to display emotional cues during consultations. Given that the recognition of emotional cues is related to higher patient satisfaction,[74] clinicians might have more difficulty reading the emotions of their male patients because the latter do not display them easily. Therefore, if male patients have the tendency to internalize their emotions, are less willing to seek help, and disclose less fear of treatment, clinicians might have to put in extra effort and sensitivity to probe more for emotional cues if they want to provide patient-centered care, adequate treatment, and accurate diagnosis of emotion-related disorders. For practitioners, possessing emotional skills such as emotion recognition is thus essential not only when dealing with male patients but also more generally within the healthcare context.

■ GENDER DIFFERENCES IN EMOTIONAL INTELLIGENCE

Mayer and Salovey[75] define emotional intelligence (EI) as the ability to accurately recognize, use, understand, and regulate emotions. According to EI theories, accuracy in emotion recognition, using emotion to facilitate cognitive functioning, and understanding and managing emotions are essential for social functioning.[76] Despite the popular belief that women are more skilled than men when it comes to EI,[77] a review of the literature points out that there is no clear conclusion on whether women or men have stronger EI.[78]

As in the general population, studies on differences in EI between female and male healthcare providers have reported mixed results that seem to depend on the instrument used to measure EI. A group of studies using the Mayer–Salovey–Caruso EI Test, the EI Scale, and self-developed EI measures concluded that female medical students have an overall higher EI score compared to male students,[79–81] but other studies conducted on healthcare providers (i.e., psychiatrists, surgeons) and medical students in different medical fields (i.e., nursing, dental, mental health work) with the Bar-On Emotional Quotient Inventory and the Schutte Emotional Intelligence found no gender differences.[82,83] These contradictory findings might be due to the use of different EI questionnaires and suggests that gender differences in EI actually appear in specific domains of EI. A study confirms that female surgeons, pediatricians, and pathologists scored higher in "relationships" (being able to have satisfactory social relationships) and "impulse control" (being reflective and less likely to surrender to one's own drive),[84] whereas their male counterparts scored higher in "emotion management" (being able to affect other people's feelings) and "stress management" (being able to cope with pressure and regulate stress) subscales of the Trait Emotional Intelligence Questionnaire.[84] This observation reflects again gender stereotypes with women being more skilled in relationship-related abilities and men being better in exerting control over the situation. This highlights different general strengths of male and female clinicians and areas in which each can strive for improvement. Because gender differences in EI seems to vary depending on the subdomains studied, we will now focus on two specific subdomains of EI that consistently show gender differences: emotion recognition and emotion regulation (see also Chapter 5, Perception of Emotion in the Medical Visit, and Chapter 7, Emotion Regulation in Patients, Providers, and the Clinical Relationship).

Emotion Recognition

Emotion recognition is an important dimension of emotional intelligence. Accuracy in recognizing emotions has been shown to be beneficial in the workplace as it relates to more positive outcomes in sales, negotiations, and interactions with clients.[85] The first study measuring emotion recognition accuracy using performance tests (i.e., accuracy in recognizing the emotions displayed in portraits) took place in the 1920s and showed a gender difference favoring women.[86] This finding was later confirmed in meta-analyses and we now know that women are not only better but also faster at recognizing others' emotions correctly compared to men.[87,88] This gender difference is observed across different nonverbal channels (i.e., face, body, and voice), cultures,[89] age categories,[90] and specific emotions with the difference being larger for negative emotions and especially for anger and sadness.[91]

Emotion recognition plays an important role in the medical encounter. The ability of physicians to read nonverbal or emotional expressions is linked to positive patient outcomes in the clinical setting[92] such as patient satisfaction,[74] appointment keeping,[93] and evaluation of medical care.[94] The few studies that have compared emotion recognition of male and female physicians find that female medical students and residents have better emotional and nonverbal recognition skills than male physicians as measured with several validated tests.[95,96] One study on general practitioners shows that male and female physicians do not differ in their emotion recognition skills.[97] However, the results of this study indicate that female physicians with higher emotion recognition skills adapted their communication behaviors (speaking time, smiling, nodding, loudness of voice) to their patients' communication preferences, whereas for male physicians, there was not a link between emotion recognition accuracy and the extent to which they adapted their communication style to their patients' preferences.[97] Another study further suggests that the relation between accuracy in identifying emotional cues (measured with standard tests of emotion and nonverbal behavior recognition skills[98,99]) differs for male and female medical students.[100] Results showed that both female and male medical students who are better at recognizing emotions were evaluated as more likeable and compassionate. Male physicians with better emotion recognition skills were additionally rated not only as warmer and more engaged and female physicians as more interested and less distressed, but also as more irritated and more dominant. Female physicians with better emotion recognition skills elicit more mixed impressions, maybe because they are more authentic, whereas for male physicians, being able to accurately read the patients' emotions exceeds the expectations harbored for them in a positive sense and they are thus perceived as particularly warm and engaged. Overall, being able to accurately read emotions can have beneficial impacts for both female and male clinicians and research shows that emotion recognition skills can be improved successfully with short training sessions combining feedback and practice.[101] Clinical curricula could thus include an emotion recognition training to improve clinicians' ability to read, understand, and react to their patients' emotions.

Emotion Regulation

The ability to regulate or manage emotions is another essential dimension of emotional intelligence. It is defined as the way "individuals influence which emotions they have, when they have them, and how they experience and express these emotions."[102] Emotion regulation is essential for healthcare providers because they need to deal with several negative emotions (e.g., pain, fear, disgust) on a daily basis. Moreover, it has been suggested that too much emotional involvement can disrupt medical objectivity[103] and lead to compassion fatigue.[61] Healthcare providers have been shown to use emotional engagement or disengagement strategies to regulate emotions in their work.[104] However, to the best of our knowledge, no existing research focuses on gender differences in the emotion regulation strategies applied by healthcare providers. Nevertheless, studies in the field of emotional labor give more insights into gender differences in healthcare providers' emotion regulation.

Emotional labor is a form of emotion regulation that refers to regulating felt and displayed emotion at work to maintain an image in line with the workplace requirements.[105] It implies the downplaying of work-inappropriate felt emotions while displaying other emotions that are not necessarily felt.[106] Studies on emotional labor originally focused on women who are required to portray positive emotions to clients (i.e., paralegals, flight attendants) and men who are required to display negative emotions like anger and emotional detachment (i.e., tax collectors).[107,108] Female and male professionals show-ing positive emotions while suppressing negative ones reported high feelings of inauthenticity, but for female professionals, showing negative emotions while suppressing positive ones was experienced as even more inauthentic.[109] Because women are generally more emotionally expressive than men[110] and gender role norms support free emotion expression for women (and emotion suppression for men),[111] women typically experience more emotional disso-nance than men when performing emotional labor.[112]

Emotional labor is an important part of the professional lives of nurses, physicians, and clinical psychologists.[113] Professional and social obligations of healthcare workers require them to suppress feelings of anger and frustration and instead express agreeableness and friendliness, even when encountering hostile behavior from patients.[107] The few studies on gender differences in emotional labor in the healthcare context report mixed findings. One study including a pooled sample of physicians and nurses found that female and male healthcare providers did not differ in terms of self-reported emotional labor.[114] Regarding nursing care, male nurses reported performing emotional labor less often than female nurses, which resulted in higher self-reported job satisfaction than their female colleagues.[115] The authors suggest that male nurses benefit from a so-called "status shield"[115]: They receive fewer emo-tional displays in the workplace, because being a male is stereotypically asso-ciated with higher status and it is not socially accepted to share one's emotions with high status individuals.[105] Thus, female nurses encounter more negative emotional interactions directed toward them at work, forcing them to use more emotional labor and leading to lower job satisfaction.[115]

In sum, emotional labor is a given necessity in healthcare professions and has the potential to heighten the emotional dissonance and stress of health-care providers, and emotional labor seems to have a stronger negative effect on job satisfaction for female than male providers.[116] Emotional labor can be faced using different strategies, either surface or deep acting. In surface act-ing, individuals will simply enact the behavior that portrays a required stance without trying to change or adapt how they actually feel. For instance, a nurse who actually feels happy and energetic will put on a face that shows concern and will hide their happiness when interacting with a depressed patient. In deep acting, the nurse would actually try to work on their emotions and try to feel concerned. Thus, people using deep acting will try to change how they feel in order to be aligned with the emotions they are expected to display.[117]

Deep acting has been shown to relate to lower levels of stress for professionals than just suppressing felt emotions to display expected emotions (surface acting).[117] There is evidence that female physicians engage in more deep acting than male physicians.[118] Learning how to regulate one's emotion through deep acting is thus an avenue to lower the detrimental effect of emotional labor.[119] Healthcare providers, and especially female providers, would benefit from a more consistent use of deep acting strategies. For the sake of maintaining good physical and mental health for clinicians, clinical curricula might want to focus more on teaching emotion regulation strategies because findings have shown that providing service training programs as well as being mentored by more experienced colleagues encourages the use of deep acting.[120]

■ GENDER DIFFERENCES IN BURNOUT

Maslach defined burnout as a psychological syndrome encompassing emotional exhaustion, depersonalization (i.e., treating other people like objects), and a diminished sense of personal accomplishment (i.e., reduced productivity or capability and low morale) due to long-lasting interpersonal stressors at work.[121] Similar to depression and anxiety,[122] women are more prone to experience burnout.[123] Nevertheless, burnout or depression might go undetected in men because the social norms for reporting them puts men at a disadvantage. Moreover, men are more prone than women to experiencing alexithymia, a condition in which people experience difficulties in detecting and describing feelings in words.[124] So, if men are less emotionally expressive, more reluctant to report feelings related to burnout, and at higher risk for having impaired access to their own inner feelings (i.e., alexithymia), it is not surprising that even trained physicians and clinicians are more likely to diagnose female patients with depression and anxiety disorders than male patients.[125] Thus, men risk not receiving appropriate treatment when subject to burnout.[126] Even when burnout is detected, men and women experience it differently. Women suffering from burnout report more emotional exhaustion while men report more depersonalization (see Chapter 16, Striving and Thriving: Challenges and Opportunities for Clinician Emotional Wellness for more on clinician wellness).[127] Clinicians might thus want to be particularly attentive to gender when screening their patients for burnout as this condition and other emotionally related conditions might be more difficult to detect in male patients and might manifest differently in male compared to female patients.

Burnout can occur as a consequence of intense emotion regulation. Indeed, the psychological strain of regulating one's emotions and the potential resulting emotional dissonance can eventually lead to burnout.[123] This can be especially pronounced in work, which is intense in emotional labor such as healthcare professions.[128] The association of emotional dissonance and emotional exhaustion is more pronounced for women than for men.[112] Research suggests that female physicians experience more emotional strain at work, because they show more emotional exhaustion and feel less valued by their colleagues and patients compared to male physicians.[61] Studies on burnout in physicians report that there is either no gender difference[129,130] or that female physicians are more prone to burnout than male physicians.[131,132] In nursing care, studies showed that female and male nurses report similar levels of burnout[133] and exhaustion.[134] Knowing that women in men-dominated professions take more days of sick leave[135] and self-report poorer health and more psychological distress than women in female-type professions,[136] and knowing that men working in a profession stereotypically considered as female take more days of sick leave than men working in other jobs,[135] one can conclude that working in gender-dissonant jobs is likely to take its toll on health and well-being. Thus, female physicians (gender dissonant occupation) might be more at risk of burnout than male physicians (gender congruent occupation), whereas female nurses (gender congruent occupation) are less at risk of depersonalization than male nurses (gender dissonant occupation). A further potential explanation for gender differences in burnout is that female physicians engage in more communication, on average, with patients and have longer patient visits,[58] which can result in increased stress due to heavier workload. Moreover, female clinicians are more subject to physical, verbal,[137] and sexual harassment[138] in their workplace than their male peers. Finally, female physicians experience more difficulty integrating work and domestic responsibilities,[139] as studies have shown that on average, female physicians spend 8.5 more hours per week on domestic activities than their male counterparts.[140] These results indicate that additional support for mitigating burnout is needed, particularly for women clinicians, as evidence suggests that they face additional demands for emotional responsiveness and emotion regulation that exceed those of their male colleagues.

■ CONCLUSION

By reviewing the literature regarding gender differences in emotional experience, expression, and social perception, this chapter highlights the pervasive influence of gender stereotypes. Consequently, male patients have the tendency to express less emotion and especially less sadness and fear. Therefore, extra effort is needed to elicit emotional cues from male patients. Moreover, the reviewed studies show that displaying gender-incongruent emotions is typically punished through social exclusion. Thus, female patients expressing anger might be more easily labelled as "difficult patients" than male patients displaying the same level of anger. Similarly, male patients' displaying stereotypically female emotions such as sadness might trigger more discomfort in clinicians. Moreover, gender stereotypes still influence the way male and female clinicians are evaluated. For instance, female clinicians' anger is evaluated more harshly and they need to show more prosocial emotions than men in order to benefit from more positive patient outcomes.

On the provider side, a summary of studies showed that female physicians are generally evaluated more favorably than male physicians, but the difference is so small that it is negligible.[141] With an increasingly gender-equal society, gender stereotypes might slowly change. For instance, studies show that fear is still an emotion understood as stereotypically female with women feeling and displaying more of it than men, but women and men are not necessarily perceived differently when they express fear. This might be a sign of societal evolution toward a more egalitarian perception of displayed emotions. Considering evidence for female physicians' superior communication behaviors and patient health outcomes,[58,142] as well as the normalization of women in medicine due to the dramatic influx of women into medicine, one might expect that female physicians' evaluation will be less impacted by gender role stereotypes in the future and that they could in turn benefit more from their superior communication abilities.

Aligned with the stereotypical communal role of women, the reviewed studies also show that women are better than men at recognizing and regulating emotions, but these abilities seem to take a toll on women who present higher rates of emotional dissonance and burnout. Fortunately, there is indication that women use better emotional regulation strategies (e.g., deep acting) and encouraging them to use this strategy seems a good path toward building resilience in female healthcare providers. Moreover, studies show that emotion regulation can be trained and thus presents an interesting potential avenue for interventions preventing burnout in medical practice.

It is important to keep human diversity in mind in order to prevent the negative influence of gender stereotypes and discrimination based on average tendencies. As clearly highlighted in this chapter, expecting certain kinds of emotions or judging emotions based on gender stereotypes can have important clinical drawbacks. Knowing that those stereotypes can affect practitioners in how they treat patients is important to counteract the effect of such implicit stereotypes. This chapter thus serves as a basis for thinking critically about how gender influences patients' and physicians' displays of emotions and how these emotions are perceived and managed in clinical settings.

REFERENCES

1. Brody LR, Hall JA. Gender and emotion in context. In: Gross JJ, ed. *Handbook of Emotions*. 3rd ed. New York, NY: The Guilford Press; 2008:395-408.

2. Schmid Mast M, Hall JA, Klöckner C, Choi E. Physician gender affects how physician nonverbal behavior is related to patient satisfaction. *Med Care*. 2008;46(12):1212-1218.

3. Ussher JM. Diagnosing difficult women and pathologising femininity: gender bias in psychiatric nosology. *Fem Psychol*. 2013;23(1):63-69.

4. Carlström R, Ek S, Gabrielsson S. "Treat me with respect": transgender persons' experiences of encounters with healthcare staff. *Scand J Caring Sci*. 2020.

5. Mizock L, Mueser KT. Employment, mental health, internalized stigma, and coping with transphobia among transgender individuals. *Psychol Sex Orientat Gend Divers*. 2014;1(2):146-158.

6. Eagly AH, Steffen VJ. Gender stereotypes stem from the distribution of women and men into social roles. *J Pers Soc Psychol*. 1984;46(4):735-754.

7. Eagly AH, Wood W. Social role theory of sex differences. In: Naples NA, Hoogland RC, Wickramasinghe M, Wong WC, eds. *The Wiley Blackwell Encyclopedia of Gender and Sexuality Studies*. Chichester, UK: Wiley Blackwell; 2016:458-476.

8. Fischer A. Sex differences in emotionality: fact or stereotype? *Fem Psychol*. 1993;3(3): 303-318.

9. Bakan D. *The Duality of Human Existence: An Essay on Psychology and Religion*. Oxford, UK: Rand Mcnally; 1966.

10. Gross JJ, John OP. Facets of emotional expressivity: three self-report factors and their correlates. *Pers Individ Differ*. 1995;19(4):555-568.

11. Bertakis KD, Helms LJ, Callahan EJ, Azari R, Leigh P, Robbins JA. Patient gender differences in the diagnosis of depression in primary care. *J Wom Health Gend Base Med*. 2001;10(7):689-698.

12. Sollami A, Caricati L, Mancini T. Ambivalent stereotypes of nurses and physicians: impact on students' attitude toward interprofessional education. *Acta Biomed*. 2015; 86(S1):19-28.

13. MacDougall G. Caring: a masculine perspective. *J Adv Nursing*. 1997;25(4):809-813.

14. Castel ES, Ginsburg LR, Zaheer S, Tamim H. Understanding nurses' and physicians' fear of repercussions for reporting errors: clinician characteristics, organization demographics, or leadership factors? *BMC Health Serv Res*. 2015;15(326):1-10.

15. Zurlinden J. News and trends in nursing. *Nursing Spectrum Career Fitness Guide*. 1998:9-11.

16. Paterson BL, Tschikota S, Crawford M, Saydak M, Venkatesh P, Aronowitz T. Learning to care: gender issues for male nursing students. *Can J Nurs Res*. 1996;28(1):25-39.

17. Lodge N, Mallett J, Blake P, MSc IF. A study to ascertain gynaecological patients' perceived levels of embarrassment with physical and psychological care given by female and male nurses. *J Adv Nursing*. 1997;25(5):893-907.

18. Anspach R. Gender and healthcare. In: Bird CE, Conrad P, Fremont AM, Timmermans S, eds. *Handbook of Medical Sociology*, 6th ed. Nashville, TN: Vanderbilt University Press; 2010:229-249.

19. Brebner J. Gender and emotions. *Pers Indiv Differ*. 2003;34(3):387-394.

20. Schwartz GE, Brown S-L, Ahern GL. Facial muscle patterning and subjective experience during affective imagery: sex differences. *Psychophysiology*. 1980;17(1):75-82.

21. Fischer A, Manstead AS. The relation between gender and emotions in different cultures. In: Fischer A, ed. *Gender and Emotion: Social Psychological Perspectives*. Cambridge, UK: Cambridge University Press; 2000:71-94.

22. Kohnstamm GA. Temperament in childhood: cross-cultural and sex differences. In: Kohnstamm GA, Bates J, Rothbart M, eds. *Temperament in Childhood*. Oxford, UK: John Wiley & Sons; 1989:483-508.

23. Plant EA, Hyde JS, Keltner D, Devine PG. The gender stereotyping of emotions. *Psychol Women Q*. 2000;24(1):81-92.

24. Weissman MM, Olfson M. Depression in women: implications for health care research. *Science*. 1995;269(5225):799-801.

25. Borowsky SJ, Rubenstein LV, Meredith LS, Camp P, Jackson-Triche M, Wells KB. Who is at risk of nondetection of mental health problems in primary care? *J Gen Intern Med*. 2000;15(6):381-388.

26. Stoppe G, Sandholzer H, Huppertz C, Duwe H, Staedt J. Gender differences in the recognition of depression in old age. *Maturitas*. 1999;32(3):205-212.

27. Perry-Parrish C, Zeman J. Relations among sadness regulation, peer acceptance, and social functioning in early adolescence: the role of gender. *Soc dev*. 2011;20(1):135-153.

28. Lewis K. When leaders display emotion: how followers respond to negative emotional expression of male and female leaders. *J Organ Behav*. 2000;21(2):221-234.

29. Ven N van de, Meijs MHJ, Vingerhoets A. What emotional tears convey: tearful individuals are seen as warmer, but also as less competent. *Br J Soc Psychol*. 2017;56(1):146-160.

30. Whitney SN, McCullough LB, Frugé E, McGuire AL, Volk RJ. Beyond breaking bad news. *Cancer*. 2008;113(2):442-445.

31. Compton MT, Frank E. Mental health concerns among Canadian physicians: results from the 2007-2008 Canadian Physician Health Study. *Compr Psychiat*. 2011;52(5):542-547.

32. Sung AD, Collins ME, Smith AK, et al. Crying: experiences and attitudes of third-year medical students and interns. *Teach Learn Med*. 2009;21(3):180-187.

33. Arrindell WA. Phobic dimensions: IV. the structure of animal fears. *Behav Res Ther*. 2000;38(5):509-530.

34. Hutson-Comeaux SL, Kelly JR. Gender stereotypes of emotional reactions: how we judge an emotion as valid. *Sex Roles*. 2002;47(1/2):1-10.

35. Peck EY-Y. Gender differences in film-induced fear as a function of type of emotion measure and stimulus content: a meta-analysis and laboratory study. Dissertation Abstracts International Section A: Humanities and Social Sciences, Vol 61(1-A), Jul 2000: 17.

36. McLean CP, Anderson ER. Brave men and timid women? a review of the gender differences in fear and anxiety. *Clin Psychol Rev*. 2009;29(6):496-505.

37. Heikkilä J, Paunonen M, Virtanen V, Laippala P. Gender differences in fears related to coronary arteriography. *Heart Lung*. 1999;28(1):20-30.

38. Astramskaitė I, Poškevičius L, Juodžbalys G. Factors determining tooth extraction anxiety and fear in adult dental patients: a systematic review. *Int J Oral Maxillofac Surg.* 2016;45(12):1630-1643.

39. Fabes RA, Martin CL. Gender and age stereotypes of emotionality. *Pers Soc Psychol Bull.* 1991;17(5):532-540.

40. Hamama-Raz Y, Solomon Z, Ohry A. Fear of personal death among physicians. *OMEGA-J Death Dying.* 2000;41(2):139-149.

41. Livingston PB, Zimet CN. Death anxiety, authoritarianism and choice of specialty in medical students. *J Nerv Ment Dis.* 1965;140(3):222-230.

42. Rhodes-Kropf J, Carmody SS, Seltzer D, et al. "This is just too awful; I just can't believe I experienced that …": medical students' reactions to their "most memorable" patient death. *Acad Med.* 2005;80(7):634-640.

43. Saravanan C, Wilks R. Medical students' experience of and reaction to stress: the role of depression and anxiety. *Sci World J.* 2014;1-8.

44. Muller D, Ornstein K. Perceptions of and attitudes towards medical errors among medical trainees. *Med Educ.* 2007;41(7):645-652.

45. Blanch DC, Hall JA, Roter DL, Frankel RM. Medical student gender and issues of confidence. *Patient Educ Couns.* 2008;72(3):374-381.

46. Latu IM, Mast MS, Lammers J, Bombari D. Successful female leaders empower women's behavior in leadership tasks. *J Exp Soc Psychol.* 2013;49(3):444-448.

47. Fischer A, Evers C. The social basis of emotion in men and women. In: Ryan MK, Branscombe NR, eds. *The SAGE Handbook of Gender and Psychology.* London, UK: SAGE; 2013:183-198.

48. Addis ME, Mahalik JR. Men, masculinity, and the contexts of help seeking. *Am Psychol.* 2003;58(1):5-14.

49. Thomas SP. Men's anger: a phenomenological exploration of its meaning in a middle-class sample of American men. *Psychol Men Masc.* 2003;4(2):163-175.

50. Koçer E, Koçer A, Canan F. Anger management and factors that influence anger in physicians. *Balk Med J.* 2011;28(1):62-68.

51. Tiedens LZ. Anger and advancement versus sadness and subjugation: the effect of negative emotion expressions on social status conferral. *J Pers Soc Psychol.* 2001;80(1):86-94.

52. Brescoll VL, Uhlmann EL. Can an angry woman get ahead? Status conferral, gender, and expression of emotion in the workplace. *Psychol Sci.* 2008;19(3):268-275.

53. Hareli S, Shomrat N, Hess U. Emotional versus neutral expressions and perceptions of social dominance and submissiveness. *Emotion.* 2009;9(3):378-384.

54. Eagly AH. The his and hers of prosocial behavior: an examination of the social psychology of gender. *Am Psychol.* 2009;64(8):644-658.

55. Hoffman ML. Empathy and prosocial behavior. In: Lewis M, Haviland-Jones JM, Feldman Barrett L, eds. *Handbook of Emotions.* New York, NY: The Guilford Press; 2008:440-455.

56. Konrath SH, O'Brien EH, Hsing C. Changes in dispositional empathy in American college students over time: a meta-analysis. *Pers Soc Psychol Rev.* 2011;15(2):180-198.

57. Doherty RW. The Emotional Contagion Scale: a measure of individual differences. *J Nonverbal Behav.* 1997;21(2):131-154.

58. Roter DL, Hall JA, Aoki Y. Physician gender effects in medical communication: a meta-analytic review. *JAMA.* 2002;288(6):756-764.

59. Hojat M. *Empathy in Patient Care: Antecedents, Development, Measurement, and Outcomes.* New York, NY: Springer Science & Business Media; 2007.

60. Hojat M, Gonnella JS, Nasca TJ, Mangione S, Vergare M, Magee M. Physician empathy: definition, components, measurement, and relationship to gender and specialty. *AJP.* 2002;159(9):1563-1569.

61. Gleichgerrcht E, Decety J. Empathy in clinical practice: how individual dispositions, gender, and experience moderate empathic concern, burnout, and emotional distress in physicians. *PLoS One.* 2013;8(4):1-12.

62. Hojat M, Vergare MJ, Maxwell K, et al. The devil is in the third year: a longitudinal study of erosion of empathy in medical school. *Acad Med.* 2009;84(9):1182-1191.

63. Santos MA, Grosseman S, Morelli TC, Giuliano IC, Erdmann TR. Empathy differences by gender and specialty preference in medical students: a study in Brazil. *Int J Med Educ.* 2016;7:149-153.

64. Brunero S, Lamont S, Coates M. A review of empathy education in nursing. *Nurs Inq.* 2010;17(1):65-74.

65. Baron-Cohen S, Wheelwright S. The Empathy Quotient: an investigation of adults with Asperger Syndrome or high functioning autism, and normal sex differences. *J Autism Dev Disord.* 2004;34(2):163-175.

66. Penprase B, Oakley B, Ternes R, Driscoll D. Do higher dispositions for empathy predispose males toward careers in nursing? A descriptive correlational design. *Nurs Forum.* 2015;50(1):1-8.

67. Berg K, Blatt B, Lopreiato J, et al. Standardized patient assessment of medical student empathy: ethnicity and gender effects in a multi-institutional study. *Acad Med.* 2015;90(1):105-111.

68. Nicolai J, Demmel R. The impact of gender stereotypes on the evaluation of general practitioners' communication skills: an experimental study using transcripts of physician–patient encounters. *Patient Educ Couns.* 2007;69(1):200-205.

69. Hall JA, Roter DL, Blanch-Hartigan D, Schmid Mast M, Pitegoff CA. How patient-centered do female physicians need to be? Analogue patients' satisfaction with male and female physicians' identical behaviors. *Health Commun.* 2015;30(9):894-900.

70. Schmid Mast M, Kadji KK. How female and male physicians' communication is perceived differently. *Patient Educ Couns.* 2018;101(9):1697-1701.

71. Roter DL, Hall JA. Physician gender and patient-centered communication: a critical review of empirical research. *Annu Rev Public Health.* 2004;25(1):497-519.

72. Manstead ASR. Expressiveness as an individual difference. In: Feldman R, Rimé B, eds. *Fundamentals of Nonverbal Behavior.* Paris, France: Editions de la Maison des Sciences de l'Homme; 1991:285-328.

73. Brody LR. *Gender, Emotion, and the Family.* Cambridge, MA: Harvard University Press; 2009.

74. Blanch-Hartigan D. Patient satisfaction with physician errors in detecting and identifying patient emotion cues. *Patient Educ Couns.* 2013;93(1):56-62.

75. Salovey P, Mayer JD. Emotional intelligence. *Imagin Cogn Personal.* 1990;9(3):185-211.

76. Mandell B, Pherwani S. Relationship between emotional intelligence and transformational leadership style: a gender comparison. *J Bus Psychol.* 2003;17(3):387-404.

77. Nasir M, Masrur R. An exploration of emotional intelligence of the students of IIUI in relation to gender, age and academic achievement. *Bull Educ Res.* 2010;32(1):37-51.

78. Sanchez-Nunez M, Fernández-Berrocal P, Montañés J, Latorre JM. Does emotional intelligence depend on gender? the socialization of emotional competencies in men and women and its implications. *Electron J Res Educ Psychol.* 2008;6(2):455-474.

79. Todres M, Tsimtsiou Z, Stephenson A, Jones R. The emotional intelligence of medical students: an exploratory cross-sectional study. *Med Teach.* 2010;32(1):e42-e48.

80. Austin EJ, Evans P, Magnus B, O'Hanlon K. A preliminary study of empathy, emotional intelligence and examination performance in MBChB students. *Med Educ.* 2007;41(7):684-689.

81. Carrothers RM, Gregory SW Jr, Gallagher TJ. Measuring emotional intelligence of medical school applicants. *Acad Med.* 2000;75(5):456-463.

82. Stanton C, Sethi FN, Dale O, Phelan M, Laban JT, Eliahoo J. Comparison of emotional intelligence between psychiatrists and surgeons. *Psychiatr Online.* 2011;35(4):124-129.

83. Birks Y, McKendree J, Watt I. Emotional intelligence and perceived stress in healthcare students: a multi-institutional, multi-professional survey. *BMC Med Educ.* 2009;9(61):1-8.

84. McKinley SK, Petrusa ER, Fiedeldey-Van Dijk C, et al. Are there gender differences in the emotional intelligence of resident physicians? *J Surg Educ.* 2014;71(6):e33-e40.

85. Schmid Mast M, Latu I. 13 Interpersonal accuracy in relation to the workplace, leadership, and hierarchy. In: Hall JA, Schmid Mast M, West TV, eds. *The Social Psychology of Perceiving Others Accurately.* Cambridge, UK: Cambridge University Press; 2016:270-286.

86. Buzby DE. The interpretation of facial expression. *Am J Psychol.* 1924;35(4):602-604.

87. Hall JA, Gunnery SD, Horgan TG. Gender differences in interpersonal accuracy. In: Hall JA, Schmid Mast M, West TV, eds. *The Social Psychology of Perceiving Others Accurately.* Cambridge, UK: Cambridge University Press; 2016:309-327.

88. Vassallo S, Cooper SL, Douglas JM. Visual scanning in the recognition of facial affect: is there an observer sex difference? *J Vision.* 2009;9(3):1-10.

89. Kirkland RA, Peterson E, Baker CA, Miller S, Pulos S. Meta-analysis reveals adult female superiority in "Reading the Mind in the Eyes Test". *N Am J Psychol.* 2013;15(1):121-146.

90. Ruffman T, Murray J, Halberstadt J, Taumoepeau M. Verbosity and emotion recognition in older adults. *Psychol Aging.* 2010;25(2):492-497.

91. Thompson AE, Voyer D. Sex differences in the ability to recognise non-verbal displays of emotion: a meta-analysis. *Cogn Emot.* 2014;28(7):1164-1195.

92. Ruben MA. Interpersonal accuracy in the clinical setting. In: Hall JA, Schmid Mast M, West TV, eds. *The Social Psychology of Perceiving Others Accurately.* Cambridge, UK: Cambridge University Press; 2016:287-308.

93. DiMatteo MR, Hays RD, Prince LM. Relationship of physicians' nonverbal communication skill to patient satisfaction, appointment noncompliance, and physician workload. *Health Psychol.* 1986;5(6):581-594.

94. DiMatteo MR, Taranta A, Friedman HS, Prince LM. Predicting patient satisfaction from physicians' nonverbal communication skills. *Med Care.* 1980;18(4):376-387.

95. Hall JA, Andrzejewski SA, Yopchick JE. Psychosocial correlates of interpersonal sensitivity: a meta-analysis. *J Nonverbal Behav.* 2009;33(3):149-180.

96. Hall JA, Ship AN, Ruben MA, et al. The Test of Accurate Perception of Patients' Affect (TAPPA): an ecologically valid tool for assessing interpersonal perception accuracy in clinicians. *Patient Educ Couns.* 2014;94(2):218-223.

97. Carrard V, Schmid Mast M, Jaunin-Stalder N, Junod Perron N, Sommer J. Patient-centeredness as physician behavioral adaptability to patient preferences. *Health Commun.* 2018;33(5):593-600.

98. Nowicki S, Duke MP. Individual differences in the nonverbal communication of affect: the Diagnostic Analysis of Nonverbal Accuracy Scale. *J Nonverbal Behav.* 1994;18(1):9-35.

99. Rosenthal R, Hall JA, DiMatteo MR, Rogers PL, Archer D. *Sensitivity to Nonverbal Communication: The PONS Test.* Baltimore, MD: Johns Hopkins University Press; 1979.

100. Hall JA, Roter DL, Blanch DC, Frankel RM. Nonverbal sensitivity in medical students: implications for clinical interactions. *J Gen Intern Med.* 2009;24(11):1217-1222.

101. Blanch-Hartigan D, Andrzejewski SA, Hill KM. The effectiveness of training to improve person perception accuracy: a meta-analysis. *Basic Appl Soc Psych.* 2012;34(6):483-498.

102. Gross JJ. Emotion regulation: past, present, future. *Cogn Emot.* 1999;13(5):551-573.

103. Smith AC, Kleinman S. Managing emotions in medical school: students' contacts with the living and the dead. *Soc Psychol Q.* 1989;52(1):56-69.

104. Henderson A. Emotional labor and nursing: an under-appreciated aspect of caring work. *Nurs Inq.* 2001;8(2):130-138.

105. Hochschild AR. *The Managed Heart: Commercialization of Human Feeling.* 3rd ed. Berkeley, CA: University of California Press; 1983.

106. Kruml SM, Geddes D. Catching fire without burning out: is there an ideal way to perform emotional labor? In: Ashkanasy N, Charmine E, Hartel E, Zerbe W, eds. *Emotions in the Workplace: Research, Theory, and Practice.* Westport, CT: Greenwood; 2000:177-188.

107. Erickson RJ, Ritter C. Emotional labor, burnout, and inauthenticity: does gender matter? *Soc Psychol Q.* 2001;64(2):146-163.

108. Johnson H-AM, Spector PE. Service with a smile: do emotional intelligence, gender, and autonomy moderate the emotional labor process? *J Occup Health Psychol.* 2007;12(4):319-333.

109. Simpson PA, Stroh LK. Gender differences: emotional expression and feelings of personal inauthenticity. *J Appl Psychol.* 2004;89(4):715-721.

110. Briton NJ, Hall JA. Beliefs about female and male nonverbal communication. *Sex Roles.* 1995;32(1-2):79-90.

111. Ganong LH, Coleman M. Sex, sex roles, and emotional expressiveness. *J Genet Psychol.* 1985;146(3):405-411.

112. Kenworthy J, Fay C, Frame M, Petree R. A meta-analytic review of the relationship between emotional dissonance and emotional exhaustion. *J Appl Soc Psychol.* 2014;44(2):94-105.

113. Bagdasarov Z, Connelly S. Emotional labor among healthcare professionals: the effects are undeniable. *Narrat Inq Bioth.* 2013;3(2):125-129.

114. Zammuner VL, Galli C. The relationship with patients: "Emotional labor" and its correlates in hospital employees. In: Hartel CEJ, Zerbe WJ, Ashkanasy NM, eds. *Emotion in Organizational Behavior.* Mahwah, NJ: Lawrence Erlbaum Associates, Inc.; 2005:250-283.

115. Cottingham MD, Erickson RJ, Diefendorff JM. Examining men's status shield and status bonus: how gender frames the emotional labor and job satisfaction of nurses. *Sex Roles.* 2015;72(7):377-389.

116. Psilopanagioti A, Anagnostopoulos F, Mourtou E, Niakas D. Emotional intelligence, emotional labor, and job satisfaction among physicians in Greece. *BMC Health Serv Res.* 2012;12(1):463-475.

117. Mann S, Cowburn J. Emotional labour and stress within mental health nursing. *J Psychiatr Ment Health Nurs.* 2005;12(2):154-162.

118. Lovell B, Lee RT, Brotheridge CM. Gender differences in the application of communication skills, emotional labor, stress-coping and well-being among physicians. *Int J Med.* 2009;2(3):273-279.

119. Pisaniello SL, Winefield HR, Delfabbro PH. The influence of emotional labour and emotional work on the occupational health and wellbeing of South Australian hospital nurses. *J Vocat Behav.* 2012;80(3):579-591.

120. Chi N-W, Wang I-A. The relationship between newcomers' emotional labor and service performance: the moderating roles of service training and mentoring functions. *Int J Hum Resour Manag.* 2018;29(19):2729-2757.

121. Maslach C. *Burnout: The Cost of Caring.* Englewood Cliffs, NJ: Prentice Hall; 2003.

122. Kessler RC, Chiu WT, Demler O, Walters EE. Prevalence, severity, and comorbidity of 12-month DSM-IV disorders in the National Comorbidity Survey Replication. *Arch Gen Psychiatry.* 2005;62(6):617-627.

123. Maslach C, Schaufeli WB, Leiter MP. Job burnout. *Annu Rev Psychol.* 2001;52(1):397-422.

124. Levant RF. Toward the reconstruction of masculinity. In: Levant RF, Pollack WS, eds. *A New Psychology of Men.* New York, NY: Basic Books/Hachette Book Group.; 1995:229-251.

125. Wrobel NH. Effect of patient age and gender on clinical decisions. *Prof Psychol-Res Pr.* 1993;24(2):206-212.

126. Wilcox VL. Effects of patients' age, gender, and depression on medical students' beliefs, attitudes, intentions, and behavior. *J Appl Soc Psychol.* 1992;22(14):1093-1110.

127. Purvanova RK, Muros JP. Gender differences in burnout: a meta-analysis. *J Vocat Behav.* 2010;77(2):168-185.

128. Wharton AS. The affective consequences of service work: managing emotions on the job. *Work Occup.* 1993;20(2):205-232.

129. Chen K-Y, Yang C-M, Lien C-H, et al. Burnout, job satisfaction, and medical malpractice among physicians. *Int J Med Sci.* 2013;10(11):1471-1478.

130. Lemkau JP, Rafferty JP, Purdy RR, Rudisill JR. Sex role stress and job burnout among family practice physicians. *J Vocat Behav.* 1987;31(1):81-90.

131. Ratanawongsa N, Roter DL, Beach MC, et al. Physician burnout and patient-physician communication during primary care encounters. *J Gen Intern Med.* 2008;23(10):1581-1588.

132. Linzer M, McMurray JE, Visser MR, Oort FJ, Smets E, De Haes HC. Sex differences in physician burnout in the United States and the Netherlands. *J Am Med Womens Assoc (1972).* 2002;57(4):191.

133. Kandolin I. Burnout of female and male nurses in shiftwork. *Ergonomics.* 1993;36(1-3):141-147.

134. Tang CS-K, Lau BH-B. Gender role stress and burnout in Chinese human service professionals in Hong Kong. *Anxiety Stress Coping.* 1996;9(3):217-227.

135. Hensing G, Alexanderson K, Åkerlind I, Bjurulf P. Sick-leave due to minor psychiatric morbidity: role of sex integration. *Soc Psychiatry Psychiatr Epidemiol.* 1995;30(1):39-43.

136. Hunt K, Emslie C. Men's work, women's work? Occupational sex ratios and health. In: Orth-Gomer K, Chesney M, Wenger NK, eds. *Women, Stress, and Heart Disease.* Mahwah, NJ: Lawrence Erlbaum Associates, Inc.; 1998:99-118.

137. Hu Y-Y, Ellis RJ, Hewitt DB, et al. Discrimination, abuse, harassment, and burnout in surgical residency training. *New Engl J Med.* 2019;381(18):1741-1752.

138. Nielsen MBD, Kjær S, Aldrich PT, et al. Sexual harassment in care work—dilemmas and consequences: a qualitative investigation. *Int J Nurs Stud.* 2017;70:122-130.

139. Burns KEA, Fox-Robichaud A, Lorens E, Martin CM, for the Canadian Critical Care Society. Gender differences in career satisfaction, moral distress, and incivility: a national, cross-sectional survey of Canadian critical care physicians. *Can J Anesth/J Can Anesth.* 2019;66(5):503-511.

140. Jolly S, Griffith KA, DeCastro R, Stewart A, Ubel P, Jagsi R. Gender differences in time spent on parenting and domestic responsibilities by high-achieving young physician-researchers. *Ann Intern Med.* 2014;160(5):344-353.

141. Hall JA, Blanch-Hartigan D, Roter DL. Patients' satisfaction with male versus female physicians: a meta-analysis. *Med Care.* 2011;49(7):611-617.

142. Tsugawa Y, Jena AB, Figueroa JF, Orav EJ, Blumenthal DM, Jha AK. Comparison of hospital mortality and readmission rates for Medicare patients treated by male vs female physicians. *JAMA Intern Med.* 2017;177(2):206-213.

Culture and Emotions in the Medical Encounter

CHAPTER 12

Karolien Aelbrecht and Mary Catherine Beach

■ INTRODUCTION

Over the past two decades, people have migrated to and from various places in the world at an unprecedented pace,[1] leading to a heterogeneous mix of cultures within each country that requires healthcare providers to sensitively navigate cultural nuances in order to effectively deliver medical care.[2] Today, there are about 272 million migrants worldwide—51 million more than just 10 years ago—which is approximately 3.5% of the world's population.[3] This means that healthcare providers now are working in a superdiverse society, with patients and clients who come from very different sociocultural backgrounds. Furthermore, many countries, such as the United States and much of Europe, are already highly diverse due to their historical development. For the local healthcare system, and in particular primary healthcare services, which are often the first point of contact in the healthcare system, this social and cultural mixture of people entails many challenges and has direct implications when it comes to effectively navigating emotional communication during patient encounters.[4]

Recognizing and responding effectively to patients' emotions has proven difficult for many providers,[5,6] even when they share a similar cultural background with their patient. Addressing emotions in an ethnically and/or culturally discordant context is an even greater challenge in practice.[7] Therefore, the focus of this chapter will be on strategies for successfully identifying, engaging with, and appropriately responding to cultural barriers that affect emotional communication during medical encounters.

Cultural Distance in Clinical Encounters

Although the term "culture" is typically ascribed to geographic regions or countries of origin, a person's culture can be defined by many aspects of their lives, such as their age, religion, socioeconomic class, race/ethnicity, gender, sexual orientation, gender identity, disability, or immigration status. These multiple influences have a broad impact on one's life—including aspects of life that are relevant for healthcare practices and communication—such as traditions and customs, spirituality, style of communication, attitudes and beliefs about medicine and healthcare, attitudes toward personal autonomy, and family dynamics.[8]

All persons, clinicians and patients alike, have their own personal culture. In addition to the culture within which one grows up, health professionals are often acculturated in a Western medical tradition that embraces a scientific tradition with particular models of health and disease and places a high value on objectivity. With this training, clinicians take on their own "medical culture" that can create differences between their perspectives and those of the "lay culture" of patients they serve. This social or cultural distance between clinicians and patients can often create challenges for effective communication.[9-11]

■ CULTURAL NORMS FOR EMOTIONAL EXPRESSION

Clearly, individuals vary in their personal tendencies regarding emotional experience, expression, and reaction to the emotional expressions of others. While such individual differences exist, these personal experiences and behaviors also develop from absorbing the values, norms, beliefs, and habits of their cultural or ethnic group, including influences from their family of origin. For behaviors in the broad domain of emotion, cross-cultural research and medical anthropology have identified many general cultural tendencies that are relevant to clinician–patient interactions.[12]

At one point, theorists and researchers diverged sharply on the issue of cross-cultural universality (vs. cultural specificity) in how emotions are experienced, expressed, and decoded.[13] Consensus now occupies a middle ground: the answer depends on the behavior and the culture, with both extremes of the universality-cultural specificity continuum generally rejected. There are cultural differences in norms for feeling, showing, and judging emotions, yet these operate on top of at least some universal tendencies. For example, a short list of "basic" emotions (happiness, sadness, anger, fear, surprise, and disgust) shows evidence of cross-cultural similarity of expression and recognition.[14] However, a number of culture-specific patterns of emotion expression are well documented, one being the demonstration of emotion "dialects" in emotion expression that allow people to decode the emotional expressions of in-group members better than those of out-group members.[15] Understanding of these dialects is, fortunately, capable of evolving with increased exposure to the out-group culture.[16]

Cultural norms for conveying affective messages differ in countless ways. Ignorance of such norms can result in gaffes that range from the merely amusing to the seriously insulting or even life-endangering. If both parties are alert and forgiving, no harm may come; if one party attributes the other's ignorance to willful disrespect, injury may ensue. For example, a Thai family visit to a doctor ending with the doctor's affectionate pat on the head of a Thai child can be interpreted as offensive and undermine the rapport between the doctor and the family. Complications sometimes begin in the first moments of a clinical encounter, when provider and patient differ in their cultural norms for greeting.[13] If one adds in differing cultural or religious norms relating to gender and formality versus familiarity, it is clear that pitfalls exist even in the first, relatively unfraught, moments of interaction. In clinical situations the chances of emotional miscommunication only multiply from that point on. However, by learning what cues to attend to in order to more responsively navigate these cultural differences, a clinician can proactively mitigate the cultural divide.

Many nonverbal behaviors, including facial and gazing behavior, touching, and gestures with emotional meanings or impacts, differ between cultures.[17] Behaviors that are morphologically very different can carry similar meanings from one culture to another. Conversely, behaviors that look the same can carry different meanings.[18,19] Emotional expressions and behaviors that connote emotion can differ in quantity across cultures even when the underlying message is likely the same.[20,21] The frequency of smiling, interpersonal touch, preferences for personal space, and the directness of interpersonal body positioning vary across cultures, yet more smiling, more touch, smaller interpersonal distances, and more directly-facing interaction likely convey similar emotional messages of affiliation and intimacy within cultures.[17] The terms "high-contact" and "low-contact" have been applied to cultures that establish close interaction distances, touch each other frequently, and display other behaviors that imply more sensory stimulation and more permeable interpersonal boundaries.[22] Central and South America, southern Europe, and the Middle East are often classified as high-contact regions; Asia and northern Europe are viewed as low contact, as well as the United States according to some writers.[17] These are broad generalizations of course, and the existence of within-region and other subcultural differences, as well as individual differences, means one's assumptions should be held lightly.

Cultures differ in their rules for displaying emotion in different contexts;[23] for example, Japanese respondents reported more inhibition of expressing powerful emotions than respondents from Canada and the United States, and also believed that positive emotions should be expressed less than Canadians did.[24] East Asian cultures in general have overall reduced emotional expressivity compared to Western cultures. The latter difference is often connected by scholars to the values central to collectivistic (interdependent) versus individualistic cultures.[25,26]

Aside from expression, culture has a profound influence on how people assign emotion labels to their own emotional and physical experiences, depending on their appraisal of antecedent events and the explanatory models they subscribe to.[27] In the clinical context, emotional disturbances of different kinds must therefore be understood within the context of cultural background. The term "cultural idioms of distress" refers to culturally specific ways of expressing suffering, which in the clinical situation requires special awareness.[28–30] Stigma attached to mental health problems in some cultures adds further demands on clinicians to address emotional issues in ways that are not counterproductive.[31]

Culture also influences emotion regulation practices,[32] and even the same regulation strategies can have different impacts in different cultures. For example, frequency of emotion suppression—generally considered a maladaptive way of handling one's own emotions (see Chapter 7, Emotion Regulation in Patients, Providers, and the Clinical Relationship)—is more closely linked to depression in Western populations as compared with Chinese due to better skill among the Chinese in deciding when suppression is appropriate.[33]

CROSS-CULTURAL BARRIERS TO RELATIONSHIP BUILDING

Many studies have demonstrated that communication between patients and healthcare providers generally differs according to the patient's cultural background, with lower-quality communication between minority patients and their providers.[34–39] For example, studies have shown that clinicians are more verbally dominant, use less positive affective tone, engage in less socio-emotional/ psychosocial talk, and spend less time chatting with minority patients than white patients.[35,39,40] These differences in communication are thought to contribute to widespread racial/ethnic disparities in the quality of healthcare.

This lower quality communication may extend into the realm of emotional communication. In response to emotional expressions made by ethnic minority patients in Belgium, physicians more often explored the factual, medical content of the cue rather than the emotion itself, for example describing the procedure of the operation in response to a patient's distress rather than addressing the distress itself.[41] This is consistent with other studies documenting physicians' responses to patients' emotional cues and expressed concerns (see Chapter 6, Emotion Cues as Clinical Opportunities).

In response to expressions of emotion from African-American patients in the United States, two studies have found that clinicians are less likely to provide space for the patient to speak further (e.g., acknowledgment, empathy, silence, and back-channeling responses such as mmm-hmm that encourage the speaker to continue), less likely to make exploratory statements (e.g., questions and invitations to speak), and more likely to block the conversation (e.g., shut down and postpone) than with patients from other racial groups.[42,43]

There are a few studies that have examined the expression of emotion by racial/ethnic minority compared to majority cultural groups. The findings, perhaps not surprisingly, are mixed. One study found that racial/ethnic minority patients make fewer or less direct emotional statements,[43] although other studies have not shown such differences[44] and some have shown the opposite.[7] When differences in expression, perception of, and response to emotion in clinical encounters exist based on patient race/ethnicity, they may be a result of cultural differences or distance between clinicians and patients (described above), or may result from other barriers to relationship building such as language barriers, stereotyping, bias, racism, anxiety, or mistrust (described below).

Language Barriers

We also know from extensive research that a language barrier negatively impacts the quality of communication in clinical encounters, which—in turn—negatively impacts the quality of care delivered.[38,45–52] Patient–provider communication becomes even more complex when there is a language barrier. For example, Rivadeneyra et al. found that language-discordant patients with interpreters presented fewer symptoms, feelings, expectations, and thoughts and were more likely to have those comments ignored than majority language-concordant encounters.[53] Observation of dialogue in meetings that include family members in ICU settings revealed fewer incidents of physicians providing support, valuing family input, easing emotional burdens, and active listening in interpreted compared to meetings without an interpreter.[54]

With respect to emotional communication specifically, studies have similarly shown that language barriers have a profound and adverse impact.[38,44,52,55,56] In this context, underlying emotions are often veiled by language- or culture-specific norms and can thus be missed by physicians.[46,57,58] The ability to explore emotions, taking into account subtle distinctions, is a prerequisite to truly understanding the patients' narrative. In other words, if a provider is trying to apply patient- or relationship-centered care by exploring the patient's story in general and their emotions in particular using communication skills that focus mainly on partnership building, they cannot do this without a common language that both parties have sufficiently mastered.

Stereotyping, Racism, and Bias

The 2003 report of the Institute of Medicine, "Unequal Treatment: Confronting Racial and Ethnic Disparities in Health Care," documented the extent to which discrimination and inequality in healthcare exist.[40,59] Besides having difficulty accessing healthcare,[59] ethnic minority patients are more likely to experience bias and discrimination when seeking medical treatment than ethnic majority patients.[40,52,60]

Implicit bias refers to the unconscious and unintentional assumptions (attitudes and stereotypes) people make about each other.[61] Multiple studies have shown that implicit biases exist among clinicians as well as most other people, even among those who hold nonprejudicial explicit attitudes, and that these biases adversely impact healthcare quality.[62–70] Racial bias, or racism, has been referred to as the "public health crisis we can no longer ignore"[71] and is associated with mistrust among minority patients,[72] reduced preventive health screenings,[73] and delays in seeking care for life-threatening conditions.[74]

A recent systematic review of studies on the impact of implicit bias among clinicians on patient–clinician communication found that all studies showed providers with stronger implicit bias to demonstrate poorer patient–provider communication.[75] For example, one study demonstrated that unconscious racial bias among clinicians in the United States is associated with less patient-centered communication and lower ratings of care among African-American patients.[76] Other studies, both in the United States and in Europe,[52,77] have revealed that patients may experience implicit discrimination as a result of differences in their ethnic, cultural, or linguistic background relative to the clinician. For example, African-American patients seen by clinicians with greater implicit bias rated their experience lower in terms of patient-centered care and that non-Black physicians with higher levels of implicit, but not explicit, racial bias were more verbally dominant than physicians with lower levels of implicit bias, indicating that physicians with more negative implicit racial attitudes talked more than physicians with less negative racial attitudes.[77]

■ SUGGESTED STRATEGIES

Patient–Clinician Concordance

Racial/Ethnic/Cultural

There is a considerable amount of evidence that communication, relationships, and healthcare quality in general are better for racial/ethnic minority patients who are in race-concordant (i.e., when clinician and patient share the same race) compared to race-discordant (i.e., clinician and patient do not share the same race) relationships. Racial/ethnic minority patients have reported higher quality healthcare when receiving care from concordant versus discordant clinicians.[78,79] In studies that have observed dialogue, race-concordant versus discordant encounters appeared to be longer and have more patient positive affect.[35,80]

There are many possible reasons why racial/ethnic concordance may lead to better quality healthcare for racial/ethnic minority patients. First, racial/ethnic concordance may result in less stereotyping by clinicians, and less bias and racism toward and greater investment in patients from the shared culture or identity. Independent of the actual feelings or commitment toward the patients, minority patients who have experienced discrimination and bias may be more likely to trust a clinician from their own racial/ethnic group (which could explain the fact that these visits tend to be characterized by more positive patient affective tone). In this setting, perhaps patients may feel more comfortable sharing their emotions and may be more likely to believe that the clinician has their best interest at heart.

Of course, we are describing the reality of emotional reactions and not prescribing that healthcare should be segregated according to racial or cultural concordance. Healthcare providers should be able to help every person and provide equally high-quality care to all. Furthermore, patients do not always have the privilege of selecting whomever they would like as a care provider. Through increased awareness to these cultural considerations, healthcare providers can seize opportunities to create rapport, address emotion, minimize communication barriers, and demonstrate cultural humility.

Language

Language concordance with clinicians for patients who do not speak the country's majority language leads to better patient outcomes in all respects.[81,82] For example, in the United States, patients with limited English proficiency (LEP) who had language-discordant clinicians (i.e., clinician and patient do not share a common language) reported lower trust, worse communication, and more discrimination,[83,84] whereas LEP patients with language-concordant clinicians (i.e., clinician and patient share a common language) reported similar communication to English-proficient patients.[83] Furthermore, patients who do not speak the country's majority language and who interact with language-discordant clinicians are more likely to have unanswered questions[85] and pay less attention to the psychosocial aspects of care in documentation of their encounters.[86] Finally, patients disclose less when trying to communicate in a less familiar language.[87,88] A recent systematic review found that 76%

of studies evaluating the impact of language concordance on patient understanding, ratings of communication, and health outcomes found a beneficial impact on at least one of those outcomes, concluding that language concordance between patient and clinician improves healthcare quality and patient outcomes.[89]

Many mistakes happen when providers overestimate their knowledge and understanding of a common language[47,90–92] and think that *some* proficiency in a shared language is enough to conduct a consultation. Therefore, it is important for clinicians to use professional interpreters whenever possible unless the clinician is completely fluent in the patient's language.

Quality Language Interpretation

When language concordance between the patient and clinician is not possible, providing appropriate high-quality language support is critical. In many Western countries interpreter-mediated medical encounters are now a standard part of daily clinical work for healthcare professionals. In current healthcare practice, two main types of interpreters can be distinguished: (1) the trained professional interpreter and (2) the ad-hoc (informal) interpreter, such as a family member, a friend, an acquaintance, or even a passer-by who speaks and understands the language of the patient (e.g., another patient or a receptionist).

Any interpretation is better than no interpretation for patients who don't speak the majority language. Although professional interpreters are legally required in the United States by all health organizations that receive federal funds, not all health systems around the world have this resource available.[93] One group of studies has shown that interpretation leads to a better patient experience and enhanced understanding[94–97] as well as more patient disclosure of traumatic events[98] among asylum seekers. Another set of studies has shown that patients report more understanding and satisfaction for interpreted versus uninterpreted encounters (although these studies also confirmed that the best understanding and satisfaction was seen in language-concordant groups).[81,82]

Deficits in communication are alleviated to some extent by professional interpretation, although not completely. Although multiple studies have demonstrated that interpreters make many errors and omissions,[87,99] studies have also shown that professional interpreters make fewer errors[100] and lead to a better patient experience[81,93] than informal interpreters. Concerning communication of emotions, one study found that patients who had informal interpreters (family members) expressed fewer emotional concerns than those without informal interpreters, and that only half of all patients' cues were translated by the informal interpreter to the physician.[56]

Professional interpretation does not need to be on site, if the resource could be made available remotely. Studies have also shown that technology-assisted professional interpretation is not inferior and may prove better than in-person professional interpretation. For example, when professional interpretation was provided remotely versus in-person, there was more patient and clinician engagement and fewer errors.[101] Other studies have confirmed that patients were as satisfied with telephonic interpretation as with language-concordant interactions[102] and that telephonic interpretation was superior to in-person interpretation in terms of patient satisfaction.[103]

Finally, besides being aware that language support is important and which support is best to use, it is also important to know how to use the available support.[104,105] Clinicians should be trained in use of language support, which has been associated with improved patient experience.[105] Such training should include where to place the interpreter and themselves in the encounter, to always look at the patient, how to brief and debrief the interpreter, to speak slowly, and to speak in simple language and in manageable "chunks" of information.[104]

Self-Awareness

Cultural humility

In addition to the need for clinicians to be aware of the individual patient in front of them, they also must maintain awareness of their own thoughts, feelings, and even biases, toward every patient. Clinicians also must be willing to face their own ignorance about how the patient's culture and the assumptions, expectancies, and emotional experiences associated with it might be affecting the communication process as well as the patient's health. Sometimes, directly admitting ignorance and enlisting the patient as a cultural guide can promote a more trusting relationship and better exchange of information.

In response to the widespread realization of healthcare disparities and implicit biases among health professionals, there has been an increased enthusiasm for enhancing the capacity of clinicians to deliver high-quality care across cultural distance. Cultural humility is one promising approach, and is defined as a lifelong commitment to self-evaluation and self-critique, with the recognition that one's own way of thinking is not necessarily the best or only way of thinking.[106] For this, a reflective attitude is needed,[107,108] and it involves a continuous process of self-assessment. Physicians should thus be fully aware of their own background and identity, as well as their personal views of the (medical) situation and their cultural biases, which are often colored by previous experiences.[107,108]

We consider this reflective approach superior to the practice of teaching culture-specific knowledge, which tends to be generalizing and induce stereotypical ideas and consequent treatment behaviors toward patients with different sociocultural backgrounds than one's own. Given the fact that a superdiverse society is the reality in which most healthcare providers are working nowadays, a culture-specific approach is not sufficient anymore.[38] On the contrary, knowledge of generic theoretical sociological, psychosocial, and anthropological concepts of diversity theory is key to developing diversity-sensitive care. There are a number of ways to promote reflection, and mindfulness is one evidence-based practice that has been proven for practitioners to help them more effectively care for those from different cultural backgrounds.

Mindfulness

Mindfulness is a metacognitive skill involving attentional control (e.g., paying attention to one's experience in the present moment), emotional regulation, self-awareness, and a nonjudgmental and curious orientation toward one's experiences.[109,110] It has been suggested—and supported by emerging evidence—that mindfulness practice can reduce the likelihood that implicit biases will be activated, increase providers' awareness of and ability to control responses to biases, increase compassion (for oneself and for patients), and reduce internal sources of cognitive load (e.g., stress, burnout, and compassion fatigue).[111] Further, mindfulness has been shown to improve the quality of communication in clinical encounters.[112]

Several experiments involving nonclinicians have demonstrated that mindfulness can reduce biases, and there is reason to believe that this might apply to clinicians as well.[113-117] A systematic review of 29 studies (including 14 randomized controlled trials) of Mindfulness Based Stress Reduction (MBSR) or MBSR-based interventions in healthcare providers found that MBSR improved providers' self-rated skills on their ability to identify and accept their emotions, as well as to identify others' emotions.[118] Following mindfulness meditation training, brain imaging studies show changes in core regions associated with self-regulation of awareness, attention, and emotion,[109] including neural structures related to the control of prejudiced responses.[109,119] Thus, mindfulness has the potential to improve awareness of emotions and reduce biases and stereotyping.[111]

Patient-Centered Approach

The foundation of effective physician–patient communication acknowledges the patient's background, and integrates their perspectives, experiences, needs, ideas, emotions, expectations, and preferences concerning involvement in healthcare decisions.[120] By communicating in a more patient-centered style, the patient's goals, which are diverse and not easily predicted in advance, can be explored. Recognizing and responding to a patient's emotions is thus an

■ TABLE 12-1. Emotional Communication in Cross-Cultural Patient-Clinician Encounters

Cultural influences on emotional communication	General barriers to relationship-building *(with potential for impacting emotional communication)*	Suggested strategies for improving emotional communication in cross-cultural encounters
Expression of emotions *(intensity, descriptions, thresholds for expression)*	Language barriers	Concordance
Attitudes and reactions to emotions *(one's own and those of others)*	Stereotyping/bias/racism	Patient-centered approach
	Mistrust	Cultural humility, mindfulness, and self-awareness

inherent part of patient-oriented communication. See Table 12-1 for an overview of barriers and suggested strategies for improving emotional communication in cross-cultural encounters.

■ CONCLUSION

Delivering high-quality care in a superdiverse society requires appreciating cultural variation in emotion interpretation and expression. Given the evidence that patients who lack language- and culturally-concordant care face additional barriers that may compromise communication about emotional concerns and critical health information, it is necessary to provide high-quality interpretive services for language-discordant clinician and adopt reflective practices that foster cultural humility allowing for enhanced understanding of each patient as a unique person.

REFERENCES

1. Vertovec S. Super-diversity and its implications. *Ethn Racial Stud*. 2007;30(6):1024-1054.

2. Virupaksha H., Kumar A, Nirmala B. Migration and mental health: an interface. *J Natural Science, Biology and Medicine*. 2014;5(2):233.

3. Migration. UN.org. https://www.un.org/en/sections/issues-depth/migration/index.html. Published 2020. Accessed October 25, 2020.

4. Rechel B, Mladovsky P, Ingleby D, Mackenbach J, McKee M. Migration and health in an increasingly diverse Europe. *Lancet*. 2013;381(9873):1235-1245.

5. Butow PN, Brown RF, Cogar S, Dunn SM. Oncologists' reactions to cancer patients' verbal cues. *Psychooncology*. 2002;11(1):47-58.

6. Adams K, Cimino JEW, Arnold RM, Anderson WG. Why should I talk about emotion? Communication patterns associated with physician discussion of patient expressions of negative emotion in hospital admission encounters. *Patient Educ Couns*. 2012;89(1):44-50.

7. Schouten BC, Schinkel S. Emotions in primary care: are there cultural differences in the expression of cues and concerns? *Patient Educ Couns*. 2015;98(11):1346-1351.

8. Betancourt JR. Cultural competency: providing quality care to diverse populations. *Consult Pharm*. 2006;21(12):988-995.

9. Saha S, Sanders DS, Todd P, et al. The role of cultural distance between patient and provider in explaining racial / ethnic disparities in HIV care. *Patient Educ Couns*. 2011;85(3):e278-e284.

10. Saha S. The relevance of cultural distance between patients and physicians to racial disparities in health care. *J Gen Intern Med*. 2006;21:203-205.

11. Malat J. Social distance and patients' rating of healthcare providers. *J Health Soc Behav*. 2001;42(4):360-372.

12. Becker A, Kleinman A. The history of cultural psychiatry in the last half-century. In: Bloch S, Green S, Holmes J, eds. *Psychiatry: Past, Present, and Prospect*. Oxford, UK: Oxford University Press; 2014:74-95.

13. Matsumoto D, Hwang H. The cultural bases of nonverbal communication. In: Matsumoto D, Hwang H, Frank M, eds.. *APA handbook of nonverbal communication*. Washington, DC: American Psychological Association; 2016:77-101.

14. Ekman P, Friesen W, O'Sullivan M, et al. Universals and cultural differences in the judgments of facial expressions of emotion. *J Pers Soc Psychol*. 1987;53(4):712-717.

15. Elfenbein HA, Ambady N. On the universality and cultural specificity of emotion recognition: a meta-analysis. *Psychol Bull*. 2002;128(2):203-235.

16. Elfenbein H, Ambady N. When familiarity breeds accuracy: cultural exposure and facial emotion recognition. *J Pers Soc Psychol*. 2003;85(2):276-290.

17. Knapp ML, Hall JA, Horgan TG. *Nonverbal Communication in Human Interaction*. 9th ed. Dubuque, IA: Kendall-Hunt; 2021.

18. Rychlowska M, Miyamoto Y, Matsumoto D, et al. Heterogeneity of long-history migration explains cultural differences in reports of emotional expressivity and the functions of smiles. *PNAS USA*. 2015;112(19):E2429-E2436.

19. Morris D, Collett P, Marsh P, O'Shaughnessy M. *Gestures*. New York, NY: Stein and Day; 1979.

20. Talhelm T, Oishi S, Zhang X. Who smiles while alone? Rates of smiling lower in China than U.S. *Emotion*. 2019;19(4):741-745.

21. Szarota P. The mystery of the European smile: a comparison based on individual photographs provided by internet users. *J Nonverbal Behav*. 2010;34(4):249-256.

22. Hall E. *The Hidden Dimension*. New York, NY: Doubleday & Co.; 1966.

23. Matsumoto D. Cultural similarities and differences in display rules. *Motiv Emot.* 1990;14(3):195-214.

24. Safdar S, Friedlmeier W, Matsumoto D, et al. Variations of emotional display rules within and across cultures: a comparison between Canada, USA, and Japan. *Can J Behav Sci.* 2009;41(1):1-10.

25. Markus HR, Kitayama S. Culture and the self: implications for cognition, emotion, and motivation. *Psychol Rev.* 1991;98(2):224-253.

26. Matsumoto D, Yoo SH, Fontaine J, et al. Mapping expressive differences around the world: the relationship between emotional display rules and individualism versus collectivism. *J Cross Cult Psychol.* 2008;39(1):55-74.

27. Benning TB, Chen JA. Identifying and working with diverse explanatory models of mental illness. In: Trinh N-H, Chen J, eds. *Sociocultural Issues in Psychiatry: A Casebook and Curriculum.* Oxford, UK: Oxford University Press; 2019:127-144.

28. Maercker A, Heim E, Kirmayer LJ. *Cultural Clinical Psychology and PTSD.* Boston, MA: Hogrefe Publishing; 2019.

29. Bäärnhielm S, Mösko M. Cross-cultural communication with traumatised immigrants. In: Schouler-Ocak M, ed. *Trauma and Migration: Cultural Factors in the Diagnosis and Treatment of Traumatised Immigrants.* New York, NY: Springer International Publishing; 2015:39-55.

30. Kirmayer LJ, Dao THT, Smith A. Somatization and psychologization: understanding cultural idioms of distress. In: Okpaku SO, ed. *Clinical Methods in Transcultural Psychiatry.* Washington, DC: American Psychiatric Association; 1998:233-265.

31. Phillips D, Lauterbach D. American Muslim immigrant mental health: the role of racism and mental health stigma. *J Muslim Ment Heal.* 2017;11(1):39-56.

32. Butler EA. Emotion regulation in cultural context: implications for wellness and illness. In: Barnow S, Balkir N, eds. *Cultural Variations in Psychopathology: From Research to Practice.* Boston, MA: Hogrefe Publishing; 2013:93-114.

33. Chen S, Burton CL, Bonanno GA. The suppression paradox: a cross-cultural comparison of suppression frequency, suppression ability, and depression. *J Affect Disord.* 2020;274:183-189.

34. Martin KD, Roter DL, Beach MC, Carson KA, Cooper LA. Physician communication behaviors and trust among black and white patients with hypertension. *Med Care.* 2013;51:151-157.

35. Johnson RL, Roter D, Powe NR, Cooper LA. Patient race/ethnicity and quality of patient-physician communication during medical visits. *Am J Public Health.* 2004;94:2084-2090.

36. Beach MC, Saha S, Korthuis PT, et al. Differences in patient–provider communication for Hispanic compared to non-Hispanic white patients in HIV care. *J Gen Intern Med.* 2020;25:682-687.

37. Beach MC, Saha S, Korthuis PT, et al. Patient-provider communication differs for black compared to white HIV-infected patients. *AIDS Behav.* 2011;15:805-811.

38. Schouten BC, Meeuwesen L. Cultural differences in medical communication: a review of the literature. *Patient Educ Couns.* 2006;64(1-3):21-34.

39. Oliver MN, Goodwin MA, Gotler RS, Gregory PM, Stange KC, Brunswick N. Time use in clinical encounters: are African American patients treated differently? *J Natl Med Assoc.* 2001;93(10):380-385.

40. Smedley BD, Stith AY, Nelson AR, eds. Institute of Medicine (US) Committee on Understanding and Eliminating Racial and Ethnic Disparities in Health Care, Unequal Treatment: Confronting Racial and Ethnic Disparities in Health Care. Washington, DC: National Academies Press (US); 2003.

41. Aelbrecht K, De Maesschalck S, Willems S, Deveugele M, Pype P. How family physicians respond to unpleasant emotions of ethnic minority patients. *Patient Educ Couns.* 2017;100(10):1867-1873.

42. Park P, Saha S, Han D, et al. Emotional communication in HIV care: an observational study of patients' expressed emotions and clinician response. *AIDS Behav.* 2019;23:2816-2828.

43. Park J, Catherine M, Han D, Moore RD, Korthuis PT, Saha S. Racial disparities in clinician responses to patient emotions. *Patient Educ Couns.* 2020;103(9):1736-1744.

44. Maesschalck D, Deveugele M, Willems S. Language, culture and emotions: exploring ethnic minority patients' emotional expressions in primary healthcare consultations. *Patient Educ Couns.* 2011;84:406-412.

45. Schenker Y, Wang F, Selig SJ, Ng R, Fernandez A. The impact of language barriers on documentation of informed consent at a hospital with on-site interpreter services. *J Gen Intern Med.* 2007;22(Suppl 2):294-299.

46. Aelbrecht K, Pype P, Vos J, Deveugele M. Having cancer in a foreign country. *Patient Educ Couns.* 2016;99(10):1708-1716.

47. Ferguson W, Candib L. Culture, language, and the doctor-patient relationship. *Fam Med.* 2002;34(5):353-361.

48. Divi C, Koss R, Schmaltz S, Loeb J. Language proficiency and adverse events in US hospitals: a pilot study. *Int J Qual Heal Care.* 2007;19(2):60-67.

49. MacFarlane A, Glynn L, Mosinkie P, Murphy A. Responses to language barriers in consultations with refugees and asylum seekers: a telephone survey of Irish general practitioners. *BMC Fam Pract.* 2008;9(1).

50. Aelbrecht K, Hanssens L, Detollenaere J, Willems S, Deveugele M, Pype P. Determinants of physician–patient communication: the role of language, education and ethnicity. *Patient Educ Couns.* 2019;102(4):776-781.

51. Fernandez A, Schillinger D, Warton EM, et al. Language barriers, physician-patient language concordance, and glycemic control among insured Latinos with diabetes: The Diabetes Study of Northern California (DISTANCE). *J Gen Intern Med.* 2011;26(2):170-176.

52. Schinkel S, Schouten B, Kerpiclik F, Van Den Putte B, Van Weert J. Perceptions of barriers to patient participation: are they due to language, culture, or discrimination? *Health Commun.* 2019;34(12):1469-1481.

53. Rivadeneyra R, Elderkin-thompson V, Silver RC. Patient centeredness in medical encounters requiring an interpreter. *Am J Med.* 2000;108(6):470-474.

54. Thornton JD, Pham K, Engelberg RA, Jackson JC, Curtis JR. Families with limited English proficiency receive less information and support in interpreted intensive care unit family conferences. *Crit Care Med.* 2009;37(1):89-95.

55. Kale E, Finset A, Eikeland H. Emotional cues and concerns in hospital encounters with non-Western immigrants as compared with Norwegians: an exploratory study. *Patient Educ Couns*. 2011;84(3):325-331.

56. Schouten BC, Schinkel S. Turkish migrant GP patients' expression of emotional cues and concerns in encounters with and without informal interpreters. *Patient Educ Couns*. 2014;97(1):23-29.

57. Aelbrecht K, De Maesschalck S, Willems S, Deveugele M, Pype P. How family physicians respond to unpleasant emotions of ethnic minority patients. *Patient Educ Couns*. 2017;100(10):1867-1873.

58. Lorié Á, Reinero DA, Phillips M, Zhang L, Riess H. Culture and nonverbal expressions of empathy in clinical settings: a systematic review. *Patient Educ Couns*. 2017;100(3):411-424.

59. Hanssens L, Detollenaere J, Hardyns W, Willems S. Access, treatment and outcomes of care: a study of ethnic minorities in Europe. *Int J Public Heal*. 2016;61(4):443-454.

60. Johnson RL, Saha S, Arbelaez JJ, Beach MC, Cooper LA. Racial and ethnic differences in patient perceptions of bias and cultural competence in health care. *J Gen Intern Med*. 2004;19(2):101-110.

61. Gonzalez CM, Deno ML, Kintzer E, Marantz PR, Lypson ML, Mckee MD. Patient perspectives on racial and ethnic implicit bias in clinical encounters: implications for curriculum development. *Patient Educ Couns*. 2018;101(9):1669-1675.

62. Zestcott CA, Blair I V, Stone J. Examining the presence, consequences, and reduction of implicit bias in health care: a narrative review. *Group Process Intergr Relat*. 2016;19(4):528-542.

63. Paradies Y, Truong M, Priest N. A systematic review of the extent and measurement of healthcare provider racism. *J Gen Intern Med*. 2014;29(2):364-387.

64. Sabin JA, Riskind RG, Nosek BA. Health care providers' implicit and explicit attitudes toward lesbian women and gay men. *Am J Public Health*. 2015;105(9):1831-1841.

65. Hall WJ, Chapman M V, Lee KM, Merino YM, Thomas TW, Payne BK. Implicit racial/ethnic bias among health care professionals and its influence on health care outcomes: a systematic review. *Am J Public Health*. 2015;105(12):e60-e76.

66. Dovidio JF, Fiske ST. Under the radar: how unexamined biases in decision-making processes in clinical interactions can contribute to health care disparities. *Am J Public Health*. 2012;102(5):945-952.

67. van Ryn M, Burgess DJ, Dovidio JF, Phelan SM, Griffin JM, Fu SS. The impact of racism on clinician cognition, behavior, and clinical decision making. *Du Bois Rev*. 2011;8(1):199-218.

68. Burgess D, van Ryn M, Dovidio J, Saha S. Reducing racial bias among health care providers: lessons from social-cognitive psychology. *J Gen Intern Med*. 2007;22(6):882-887.

69. Dovidio JF, Gaertner SL. Aversive racism. *Adv Exp Soc Psychol*. 2004;36:1-51.

70. Devine PG, Forscher PS, Austin AJ, Cox WT. Long-term reduction in implicit race bias: a prejudice habit-breaking intervention. *J Exp Soc Psychol*. 2012;48(6):1267-1278.

71. Devakumar D, Selvarajah S, Shannon G, et al. Racism, the public health crisis we can no longer ignore. *Lancet*. 2020;395(10242):e112-e113.

72. Williamson LD, Smith MA, Bigman CA. Does discrimination breed mistrust? Examining the role of mediated and non-mediated discrimination experiences in medical mistrust. *J Health Commun*. 2019;24(10):791-799.

73. Powell W, Richmond J, Mohottige D, Yen I, Joslyn A. Medical mistrust, racism, and delays in preventive health screening among African-American men. *Behav Med*. 2019;45(2):102-117.

74. Mullins MA, Peres LC, Alberg AJ, et al. Perceived discrimination, trust in physicians, and prolonged symptom duration before ovarian cancer diagnosis in the African American Cancer Epidemiology Study. *Cancer*. 2019;125(24):4442-4451.

75. Maina IW, Belton TD, Ginzberg S, Singh A, Johnson TJ. A decade of studying implicit racial/ethnic bias in healthcare providers using the implicit association test. *Soc Sci Med*. 2018;199:219-229.

76. Cooper LA, Roter DL, Carson KA, et al. The associations of clinicians' implicit attitudes about race with medical visit communication and patient ratings of interpersonal care. *Am J Public Heal*. 2012;102(979-987).

77. Hagiwara N, Penner LA, Gonzalez R, et al. Racial attitudes, physician-patient talk time ratio, and adherence in racially discordant medical interactions. *Soc Sci Med*. 2018;87(2013):123-131.

78. Saha S, Komaromy M, Koepsell TD, Bindman AB. Patient-physician racial concordance and the perceived quality and use of health care. *Arch Intern Med*. 1999;159:997-1004.

79. Cooper-Patrick L, Gallo JJ, Gonzales JJ, Vu HT, Powe NR, Nelson, C et al. Race, gender, and partnership in the patient-physician relationship. *JAMA*. 1999;11:583-589.

80. Cooper L, Roter D, Johnson R, Ford D, Steinwachs D, Powe N. Patient-centered communication, ratings of care, and concordance of patient and physician race. *Ann Intern Med*. 2003;139(11):907-915.

81. Baker DW, Parker RM, Williams M V, Coates WC, Pitkin K. Use and effectiveness of interpreters in an emergency department. *JAMA*. 1996;275(10):783-788.

82. Baker DW, Hayes R, Fortier JP. Interpreter use and satisfaction with interpersonal aspects of care for Spanish-speaking patients. *Med Care*. 1998;36(10):1461-1470.

83. Wilson E, Chen AH, Grumbach K, Wang F, Fernandez A. Effects of limited English proficiency and physician language on health care comprehension. *J Gen Intern Med*. 2005;20(9):800-806.

84. Schenker Y, Karter AJ, Schillinger D, et al. The impact of limited English proficiency and physician language concordance on reports of clinical interactions among patients with diabetes: The DISTANCE study. *Patient Educ Couns*. 2010;81(2):222-228.

85. Green AR, Ngo-Metzger Q, Legedza ATR, Massagli MP, Phillips RS, Iezzoni LI. Interpreter services, language concordance, and health care quality. *J Gen Intern Med*. 2005;20(11):1050-1056.

86. Eamranond PP, Davis RB, Phillips RS, Wee CC. Patient-physician language concordance and lifestyle counseling among Spanish-speaking patients. *J Immigr Minor Heal*. 2009;11:494-498.

87. Marcos LR, Alpert M, Urcuyo L, Kesselman M. The effect of interview language on the evaluation of psychopathology in Spanish-American schizophrenic patients. *Am J Psychiatry*. 1973;130(5):549-553.

88. Kuo D, Fagan MJ. Satisfaction with methods of Spanish interpretation in an ambulatory care clinic. *J Gen Intern Med.* 1999;14(9):547-550.

89. Diamond L, Izquierdo K, Canfield D, Matsoukas K, Gany F. A systematic review of the impact of patient–physician non-English language concordance on quality of care and outcomes. *J Gen Intern Med.* 2019;34(8):1591-1606.

90. Landmark A, Svennevig J, Gerwing J, Gulbrandsen P. Patient involvement and language barriers: problems of agreement or understanding? *Patient Educ Couns.* 2017;100(6):1092-1102.

91. Diamond LC, Schenker Y, Curry L, Bradley EH, Fernandez A. Getting by: underuse of interpreters by resident physicians. *J Gen Intern Med.* 2009;24(2):256-262.

92. Prince D, Nelson M. Teaching Spanish to emergency medicine residents. *Acad Emerg Med.* 1995;2(1):32-36.

93. Jaeger FN, Pellaud N, Laville B, Klauser P. The migration-related language barrier and professional interpreter use in primary health care in Switzerland. *BMC Health Serv Res.* 2019;19(1):1-10.

94. Kline F, Axosta FX, Austin W, Johnson RG. The misunderstood Spanish-speaking patient. *Am J Psychiatry.* 1980;137(12):1530-1533.

95. Chan A, Woodruff RK. Comparison of palliative care needs of English- and non-English-speaking patients. *J Palliat Care.* 1999;15(1):26-30.

96. Moreno G, Tarn DM, Morales LS. Impact of interpreters on the receipt of new prescription medication information among Spanish-speaking Latinos. *Med Care.* 2009;47(12):1201-1208.

97. Bagchi AD, Dale S, Verbitsky-savitz N, Andrecheck S, Zavotsky K. Examining effectiveness of medical interpreters in Emergency Departments for Spanish-speaking patients with limited English proficiency: results of a randomized controlled trial. *Ann Emerg Med.* 2010;57(3):248-256.

98. Eytan A, Bischoff A, Rrustemi I, et al. Screening of mental disorders in asylum-seekers from Kosovo. *Aust New Zeal J Psychiatry.* 2002;36(4):499-503.

99. Price J. Foreign language interpreting in psychiatric practice. *Aust New Zeal J Psychiatry.* 1975;9(4):263-267.

100. Flores G, Laws MB, Mayo SJ, et al. Errors in medical interpretation and their potential clinical consequences in pediatric encounters. *Pediatrics.* 2003;111(1):6-14.

101. Hornberger JC, Gibson CD, Wood W, et al. Eliminating language barriers for non-English-speaking patients. *Med Care.* 1996;34(8):845-856.

102. Lee LJ, Batal HA, Maselli JH, Kutner JS. Effect of Spanish interpretation method on patient satisfaction. *J Gen Intern Med.* 2002;17(8):641-646.

103. Crossman KL, Wiener E, Roosevelt G, Bajaj L, Hampers L. Interpreters: telephonic, in-person interpretation and bilingual providers. *Pediatrics.* 2010;125(3):e631-e638.

104. Jacobs EA, Diamond LC, Stevak L. The importance of teaching clinicians when and how to work with interpreters. *Patient Educ Couns.* 2010;78(2):149-153.

105. Bischoff A, Perneger TV, Bovier PA, Loutan L, Stalder H. Improving communication between physicians and patients who speak a foreign language. *Br J Gen Pract.* 2003;53(492):541-546.

106. Tervalon M, Murray-Garcia J. Cultural humility versus cultural competence: a critical distinction in defining physician training outcomes in multicultural education. *J Health Care Poor Underserved*. 1998;9(2):117-125.

107. Teal CR, Street RL. Critical elements of culturally competent communication in the medical encounter: a review and model. *Soc Sci Med*. 2009;68(3):533-543.

108. Muntinga ME, Krajenbrink VQ, Peerdeman SM, Croiset G, Verdonk P. Toward diversity-responsive medical education: taking an intersectionality-based approach to a curriculum evaluation. *Adv Heal Sci Educ Theory Pract*. 2016;21(3):541-559.

109. Tang Y-Y, Hölzel BK, Posner MI. The neuroscience of mindfulness meditation. *Nat Rev Neurosci*. 2015;16(4):213-225.

110. Bishop SR, Lau M, Shapiro S, et al. Mindfulness: a proposed operational definition. *Clin Psychol Sci Pract*. 2004;11(3):230-241.

111. Burgess DJ, Beach MC, Saha S. Mindfulness practice: a promising approach to reducing the effects of clinician implicit bias on patients. *Patient Educ Couns*. 2017;100(2):372-376.

112. Beach MC, Roter D, Korthuis PT, et al. A multicenter study of physician mindfulness and health care quality. *Ann Fam Med*. 2013;11(5):421-428.

113. Kang Y, Gray JR, Dovidio JF. The nondiscriminating heart: lovingkindness meditation training decreases implicit intergroup bias. *J Exp Psychol Gen*. 2014;143(3):1306-1313.

114. Stell AJ, Farsides T. Brief loving-kindness meditation reduces racial bias, mediated by positive other-regarding emotions. *Motiv Emot*. 2016;40:140-147.

115. Parks S, Birtel MD, Crisp RJ. Evidence that a brief meditation exercise can reduce prejudice toward homeless people. *Soc Psychol*. 2014;45(6):458-465.

116. Lueke A, Gibson B. Mindfulness meditation reduces implicit age and race bias the role of reduced automaticity of responding. *Soc Psychol Pers Sci*. 2015;6(3):284-291.

117. Lueke A, Gibson B. Brief mindfulness meditation reduces discrimination. *Psychol Conscious Theor Res Pract*. 2016;3(1):34-44.

118. Lamothe M, Rondeau É, Malboeuf-Hurtubise C, Duval M, Sultan S. Outcomes of MBSR or MBSR-based interventions in health care providers: a systematic review with a focus on empathy and emotional competencies. *Complement Ther Med*. 2016;24:19-28.

119. Amodio DM. The neuroscience of prejudice and stereotyping. *Nat Rev Neurosci*. 2014;15(10):670-682.

120. Stewart M, Brown J, Weston W, McWhinney I, McWilliam C, Freeman T. *Patient-Centred Medicine: Transforming the Clinical Method*. London: Sage; 1995.

Emotion and Decision Making in the Clinical Encounter

CHAPTER 13

Amber E. Barnato

■ INTRODUCTION

We've been trained to believe that clinical decision making is rational and analytic; that emotions get in the way of good decision making. While considerable evidence suggests that emotions do influence decision making and that very strong negative emotional states impair information processing and reasoning, increasing evidence suggests that intuitive deliberation, which relies on affective cues, may produce better outcomes than analytical deliberation alone.

In this chapter, I will focus in particular on decision making in the context of serious illness—in part because it is most often associated with emotion—and because it is my area of clinical research and practice. However, the lessons herein apply to any high-stakes encounter, including those in the emergency room or when a primary care or specialist provider delivers unexpected bad news. Importantly, this chapter will not address other important topics involving emotion and decision making, including race-, class-, and behavior-based biases that influence clinical decision making. In this chapter, I draw on literature from psychology, neuroscience, and economics, as well as clinical medicine. I explore the influences of both patient (or surrogate) and clinician emotion on the decision making of all the parties involved. I also demonstrate how patient and clinician emotions may interact and how integrated palliative care can mitigate some of the negative impacts and thereby facilitate better decision making.

■ SERIOUS ILLNESS COMMUNICATION AND DECISION MAKING

Serious illness is defined as "[a] health condition that carries a high risk of mortality and either negatively impacts a person's daily function or quality of life or excessively strains the caregiver."[1,2] Because of the stakes and strains, communication and decision making regarding serious illness elicit strong emotions in patients, caregivers, and clinicians.

Case 1

"I have lots of patients who do really well!"

You are an oncologist seeing a patient with newly diagnosed metastatic (Stage IV) pancreatic cancer. This is your first meeting and the purpose is to establish oncologic care and discuss treatment options. You lay out the details of the currently recommended chemotherapy regimen, including details of dosing regimens, likelihood of side effects, and statistics regarding disease progression and control, citing clinical trial evidence for the newest elements of the regimen. The patient quietly asks you how much time they have, and looks like they are about to cry. You feel your hands getting sweaty and your heart beating faster. You feel the overwhelming urge to reassure them, to make them less sad and scared. You know the National Comprehensive Cancer Network (NCCN) survival statistics by heart because you just took the boards, but instead this pops out of your mouth: "I don't have a crystal ball. Everyone is different. I have lots of patients who do really well!"

This case has multiple layers. You felt anxious and panicked in response to the question about prognosis, so different from your calm and composed self a few moments earlier in the conversation. You hate when patients cry! In the moment, you reassure yourself that you are just helping the patient maintain hope and keep a positive attitude. But on your drive home you replay the conversation and feel a nagging doubt. Why did you feel so comfortable providing some of the epidemiologic statistics about changes in tumor size or frequency of side effects from chemotherapy to the patient but not other statistics, like survival? Why didn't you answer their question more honestly and directly, or did you even answer the right question—the question *under* the question? Was the patient seeking reassurance or were they signaling a need to talk about their fears and worries? Why weren't you open to exploring the emotion you saw there? As you turn into your driveway, you make a mental note to ask your nurse to refer the patient to your palliative care colleague for comanagement and hope that you might do a little better next time.

Case 2

"They just don't get it!"

You are a palliative care clinician and your critical care colleague consults you to participate in a family meeting to discuss "goals of care" with a patient in the ICU. The provider describes the clinical context: The patient is not improving despite more than a week of maximal life-supporting treatment. The family members want to continue treatment even though the patient has a well-documented advance directive that, in the provider's judgment, runs counter to the family's choice for the patient. In wrapping up the case summary, the provider exhales loudly, rolls their eyes, shakes their head, and shrugs their shoulders, concluding with a conspiratorial, derisive tone: "They just don't get it!"

There are many layers of emotion in this clinical scenario. The referring provider is frustrated. Under that frustration may lie nonconscious defensiveness at having their plan of care rejected by the family, a feeling of grief or inadequacy at not being able to reverse the patient's illness, or perhaps a feeling of moral distress at delivering treatment to the patient that the patient may not have wanted. You haven't met the family yet, but the apparent disconnect between their expressions of treatment preferences and the patient's documented advance directive allows you to develop a differential diagnosis in your mind, including how the family members' emotions may be influencing their "decision making." You appreciate, in particular, that you have work to do in order to differentiate between their distress-driven expressions of wants and deliberative substituted judgment—making the decision that the patient would have made if he or she were able to make decisions. And you know that strong emotion can influence information processing. Of course you may be experiencing some of your own emotions, like some disgust with your colleague for talking about a grief-stricken family so derisively. Luckily, you've honed your self-awareness skills enough to check this reflexive reaction and shift instead to a more curious, nonjudgmental, and compassionate mindset. You remember yourself as an early career physician being drawn toward the specialty of palliative care by similar frustrations. You recognize the emotions your colleague, the critical care team, and the family may be feeling and how knowing the causes and consequences of these emotions will help you support and facilitate a decision-making process that both best reflects the decisions that the patient would make for themselves if they could and that mitigates the distress associated with the decision-making process for everyone involved.

Advance Care Planning and End-of-Life Care

Many people do not receive the end-of-life care they would prefer. Approximately 20% of Americans die in hospital intensive care units, despite the fact that 90% say they would prefer to die at home.[2] More than half of patients dying in the hospital or intensive care unit (ICU) have significant pain at the end of life.[3] For patients with serious illness, the use of life-sustaining treatments may only briefly extend the length of life at the cost of quality of life. This has led to multiple national initiatives to improve the frequency and quality of serious illness conversations, such as Ariadne Labs' Serious Illness Conversation Guide and implementation program,[4] Vital Talk's communication skills training program,[5] and the Respecting Choices program.[6] Each of these initiatives emphasizes the best practice of attending to patient emotion. This strategy both builds trust and rapport between the provider and the patient or their surrogate, but also serves to help diffuse heightened emotion. By so doing, the provider can surface underlying goals, values, fears, and worries and facilitate a better alignment between patient preferences and current or future life-sustaining treatment decisions and can reduce negative mental health impacts of end-of-life decision making.[7-9]

Decisions about life-prolonging treatments in many clinical contexts such as critical care and oncology are rife with emotions precisely because they evince the very real possibility of dying. Acute anxiety and existential distress associated with mortality salience and fear of pain and other distressing symptoms often outstrip standard coping strategies.[10] Decisions are often made while the patient or surrogate decision maker is in a heightened emotional, or "hot," state. Indeed, the vast majority of family members (73%) and spouses (84%) of ICU patients exhibit signs of anxiety or depression while their loved one is in the ICU.[7-9] Rates of persistent anxiety and depression three months later are highest for family members who share in decision making (48%), particularly when end-of-life decisions are involved (82%).[7] In cancer care, a diagnosis elicits frustration, powerlessness, vulnerability, uncertainty, and shock.[11,12] Anxiety about the future and fear of pain and other distressing symptoms predominate.[12,13]

Yet advance directives are typically completed and/or discussed with loved ones when both the surrogate and patient are in a neutral, or "cold," emotional state. Experimental research demonstrates that people make different decisions when in hot compared to cold states and that hot neural processing bypasses the prefrontal centers we associate with rational (actuarial) decision making.[14] Commonly observed discord between patients' advance care plans and surrogate decisions on their behalf[15,16] is likely due, in part, to this "hot-cold gap."

To improve medical decision making it is important to acknowledge that people may not make decisions rationally and that emotions impact decisions.[14] The premise that surrogates are rational decision makers underlies most of the (failed) efforts at improving these decisions, ranging from documenting living wills[17] to addressing innumeracy—the ability to understand and work with numbers by using pictographs when providing prognostic estimates. These efforts have failed because, even when perfectly informed, people do not always behave rationally by dispassionately weighing costs and benefits and choosing the best option. If they did, many decisions could be improved by simply providing decision makers with the right information. Unfortunately, this is not the case.[18] For example, researchers who study the use of living wills have repeatedly observed that surrogates sometimes agree to treatments that the patient's living will suggests they might not have wanted.[17] Even when surrogates are provided with more information about their loved one's preferences by allowing the surrogate and patient to discuss the patient's living will, surrogates are no more likely to choose treatments that are aligned with the patient's preferences.[16] By incorporating what we know about how people actually make decisions, and, in particular, the role that emotions play in decision making, we have the potential to improve these decisions.

■ BASIC SCIENCE OF EMOTION AND DECISION MAKING

Emotions Influence Decisions

Basic behavioral and social science research has consistently demonstrated that emotions influence decisions, regardless of whether they are integral (experienced feelings about a stimulus) or incidental (feelings such as mood states that are independent of a stimulus but can be misattributed to it or can influence decision processes).[14,19–25] Preferences differ depending upon whether the decision maker is in an emotionally aroused ("hot," or emotionally charged) or unaroused ("cold" or neutral, calm or relaxed) affective state.[14,19–25] Furthermore, decision makers in an emotionally unaroused state suffer from what is called a "hot-cold empathy gap." They are unable to empathize with others in a different state or with their future selves in that state. They are unable to accurately predict their preferences in the aroused state, known as *projection bias*—they project their current cold state preferences onto their future hot state selves.[14,26,27] Perhaps the most intuitive example is when we start the day dieting and have an erroneous prediction about the desires of our future self when faced with a fresh chocolate chip cookie later that afternoon. A related concept is affective forecasting, or the estimates individuals make about their future feelings and the biases that influence these estimates.[28,29] End-of-life decisions are particularly susceptible to these biases.[30,31] Drawing on Case 2 earlier in this chapter, the critical care clinician cannot empathize with the emotionally wrought surrogate decision maker—an interpersonal gap. And the individual surrogate decision maker likely could not have predicted when they calmly filled out the advance directive with their now critically ill family member 2 years ago that the agreeing to "pull the plug" would feel like signing a death warrant—an intrapersonal gap.

Negative emotions, such as the anxiety and fear of loss seen in surrogates, have been shown to cause people to avoid making decisions (sticking instead with the status quo), particularly when the decision itself generates negative emotion.[32] Different negative emotions, such as fear, anger, depression, sadness, and anxiety, may have different effects on decisions. Fear and anger, whether naturally occurring or experimentally induced, have been shown to differentially influence risk perceptions and risk preferences.[33] Fear increases risk perceptions and leads to more risk-averse choices. Anger has opposite effects.[20,33] Depression has been linked with slower decision making.[34] Likewise, time preference—one's relative valuation of receiving a good now versus later—has been linked to emotion.[35] Negative emotions, such as fear and anger, are linked with greater impulsivity, that is, putting lower weight on future outcomes more than immediate ones.[14]

Of particular relevance to medical decision making is the relationship between uncertainty and emotion.[36] Uncertainty is aversive[37]; people are willing to pay to reduce it.[38] In animal models, a part of the brain called the behavioral inhibition system is activated by novel or unexpected events, which causes anxiety.[39] Indeed, rats will choose more frequent electrical shocks that come in regular intervals to less frequent, unpredictable shocks. In humans, some of the aversive aspects of uncertainty are due to our tendency toward imagining negative outcomes more than positive outcomes, when faced with uncertainty.[40]

There are many individual differences that influence individuals' affective responses to stimuli, and to uncertainty in particular.[41] Some of these, including emotion perception, emotional awareness, emotion regulation, and burnout have been discussed in other chapters (see Chapter 5, Perception of Emotion in the Medical Visit; Chapter 6, Emotion Cues as Clinical Opportunities; Chapter 7, Emotion Regulation in Patients, Providers, and the Clinical Relationship; and Chapter 16, Striving and Thriving: Challenges and Opportunities for Clinician Emotional Wellness). Other individual differences, such as uncertainty tolerance,[42] trait optimism,[43] trait anxiety,[44] and other factors[45] are known to influence responses to uncertainty and subsequent decision making.

Emotions Undermine Analytic Decision Making

Rational choice theory assumes that decision makers select the optimal choice by calculating expected benefits and being guided by consistent personal values. Yet there is a considerable literature from behavioral decision science that under conditions of uncertainty, stress, and anxiety, people decrease information processing and instead form quick, "intuitive" judgments.[25,46,47] This has led to a theory of cognition that involves two systems of information processing, *System* 1, which is nonconscious, intuitive, associative, and fast, relying on heuristics, and *System* 2, which is slower, follows rule-based algorithms, and is therefore more deliberative and analytic.[48] These behavioral observations have been corroborated by neuroimaging studies. Specifically, "hot" neural processing bypasses the prefrontal centers we associate with rational (actuarial) decision making.[14] Thus, in addition to our sense that patients or families may be "flooded" with emotions such as anxiety, fear, and sadness that distract them and prevent encoding and processing of, say, prognostic or treatment choice information, these emotions likely increase reliance on System 1 processing and its biases.[25]

Emotions as Cognition

Yet emotion itself may be a form of information processing. Affect—the sense of feeling which changes from unpleasant to pleasant (valence), and from agitated to calm (arousal), and which may be less consciously appraised—and emotions—more specific, conscious labels that we give our affect—serve an adaptive function; they guide attention, cognition, and action. The field of behavioral decision science, which previously focused on biases—or mistakes—introduced by affect in decision making, increasingly recognizes "affective rationality."[49] Several theories posit that affect is its own type of information processing and therefore a form of cognition.[50] *Affect-as-information theory* suggests that people can use their transient emotions as information which can guide choices.[51] The *affect heuristic theory* posits that mental representations of objects, events, and options are associated with affective tags and that, taken together, can create a "gist" impression of different options.[52] The *somatic marker hypothesis* goes further and posits that it is the sympathetic and parasympathetic neuroendocrine systems' manifestation of heart rate, blood pressure, and gut activity that give the affective signals that help people make choices and take action.[53] All of these theories map onto the familiar phrase: "I'm going with my gut." Interestingly, recent work in the area of patient decision aids suggests that intuitive decisions may be better[54] and that too much deliberation—the kind that many decision aids facilitate—may undermine the informational value of affect-based intuition and ultimately interfere with patients making value-aligned choices.[55] Specifically, there is likely relevant information influencing the decision that is not codified in the decision aid.

Ellen Peters and colleagues lay out four separate roles for affect in judgment and decision-making processes.[56] First, as above, emotions act as information ("How do I feel about this?"), which provides a guide. Second, emotions can serve as a "common currency" in which one is able to compare our preferences for different options based on the emotion they evoke in us, which makes comparisons among a complex set of options easier. That is, affective information can be easier to integrate than less affective information about the choice set (i.e., integration). Third, affect also cues attention—the stronger the emotional response, the more likely the decision maker is to seek out or attend to additional information on which to base a decision. Finally, affect motivates behavior, particularly since individuals seek to return to a "homeostasis" involving more positive mood states, which uncertainty or ambiguity (indecision) typically undermines. Keltner and Lerner have proposed an "emotion-imbued choice model" of judgment and decision making.[57,58] This model updates rational choice models by adding incidental influences (including mood and carryover effects from incidental emotion) and current emotion that are integral to the decision at hand. Whether a specific emotion improves or impair judgment depends on how the emotion affects content of thought, depth of thought, and the content of implicit goals.

Emotions—whether experienced explicitly (consciously) or implicitly (nonconsciously)—similarly provide a cognitive resource to clinicians' decision making. A recent review of the role of emotion in clinical reasoning and clinical decision making noted that, while there is substantial evidence of the relationship between clinician emotion and clinical reasoning and decision making, the dominant models used in medical education exclude emotion.[59] Clinical decision making is described as a "hypothetico-deductive process of determining patients' problems"[60] using a Bayesian approach to developing hypotheses (differential diagnoses) and estimating probabilities, or likelihood, of different conditions.[61] The evolution of a novice to an expert progresses from a reliance on "analytical" to "intuitive" processes based upon calibrating an experience-feedback loop in support of pattern recognition.[62] Only Croskerry's "Universal Model of Diagnostic Reasoning" mentions emotion, including affect in *System* 1 (intuitive) clinical decisions but not in *System* 2 (analytical) decision.[63] In addition to insights from basic behavioral science that suggest emotion may be more involved in decision making than clinicians believe,[14,58] the clinical literature clearly demonstrates that a clinician's ability to recognize, understand, and manage or regulate emotions during clinical consultations correlates with patient trust and satisfaction with care.[64] Further, emotions are central to motivating "holistic" care and guiding moral or ethical clinical judgments.[65]

■ INTERVENTIONS

Addressing Emotion in the Clinical Encounter

There are several best practices in patient–provider communication in serious illness.[4,5] These include asking about illness understanding before providing medical and prognostic information, asking about information preferences and permission to disclose prognosis, simplifying medical and prognostic information, reassessing understanding, exploring the meaning of words and phrases, and attending to emotion in the clinical encounter. Additionally, in surrogate decision making, an additional best practice is to frame the decision as the (incapacitated) patient's, not the surrogate's.

I advance a model of patient–clinician communication and decision making in which patient (or surrogate) emotion has both direct and indirect effects on decision making (see Fig. 13-1). Specifically, a patient's (or surrogate's) emotional state influences decisions directly, since emotions have been shown to evoke specific "action tendencies"[66] and "appraisal tendencies."[19,20] Their emotional state also influences decisions indirectly, since emotions could generate high levels of arousal that interfere with the surrogate's ability to retain and process information from the clinician, thereby impacting comprehension. Many clinician communication best-practices, such as assessing illness understanding and simplifying medical and prognostic information, directly influence comprehension, which may influence emotion (i.e., bad news, if understood, will evoke emotion). Attending to emotion directly influences the surrogate's emotional state. Framing the decision as the patient's, not the surrogate's, directly influences the surrogate's emotional state (since framing the decision as the surrogate's is more stressful) and directly influences the decision (i.e., "Do you want us to do X for your mother" is a fundamentally different question than "Would your mother want us to do X?"). In the case of surrogate decision making, which has been associated with long-term mental health impacts including anxiety, depression, and posttraumatic stress symptoms,[7-9] the decision (and the surrogate's comprehension and emotional state when involved in the decision) influence decisional conflict and, ultimately, these longer-term mental health outcomes.[67]

There are many interventions designed to help clinicians recognize, understand, and manage or regulate emotions during clinical encounters. This includes communication skills training such as the Serious Illness Conversation Guide[4] and VitalTalk,[5] as well as any number of mindfulness practices designed to increase awareness of one's own internal states.[68] The most effective communication skills training programs provide both mental roadmaps for conversations and "words that work" and reinforce biofeedback through simulation-based skills practice. Specifically, through role-play

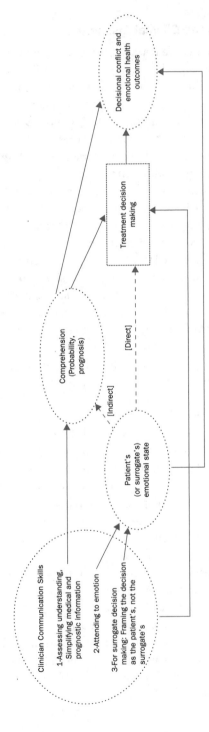

FIGURE 13-1. Clinician communication behaviors and patient (or surrogate) emotion and decision making. The figure describes the relationships I hypothesize between clinician's communication behaviors, patient/surrogate emotion, comprehension, treatment decisions, and decisional conflict. I hypothesize that the patient's (or surrogate's) emotional state influence treatment decisions. This influence may be direct; emotions have been shown to evoke specific "action tendencies"[66] and "appraisal tendencies"[19,20] —propensities to perceive the world in specific ways. Or this influence may be indirect; emotions could generate high levels of arousal that interfere with the patient's (or surrogate's) ability to retain and process information from the clinician, thereby impacting comprehension.

Further, I hypothesize that if communication best-practices "work," they do so principally by influencing *emotion*, rather than by influencing comprehension of *information*. Among these best practices, simplifying medical and prognostic information directly influences the surrogate's comprehension of the prognosis and treatment options. Comprehension then influences emotion. Attending to emotion directly influences the surrogate's emotional state. In the case of surrogate decision making when the patient is incapacitated, such as in the case of life-sustaining treatment decisions for patients in the intensive care unit, framing the decision as the patient's, not the surrogate's, directly influences the surrogate's emotional state (since framing the decision as the surrogate's is more stressful) and directly influences the decision (i.e., "Do you want us to do X for your mother" is a fundamentally different question than "Would your mother have wanted us to do X?"). To extend the model beyond the specific treatment decision to longer-term emotional health outcomes, the decision (and the patient's (or surrogate's) comprehension and emotional state/level of distress when involved in the decision) influence decisional conflict and such outcomes as anxiety, depression, and posttraumatic stress symptoms.

clinicians can experience and successfully manage the discomfort associated with discussing emotion-laden topics, interacting with emotional patients, and managing their own intrapersonal emotional responses. Simulation and role-play, therefore, can be seen as a kind of exposure therapy. Together with a cultivation of self-awareness through mindfulness practice, these individual-level interventions can further support clinicians in differentiating their own value-driven "intuitive" judgments from the patient's values in order to better support patient-centered deliberation and decision making.

There are some systems-level interventions, such as requiring or encouraging multidisciplinary care teams that include social work and psychology input to manage complex or serious illnesses. This includes systems-level integration of palliative care consultation or comanagement for patients with serious illness. These interventions support the integration of emotion into clinical decision making. Multidisciplinary care teams enable better understanding and support of patients' and family members' emotion, and—when functioning optimally—bring to light the role that team members' emotions are playing in clinical decision making.[69] Individual team members, such as lay navigators, scribes, chaplains, social workers, and palliative care providers may add value through sharing of affective labor with the primary clinical team, although this has never been studied. Affective labor—work carried out that is intended to produce or modify emotional experiences in people—has primarily been studied by feminist theorists to describe the gendered roles that women play at work and at home.[70] Team members' affective labor may be performed directly with patients, for example, when a social worker, chaplain, lay navigator, or palliative care clinician has an empathic conversation or discusses advance care planning, thereby relieving the primary clinical team of that duty. Or the affective labor may be performed with the primary clinical team by helping them process a particular case or encounter, such as when a scribe, chaplain, or palliative care provider discusses a case with the primary clinical team in an effort to understand the patient's reactions and/or debrief their feelings about the encounter.

■ CASE DISCUSSION

Case 1: Discussion—Managing Your Own Emotions

Case 1 at the beginning of this chapter may feel familiar to those who practice in primary care or other specialties. We have all had the experience of saying something reflexively to reassure a distressed patient; or, indeed, any distressed person. It is easy to rationalize evasiveness like "I don't have a crystal ball. Everyone is different. I have lots of patients who do really well!" or even false reassurance as "Everything is going to be fine!" as simply responding to distress with the goal of making someone feel better. However, such responses do not create the holding space that distressed patients need to feel heard and understood.[71] Interestingly, these reactions are often motivated by our own sense of discomfort with the patient's distress. That is to say, we are having an emotional response to the patient's emotion—or to the emotion that we anticipate them having if we disclose prognostic news. Holding space involves listening deeply and avoiding going into "problem-solving" mode.[72] There are several concrete tools a clinician can use, but the very first tool is mindful awareness of the situation. When the patient tearfully asks "How much time do I have left?" what emotions do you notice coming up in yourself? The oncologist noticed sweaty palms and rapid heartbeat, but wasn't able to slow down enough in the moment between reaction and response before blurting out something falsely reassuring. With practice, one can begin to classify one's own emotions (anxiety, dread) and take deep breaths in order to recenter on the patient, away from one's own anxiety and the associated reflexively reassuring or evasive response. Silence, eye contact, and an open body posture can be helpful here as you attend fully to the patient in front of you to look for clues. Is the patient tearful? What is their body posture? What is your "gut" telling you about how they are feeling? Your own emotions in response to another person's emotions are highly diagnostic. If you were compelled to reassure, then you clearly noticed distress (in yourself as well as in the patient). I teach my learners that if they feel a compulsion to say something, stop! I use the metaphor of a fish being faced with a hook and a dangling worm. Our reflexive response is to bite, and then we are caught! Instead, notice your compulsion, see the hook, examine it closely. This brings me to the second tool: Pausing to develop a differential diagnosis of the question (hook). Specifically, is this an "emotion cue" or an "information cue?"[73,74] Assuming that the statement is an emotional cue—a question that, on first blush, seems like a request for information but is actually a manifestation of emotion—is a safe bet. I start there because (a) it's usually correct, (b) starting there will allow me to gather data to inform my differential, and (c) it buys me some time to manage the situation. Using a mnemonic like NURSE: N(ame) U(nderstand) R(espect) S(upport) E(xplore) emotions is helpful.[73,74] You might say "I imagine you are very worried," or "This must feel really scary" to name the emotion (worry, fear) and "Tell me what most worries you?" to explore the emotion. Typically, this will lead to the patient expressing their concerns, providing you with more information about the "question behind the question," and preparing you for the next steps in the conversation. By slowing things down, you can discharge some of the patient's emotion before you provide information, thereby increasing the likelihood they will retain it. The third tool is disclosing prognostic information using the "ask-tell-ask" approach. You might say, "You asked how much time you have left, would it be helpful to talk about that now?" (asking for permission) You can also ask if they want detailed data or big picture information (asking for information preferences). Finally, you can ask the patient what they have heard or read already (if they haven't already told you) so you have a starting point (asking about what they already know). Then you can tailor your answer to their needs, being as data informed as possible, while also acknowledging prognostic uncertainty (tell). Develop a simple "headline", deliver the information, and use silence as the patient absorbs the information, and be ready for more emotion. Finally, you can check that the patient understood (ask). While these are primary palliative care skills, one way to build your capacity is to comanage some of your patients with a palliative care clinician, and consider having some joint meetings with patients while sharing prognosis in order to receive their coaching.

Case 2: Discussion—Working with a Palliative Care Team

Returning to Case 2 at the beginning of this chapter, how might a palliative care provider support the patient's family and the critical care team in medical decision making for the patient, given what we know about emotion and decision making? The critical care provider conceptualizes the problem as principally being one of information exchange—the family simply does not understand the prognostic information that the critical care provider and their team have provided; namely, that the patient is not recovering and is therefore dying. Best practices in critical care communication encourage simplifying medical and prognostic information, reducing it to a "headline." It is certainly possible that jargon such as "multisystem organ failure" and statements like the patient is "not showing any progress" aren't decoded by the family in the way that they are decoded by the medical team. Thus, encouraging the team members to name that the patient is "dying" is one way to support the team's goal to communicate prognostic information. Another is to encourage them to offer global, functional prognostic statements guided by the "best case, worst case, and most likely case" scenario, rather than discussing individual, disarticulate organ functions and laboratory values.[75] Commonly, a palliative care consultant might do this through prebriefing with the team prior to a family meeting in order to discuss global prognosis, obtaining input from additional specialists as needed, and agreeing on the structure for the family meeting.

During this prebriefing, the palliative care provider accomplishes several things. First, they are cocreating the prognostic statement with the referring provider and other consultants, and in so doing, are sharing the affective burdens associated with prognostic uncertainty. Second, they are rehearsing the meeting structure and content, thereby decreasing the ambiguity and associated anxiety of team members. Third, they are reminding the team to expect strong emotion from the family—the emotion is an indication that they have heard the terrible news that their loved one is dying—and offering reassurance that the palliative care provider will be there to help provide emotional support to the family. Fourth, by sharing ideas for how to respond to emotion—or modeling these strategies during the meeting—it may increase the team's compassion for the family. For example, saying "This isn't what you were hoping to hear" or "It must be impossible to imagine your life without [the patient]" lays bare why "getting it" is so hard for the family. Best practices in serious illness communication involve this kind of attending to patient/surrogate emotion. The use of silence and communication strategies such as naming, understanding, respecting, supporting, and exploring emotion are effective.[74] However, as noted in Chapter 7 (Emotion Regulation in Patients, Providers, and the Clinical Relationship), a prerequisite to using these communication strategies is the emotional self-regulation necessary to manage one's own emotional response in reaction to the emotions of others.[74] These emotion handling behaviors can serve to increase the family members' trust through feeling heard and understood.[71] It also discharges and diffuses emotion, which may allow surrogates to shift closer to an unaroused ("cold") state in order to engage in the values elicitation and deliberation stage of a family meeting.

The next best practice in serious illness communication is to identify goals, values, fears, and worries, and then link these to what is medically achievable by the available treatment options. When family members are acting as surrogates, the palliative care provider can provide explicit orientation to the family that their role is to share with us what they know about the patient's goals and values, and to distinguish these from their own wants and wishes. Often this can involve explicitly naming the wish that the family likely has: that the patient fully recovers and returns to the way they were before they became so sick. When the palliative care provider integrates all of the information in the room—what the family has shared about goals, values, fears, and worries—and what the critical care team has shared regarding prognosis and what is medically achievable—they can offer to make a recommendation regarding a plan. Recommending a comfort-focused plan of care requires a particular capacity for emotion regulation and self-awareness, since one must avoid value projections[71] and overcome the reflexive conditioning of clinical medicine to "fix" things.[76]

Throughout this process, the palliative care provider is showing, not telling, the referring critical care provider why a family might not "get it" and what explicit steps, informed by knowledge regarding the role of emotions in decision making, can support the family to understand prognosis, engage with and grieve the terrible news, and to make a plan that is consistent with the patient's goals, values, and preferences in that context. If possible, a debriefing with the critical care team can make explicit some of these phenomena, normalize them, and reinforce the specific strategies the palliative care provider used during the meeting that were most helpful in resolving what seemed, at first glance, a conflict between the family and the care team.

Therefore, when integrated into clinical practice, palliative care providers use intrapersonal and interpersonal emotion perception, emotional awareness, and emotion regulation to interpret and respond to both patient/caregiver emotion and provider emotion in the service of improving clinical communication and decision making in serious illness.

◼ CONCLUDING PRACTICAL ADVICE

So, what is my advice for the practicing clinician? First, expect emotion—in the patient (or surrogate) and in yourself. Practice mindful awareness of these emotions and treat them with curiosity and respect, rather than judgment. Once you are aware of these emotions, manage them. In yourself, that means introducing space between your (internal) reaction and (external) response. In the patient, that means addressing them directly. Finally, recognize how the emotion is impacting decision making. There will be times that emotion degrades decision making and others when emotions provide valuable information that can enhance decision making. And, finally, remember that without practicing, you can't get better at anything.

ACKNOWLEDGMENTS

My interest in the area of emotion and medical decision making was supported by a midcareer faculty K18 Career Enhancement Award (K18NR012847) during which I received training and mentorship from Robert Arnold and George Loewenstein. I also learned a great deal from colleagues who participated in the National Cancer Institute's "Affect and Decisional Processes Network," an 18-month initiative to facilitate scientific engagement between fundamental affective and decision scientists and clinical palliative care researchers, many whose work I cite heavily in this chapter, including Jennifer Lerner and Paul Han. Finally, financial support from the Susan J. and Richard M. Levy Distinguished Professorship to complete a 12-month fellowship in Hospice and Palliative Medicine at Dartmouth-Hitchcock Medical Center provided a rare opportunity for me to integrate insights from behavioral decision research with meta-observations of clinical education and practice.

REFERENCES

1. Kelley AS, Bollens-Lund E. Identifying the population with serious illness: the "Denominator" challenge. *J Palliat Med.* 2018;21(S2):S7-S16.

2. Angus DC, Barnato AE, Linde-Zwirble WT, et al. Use of intensive care at the end of life in the United States: an epidemiologic study. *Crit Care Med.* 2004;32(3):638-643.

3. SUPPORT Investigators. A controlled trial to improve care for seriously ill hospitalized patients: the study to understand prognoses and preferences for outcomes and risks of treatments (SUPPORT). *JAMA.* 1995;274(20):1591-1598.

4. Ariadne Lab, Serious Illness Care Program. https://www.ariadnelabs.org/areas-of-work/serious-illness-care. Accessed October 15, 2020.

5. VitalTalk. https://www.vitaltalk.org. Accessed October 15, 2020.

6. Respecting Choices: Patient-Centered Care. https://respectingchoices.org. Accessed October 15, 2020.

7. Azoulay E, Pochard F, Kentish-Barnes N, et al. Risk of post-traumatic stress symptoms in family members of intensive care unit patients. *Am J Respir Crit Care Med.* 2005;171(9):987-94.

8. Pochard F, Azoulay E, Chevret S, et al. Symptoms of anxiety and depression in family members of intensive care unit patients: ethical hypothesis regarding decision-making capacity. *Crit Care Med.* 2001;29(10):1893-7.

9. Pochard F, Darmon M, Fassier T, et al. Symptoms of anxiety and depression in family members of intensive care unit patients before discharge or death: a prospective multicenter study. *J Crit Care.* 2005;20(1):90-6.

10. Becker E. *The Denial of Death.* New York, NY: Simon & Schuster; 1973.

11. Pedersen AE, Hack TF, McClement SE, Taylor-Brown J. An exploration of the patient navigator role: perspectives of younger women with breast cancer. *Oncol Nurs Forum.* 2014;41(1):77-88.

12. Smith WB, Gracely RH, Safer MA. The meaning of pain: cancer patients' rating and recall of pain intensity and affect. *Pain.* 1998;78(2):123-129.

13. Halkett GK, Kristjanson LJ, Lobb EA. "If we get too close to your bones they'll go brittle": women's initial fears about radiotherapy for early breast cancer. *Psychooncology.* 2008;17(9):877-84.

14. Loewenstein G, Lerner JS. The role of affect in decision making. In: Davidson RJ, Scherer KR, Goldsmith HH, eds. *Handbook of Affective Sciences.* Oxford, UK: Oxford University Press; 2003.

15. Fagerlin A, Ditto PH, Danks JH, Houts RM, Smucker WD. Projection in surrogate decisions about life-sustaining medical treatments. *Health Psychol.* 2001;20(3):166-75.

16. Ditto PH, Danks JH, Smucker WD, et al. Advance directives as acts of communication: a randomized controlled trial. *Arch Intern Med.* 2001;161(3):421-30.

17. Fagerlin A, Schneider CE. Enough: the failure of the living will. *Hastings Cent Rep.* 2004;34(2):30-42.

18. Fischhoff B, Barnato AE. Value awareness: a new goal for end-of-life decision making. *MDM Policy Pract.* 2019;4(1):2381468318817523.

19. Lerner JS, Keltner D. Beyond valence: toward a model of emotion-specific influences on judgment and choice. *Cogn Emotion.* 2000;14(4):473-493.

20. Lerner JS, Keltner D. Fear, anger, and risk. *J Pers Soc Psychol.* 2001;81(1):146-59.

21. Lerner JS, Gonzalez RM, Small DA, Fischhoff B. Effects of fear and anger on perceived risks of terrorism: a national field experiment. *Psychol Sci.* 2003;14(2):144-50.

22. Lerner JS, Small DA, Loewenstein G. Heart strings and purse strings: carryover effects of emotions on economic decisions. *Psychol Sci.* 2004;15(5):337-41.

23. Lerner JS, Tiedens LZ. Portrait of the angry decision maker: how appraisal tendencies shape anger's influence on cognition. *J Behav Decision Making.* 2006;19(2):115-137.

24. Kahneman D, Schkade D, Sunstein CR. Shared outrage and erratic awards: the psychology of punitive damages. *Risk Uncertainty.* 1998;16:49-86.

25. Kahneman D. *Thinking, Fast and Slow.* New York, NY: Farrar, Straus and Giroux; 2011.

26. Loewenstein G. Hot-cold empathy gaps and medical decision making. *Health Psychol.* 2005;24(4S):S49-56.

27. Loewenstein G. Projection bias in medical decision making. *Med Decis Making.* 2005;25(1):96-105.

28. Wilson TD, Gilbert DT. Affective forecasting. *Adv Exper Social Psychol.* 2003:345-411.

29. Wilson TD, Gilbert DT. Affective forecasting: knowing what to want. *Curr Direct Psychol Sci.* 2005;14:131-134.

30. Ellis EM, Barnato AE, Chapman GB, et al. Toward a conceptual model of affective predictions in palliative care. *J Pain Symptom Manage.* 2019;57(6):1151-1165.

31. Halpern SD. Shaping end-of-life care: behavioral economics and advance directives. *Semin Respir Crit Care Med.* 2012;33(4):393-400.

32. Volandes AE, Paasche-Orlow M, Gillick MR, et al. Health literacy not race predicts end-of-life care preferences. *J Palliat Med.* 2008;11(5):754-62.

33. Loewenstein GF, Weber EU, Hsee CK, Welch ES. Risk as feelings. *Psychol Bull.* 2001; 127:267-286.

34. Reyna VF. How people make decisions that involve risk: a dual-processes approach. *Curr Direct Psychol Sci.* 2004;13:60-66.

35. Zhang S, Peng J, Qin L, Suo T, Feng T. Prospective emotion enables episodic prospection to shift time preference. *Br J Psychol.* 2018;109(3):487-499.

36. Anderson EC, Carleton RN, Diefenbach M, Han PKJ. The relationship between uncertainty and affect. *Front Psychol.* 2019;10:2504.

37. Carleton RN. Into the unknown: a review and synthesis of contemporary models involving uncertainty. *J Anxiety Disord.* 2016;39:30-43. (In eng).

38. Lovallo D, Kahneman D. Living with uncertainty: attractiveness and resolution timing. *J Behav Decision Making.* 2000;13:179-190.

39. Gray JA, McNaughton N. *The Neuropsychology of Anxiety: An Enquiry Into the Functions of the Septo-Hippocampal System*. 2nd ed. New York, NY: Oxford University Press; 2000.

40. Killingsworth MA, Gilbert DT. A wandering mind is an unhappy mind. *Science.* 2010;330(6006):932.

41. Stanovich KE, West RF. Individual differences in reasoning: implications for the rationality debate? *Behav Brain Sci.* 2000;23(5):645-65; discussion 665-726.

42. Hillen MA, Gutheil CM, Strout TD, Smets EMA, Han PKJ. Tolerance of uncertainty: conceptual analysis, integrative model, and implications for healthcare. *Soc Sci Med.* 2017;180:62-75.

43. Zhao X, Huang C, Li X, Peng J. Dispositional optimism, self-framing and medical decision-making. *Int J Psychol.* 2015;50(2):121-7.

44. Hirsh JB, Inzlicht M. The devil you know: neuroticism predicts neural response to uncertainty. *Psychol Sci.* 2008;19(10):962-7.

45. Jaśko K, Czernatowicz-Kukuczka A, Kossowska M, Czarna AZ. Individual differences in response to uncertainty and decision making: the role of behavioral inhibition system and need for closure. *Motiv Emot.* 2015;39(4):541-552.

46. Kahneman D, Slovic P, Tversky A. *Judgment Under Uncertainty: Heuristics and Biases.* Cambridge, UK: Cambridge University Press; 1982.

47. Tversky A, Kahneman D. Judgment under uncertainty: heuristics and biases. *Science.* 1974;185(4157):1124-31.

48. Kahneman D. A perspective on judgment and choice: mapping bounded rationality. *Am Psychol.* 2003;58(9):697-720.

49. Slovic P, Finucane ML, Peters E, MacGregor DG. The affect heuristic. In: Gilovich T, Griffin D, Kahneman D, eds. *Heuristics and Biases: The Psychology of Intuitive Judgment.* New York, NY: Cambridge University Press; 2002:397-420.

50. Duncan S, Barrett LF. Affect is a form of cognition: a neurobiological analysis. *Cogn Emot.* 2007;21(6):1184-1211.

51. Schwarz N, Clore GL. Mood, misattribution, and judgments of well-being: informative and directive functions of affective states. *J Pers Soc Psychol.* 1983;45:513-523.

52. Slovic P, Finucane ML, Peters E, MacGregor DG. The affect heuristic. *Eur J Oper Res.* 2007;177:1333-1352.

53. Damasio AR. The somatic marker hypothesis and the possible functions of the prefrontal cortex. *Philos Trans R Soc Lond Ser B Biol Sci.* 1996:1413-1420.

54. Usher M, Russo Z, Weyers M, Brauner R, Zakay D. The impact of the mode of thought in complex decisions: intuitive decisions are better. *Front Psychol.* 2011;2(37).

55. de Vries M, Fagerlin A, Witteman HO, Scherer LD. Combining deliberation and intuition in patient decision support. *Patient Educ Couns.* 2013;91(2):154-60.

56. Peters E, Västfjäll D, Gärling T, Slovic P. Affect and decision making: a "hot" topic. *J Behav Decision Making.* 2006;19:79-85.

57. Keltner DT, Lerner JS. Emotion. In: Gilbert DT, Fiske ST, Lindzey G, eds. *The Handbook of Social Psychology.* New York, NY: Wiley; 2010:317-352.

58. Lerner JS, Li Y, Valdesolo P, Kassam KS. Emotion and decision making. *Annu Rev Psychol.* 2015;66:799-823.

59. Kozlowski D, Hutchinson M, Hurley J, Rowley J, Sutherland J. The role of emotion in clinical decision making: an integrative literature review. *BMC Med Educ.* 2017;17(1):255.

60. Lauri S, Salanterä S. Developing an instrument to measure and describe clinical decision making in different nursing fields. *J Prof Nurs.* 2002;18(2):93-100.

61. Fischhoff B, Beyth-Marom R. Hypothesis evaluation from a Bayesian perspective. *Psychol Rev.* 1983;90(3):239-60.

62. Elstein AS, Schwartz A, Schwarz A. Clinical problem solving and diagnostic decision making: selective review of the cognitive literature. *BMJ.* 2002;324(7339):729-32.

63. Croskerry P. A universal model of diagnostic reasoning. *Acad Med.* 2009;84(8):1022-8.

64. Tulsky JA, Arnold RM, Alexander SC, et al. Enhancing communication between oncologists and patients with a computer-based training program: a randomized trial. *Ann Intern Med.* 2011;155(9):593-601.

65. Marcum JA. The role of emotions in clinical reasoning and decision making. *J Med Philosophy.* 2013;38(5):501–519.

66. Frijda NH. *The Emotions.* New York, NY: Cambridge University Press; 1986.

67. Lautrette A, Darmon M, Megarbane B, et al. A communication strategy and brochure for relatives of patients dying in the ICU. *N Engl J Med.* 2007;356(5):469-78.

68. Epstein R. *Attending: Medicine, Mindfulness, and Humanity.* New York, NY: Scribner, 2018.

69. Larson JR. *In Search of Synergy in Small Group Performance.* New York, NY: Taylor and Francis Group; 2019.

70. Hardt M. Affective labor. *Boundary.* 1999;26(2):89-100.

71. Gramling R, Stanek S, Ladwig S, et al. Feeling heard and understood: a patient-reported quality measure for the inpatient palliative care setting. *J Pain Symptom Manage.* 2016;51(2):150-4.

72. Kelemen AM, Kearney G, Groninger H. Reading the room: lessons on holding space and presence. *J Cancer Educ.* 2018;33(6):1362-1363.

73. Back AL, Anderson WG, Bunch L, et al. Communication about cancer near the end of life. *Cancer.* 2008;113(7 Suppl):1897-910.

74. Back AL, Arnold RM, Tulsky JA. *Mastering Communication with Seriously Ill Patients: Balancing Honesty with Empathy and Hope.* New York, NY: Cambridge University Press; 2009.

75. Kruser JM, Nabozny MJ, Steffens NM, et al. "Best Case/Worst Case": qualitative evaluation of a novel communication tool for difficult in-the-moment surgical decisions. *J Am Geriatr Soc.* 2015;63(9):1805-11.

76. Lynn J, DeGrazia D. An outcomes model of medical decision making. *Theor Med.* 1991;12(4):325-43.

Emotions in the Culture of Medicine

Teaching about Emotions in Healthcare

CHAPTER 14

Caitlin Holt Siropaides, Martha Howell, and Calvin L. Chou

■ INTRODUCTION

Clinicians often partake in patients' most vulnerable moments, such as receiving difficult news or coping with how an illness affects "patients' lives". Therefore, clinicians carry the responsibility of both recognizing and handling the emotions elicited by those experiences, skills that we typically do not learn explicitly and that do not always come naturally. Teaching these skills effectively requires expertise and patience, in addition to self-awareness.

Research shows that clinicians often deprioritize responding to emotion in favor of more concrete skills such as history taking or venipuncture.[1] Educators must consider recognizing and responding to emotion as critical communication skills similar in importance to traditional technical skills. We will first describe some of the core educational theories that support successful skill development in recognizing and handling emotions, and then we will enumerate effective teaching techniques. We have included both guidance from evidence-based approaches to education, as well as our collective experience teaching communication skills to health professions learners for more than 40 years.

■ OVERVIEW OF LEARNING THEORY

Why do medical students balk at the notion of mandatory attendance to lectures they could watch on YouTube? Why do smartphone apps and other social media videos resonate so much with so many? How can one learn from these various experiences? Andragogy, or adult learning theory, stresses the importance of tapping into prior experiences in order for learning to be achieved.[2] It is through these experiences that learners determine whether content is meaningful or irrelevant. Effective training must not only be learner-centered but also skills-focused, oriented to one's own practice.[3] In addition, efficacy of communication skills training depends on the degree of active and interactive strategies, namely, role-play, feedback, and small group discussions that provide and build off learner experiences, rather than didactic sessions.[4] Moreover, "learner-centered" instructional techniques value formation of learner–educator relationships, address unique learner needs, and parallel what occurs in patient–clinician relationships.[2,5,6] In order to learn effectively from experiences, one must trust the support of others and have a sense of confidence in one's abilities. Otherwise, fear, manifesting through behaviors and emotions such as perfectionism or anger, can block learning.[7]

In addition to positive perceptions of learning, *situated learning* posits that learners learn more effectively if they can envision application to relevant practice settings.[8] A common example of situated learning is case-based learning, where familiar materials and presentation structures lend accessible context. If groups of participants share a learning experience, this situated learning can generalize to interactions in a social network. *Social Cognitive Theory*, developed by psychologist Albert Bandura, affirms that humans learn most behaviors through observation, imitation, and/or modeling of social interactions.[9] Particularly relevant in adult learning, social cognitive theory takes into account both the learner and the environment in which they operate, stressing the importance of context as well as how learners interface in their environments.[10]

Learners acquire new skills and knowledge when actively involved and engaged with the learning materials, and when they have meaningful experiences. These meaningful experiences must allow learners to relate to their environments while socially interacting within a context that provides a clear learning goal. *Scaffolding* is a process through which learners can contextualize active learning by referring to previously introduced concepts and skills. Therefore, effective educators practice eliciting the learners' experiences and offer connections to build on those experiences and knowledge during skill development.[11,12] Short frameworks presented on cards or apps enhance learning retention by providing reminders of information previously taught.

The final theory that pervades effective teaching of emotions is the "learning ladder," which highlights two factors learners must take into account when learning new skills: awareness and competence. According to the model, learners move through four stages in order to adopt new skills. The first, *unconscious incompetence*, is a stage where a learner does not know what they don't know. This stage requires work to help the learner develop recognition that this learning is important, and motivation to learn something new. Educators leading unconsciously incompetent learners must provide a welcoming learning environment that both allows for learners to freely voice skepticism or dismissal, and gently guides learners toward new learning. The second stage is *conscious incompetence*, in which the learner recognizes they do not have the requisite knowledge and/or skill to accomplish what they need to do. Here, educators encourage learning by facilitating structured exercises and reminders of skills to learn. The third stage is *conscious competence*, when learners are consciously aware of having knowledge or skill but do not yet feel adept enough with it to practice confidently. They value using rubrics, frameworks, checklists, and other memory aids to aid in their practice. At each of these first three stages, the role of an educator is to provide enough psychological safety for learning to occur while simultaneously placing just the right amount of pressure to maximize learning while neither flooding the learner nor making learning activities so rudimentary as to cause boredom. Finally, the fourth stage is *unconscious competence*, evinced by experts whose learning has become automatic and incorporated into practice.[13]

In the rest of the chapter, we will refer to all of these dynamics and how they factor into effective teaching of emotion to clinical learners.

■ WHAT IS REQUIRED: BUILDING BLOCKS FOR EFFECTIVE TEACHING OF EMOTIONS IN HEALTHCARE

Most of us have developed ways to recognize and respond to emotion in social situations, predominantly with people with whom we intersect regularly, without having received explicit instruction. However, clinicians regularly encounter numerous people from diverse backgrounds and therefore can benefit from a practical approach. Somewhat paradoxically, one can distill the skills of responding to emotion into a cognitive framework, which can provide for deeper and more enduring learning. Conversely, rote memorization, arguably the most commonly used approach in traditional medical education, affords learners a limited resource. Hence, as noted in the educational theory section above, using learners' experiences (both from the past and those emerging in the context of simulation exercises or real-time interactions) will enhance understanding more deeply than cognitive knowledge alone. Before we discuss a practical approach to teaching the skills of responding to emotion, we must first address the crucial importance of personal awareness in this work, and the associated critical skill of emotion recognition.

Personal Awareness

Often when patients exhibit strong emotions, clinicians report experiencing strong emotions themselves.[14,15] For instance, if a patient becomes angry, one human instinct is to feel defensive. As reviewed in Chapter 7 on Emotion

Regulation in Patients, Providers, and the Clinical Relationship, clinicians can more effectively respond to these emotions if they attune to personal awareness of their own emotions, responses, and behaviors. With this more purposeful ownership of their emotions and ability to act on their own responses, biases, and behaviors, clinicians can decide how to respond evenly in an emotionally charged patient encounter, rather than merely reacting in the moment.

Clinicians often think of how personal awareness and authenticity apply to patient–provider interactions, but a parallel process occurs for learner–educator experiences. Ideally, in an effective learning environment, both the learner and educator deepen personal awareness by observing and analyzing responses to both a patient and the learning experience. We often find that the connection to the content of the conversation, as well as the multiple relationships, facilitates insight for optimal learning to occur. Generally, educators frame this in terms of "psychological safety," but personal awareness also requires active engagement through reflection, enough to be challenging and thought-provoking.[16] The emotional awareness that emerges forms part of a skill set of "emotional intelligence" that learners can develop.[17] With awareness of one's own emotional landscape, clinicians can then respond more effectively, and importantly, with authenticity, to others' emotional states.

Particularly with regard to developing emotional intelligence, we find that educators must take great care to recognize learners' emotional experiences of the encounter, to help them navigate potentially vulnerable situations. Educators also often experience emotional responses to a learner or situation, and thus personal awareness becomes highly important to their ability to facilitate a safe and effective educational environment.

> *An educator introduces a case to a group of learners. A white male patient is angry about a 1-week delay in medication refill. The educator discusses how a clinician can respond and explore the patient's point of view. A learner states that they would simply refuse to talk with the patient because that is disrespectful behavior and would fire the patient from clinic. Upon further discussion of alternative ways to handle the situation, the learner starts to raise their voice and assert they can run their clinic however they want.*

Educators will need to employ certain skills in order to effectively navigate challenging situations. They must mindfully decelerate a rapid natural emotional reaction into the following individual steps:

1. Recognize and name their own emotions.
2. Contemplate why and how they are experiencing these feelings.
3. Consider why that learner may be behaving or thinking in such a way.
4. Determine how their response will positively impact the learner.

Then, and only then, can an effective educator respond to the situation in a way that benefits the learner.

> *The educator may recognize that they are frustrated or angry with the learner for being argumentative or raising their voice. They may recognize they feel that the learner presents a challenge to their own expertise or to the group's learning. The educator then imagines the perspective of the learner, who has perhaps experienced implicit or explicit bias against them, or finds anger a difficult emotion to manage. Thus with this new perspective, the educator better understands the learner's standpoint and also develops a strategic response: a calm recognition of differences of opinion and redirection, and an acknowledgement that people may have different professional limits on what they feel is acceptable behavior, adding that responding to emotion first may be a valid first step.*

Most educators will find that these skills require attention, development, and deep reflection on one's teaching. As depicted above, personal awareness is valuable on the part of both the learner to develop skills of emotional response, and the educator to facilitate these potentially emotionally charged situations. In addition, it affords the educator an opportunity to demonstrate the skills necessary to defuse emotionally charged situations.

> *Educator:* *I am sensing that you are finding this situation frustrating.*
> *Learner:*   *[purses lips]*
> *Educator:* *I am really grateful that you are sharing your perspective, which I find truly valuable. Sometimes it is very important to be clear about boundaries. [brief pause to let these words sink in] In this case, I also wonder what we might learn by inquiring about the patient's perspective. Can you imagine a way of doing that?*

The learner may recognize the educator's skilled response to their own anger by naming their emotional state, relating to their point of view, and negotiating a resolution in a calm way.

Emotion Recognition

As we've reviewed, personal awareness is critical to effective observation and development of responding to emotion in both clinical and teaching environments. However, evidence has shown that clinicians often miss and do not address patients' emotional cues.[18,19] (See Chapter 5, Perception of Emotion in the Medical Visit, and Chapter 6, Emotion Cues as Clinical Opportunities for additional details on this topic.) This regularly occurs when clinicians focus solely on the "task at hand" such as a patient's complaint or symptom and thus miss the opportunity to detect and respond to emotion. Often, we find that clinicians fail to recognize the emotional driver underpinning patients' questions and, as a consequence, answer questions cognitively rather than considering how those questions have emotional resonance for the patient.

> *A clinician tells a 60 year old patient that they have diagnosed significant iron deficiency anemia and recommend a colonoscopy. The patient asks, "Isn't there anything else we can do first?" Instead of providing a direct answer that addresses other options, the clinician explores the patient's question further, revealing that the patient's father died at 65 years old from colon cancer and fears the same diagnosis.*

Furthermore, visits with providers (both internists and surgeons) who verbally address emotional cues are *shorter* than those without these verbal expressions.[18] Though initially counterintuitive, this observation makes more sense when considering what occurs when patients discern that their provider is not addressing their emotions. Patients often will reiterate the emotion until the provider provides an explicit verbal response. They may also resist a treatment plan due to that emotion or, in the worst case of continued lack of recognition by the provider, give up on attempting to communicate the emotion.[19] Using situated learning (see above), educators can create learning opportunities through simulation exercises, video review, or debriefing real-time clinical interactions, to raise learners' awareness of how patients' underlying emotions may impel interactions and behavior.

Perspective-Taking

Another strategy for improving personal awareness, emotional intelligence, and empathy is perspective-taking. Taking others' perspectives allows learners and educators an opportunity to think about how another individual might feel in the situation, and the primary drivers behind what they might do or say. This tool is used in many fields, such as teaching patient-centered care, team leadership, and professionalism, and it complements the other teaching approaches we have mentioned thus far. We mentioned earlier the importance of authentic responses. However, these can backfire. For example, if a clinician feels anger toward a patient, yelling at the patient, though authentic, may lead to unintended consequences. By taking the other person's perspective, a clinician can deepen their sense of understanding and respond more thoughtfully. Several exercises can build this important skill. Educators may ask learners to provide a written narrative of a patient's experience or role play the part of the patient ("reverse role-play") to help them better understand why a patient feels or acts a certain way. In addition, case discussions that deepen understanding of patient–clinician relationships (for e.g. in Balint groups or Schwartz Rounds) can enhance awareness of the perspectives of all contributors to a patient's care and has an additional possibility of decreasing clinician burnout.[20–22]

APPROACHES TO TEACHING COMMUNICATION SKILLS

Cognitive Framework

The primary steps of teaching how to respond to emotion consist of: (1) building the recognition of nonverbal and verbal expressions of emotion, (2) naming the emotions detected, and (3) verbally and carefully responding to those emotions. We use a framework to respond verbally to emotions called PEARLS© as illustrated in Table 14-1.

Some may balk at the concept of teaching emotion as a framework, maintaining it can feel robotic. Nevertheless, using the concept of scaffolding (see above), providing explicit examples of phrasing can allow learners to practice new expressions and using their own words to make their responses most genuine (see Table 14-1). As learners and educators develop skills to recognize and categorize types of verbal expressions of empathy, they can integrate the cognitive framework with the personal awareness and perspective-taking work we highlighted above. Through this combination of skills, learners can recognize when certain responses may be most effective and adapt those examples into their own practice to feel more authentic. This authenticity in

■ TABLE 14-1. PEARLS©: Verbal Expressions of Empathy

Skill	What you can say
Partnership with the patient	*"Let's work together on this."*
Naming **E**motion	*"I can imagine how frustrating this is for you."*
Apology/**A**ppreciation	*"I'm sorry that I upset you."*
	"I give you a lot of credit for going through this as you have."
Respect	*"This has been a difficult time for you."*
	"You've done an amazing job following the doctor's instructions."
Legitimization	*"Most people in your position would feel the same way."*
Support	*"I'll be here each step of the way."*

Source: Used by permission of the Academy of Communication in Healthcare.

turn builds both clinician confidence and comfort in their own skills, which patients recognize. Educators can introduce cognitive frameworks with in-person demonstrations, video exemplars, or repetitive drill-based exercises which utilize the theories reviewed, require minimal learner vulnerability, and limited teaching time.

Individual Coaching and Affective Approaches

Individual coaching and affective approaches to teaching communication skills and emotional responses such as simulation or role-play seem to produce the most effective learning and behavior change.[3] Experimentation through role-play or simulation can further empower learners to adapt language and behaviors to their own personality and gain confidence in such skills. We will review some basic approaches here, with the strong caveat that this chapter cannot act as a substitute for training toward expertise in teaching. Educators may notice core principles of experiential learning found throughout medical education, though there are additional nuances in teaching communication skills.[23] These strategies remain largely consistent, whether applied one-on-one (educator/learner) during a patient encounter, utilizing a standardized or simulated patient, in individual role-play, or in group learning.

To initiate the individual coaching process, we recommend eliciting a learner's vision and their perceived strengths to facilitate an open discussion about their prior experiences. This support helps build a learner's self-assurance as well as reinforce already identified positive behaviors. Second, situating their learning by eliciting learner-driven, observable, and actionable objectives helps engage and focus learners toward a goal that is meaningful to their practice. Next, prior to the simulated, recorded, or real-time encounter, we suggest setting expectations for logistics to support a safe learning environment. For instance, we might agree on what a learner can do if they feel uncertain and discuss how an educator might interject or redirect the patient encounter or "time out" if in simulation or role-play. Lastly, high-quality feedback can provide highly impactful learning. We find that learners, particularly those who are self-aware or high functioning, will focus on their negative or "bad" behaviors. We prefer first to focus on the successes of the learner, which both reinforces those positive behaviors and also helps identify skills which the learner may not have recognized as exemplary. Subsequently, we typically identify the one or two opportunities we deem most important for improvement, ideally related to their original learning goals. The astute reader will note that this learner-centered approach reflects many of the educational theories we outlined earlier in this chapter.

Group Learning

Group learning has the advantage of some efficiency, given that multiple learners can learn from each other, highlighting the benefits of social cognitive theory (see above). Though learning in groups certainly adds complexity, it can also provide rewards for both the educator and learners. Overall, the steps to facilitating a group practice for responding to emotion parallels the individual coaching process: optimizing the learning environment and enumerating goals; running an exercise; and debriefing using effective feedback principles. The part of the patient can be played by another learner, a standardized or simulated patient, or possibly, under circumstances that do not interfere with their care, a real patient.

Critically, teachers must recognize the vulnerable nature of this work, where learners perform in front of their peers during often highly emotional simulated experiences. Therefore, the physical and emotional learning environment can make or break a group exercise. We have found that an intimate physical layout of the group, as shown in Fig. 14-1, helps to clearly identify roles and facilitate open discussion. As with most educational experiences, individual and group learner dynamics can produce a challenging environment. In our experience, educators with limited facilitation experience will have the most success in a group no larger than five to six learners. Those with more experience may successfully facilitate a group of seven to eight, with larger groups potentially presenting additional challenges.[24] Recognizing the impact of implicit and explicit biases, attending to the characteristics of both the participants and facilitator can further contribute to a safe and effective

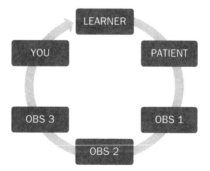

FIGURE 14-1. Physical layout for role-play in in-person small groups. Positioning of learners for role-play in an in-person group training context. "YOU" signifies the facilitator, placed alongside the learner for ease of intervention and for providing literal hand-on-shoulder support when necessary. The learner plays the role of themselves in an authentic clinical situation; a participant (or standardized patient, in some cases) portrays a patient; when invited by the facilitator, three participants (Obs1, Obs2, Obs3) provide observations and feedback to the learner. (Copyrighted figure used by permission of the Academy of Communication in Healthcare.)

learning environment. For instance, differences in hierarchy, race and ethnicity, level of trainees, gender identity, and profession can all impact individual and group dynamics and should be recognized and balanced if possible. To help establish a comfortable and productive atmosphere, educators can engage learners by encouraging participation in introductions and a form of "ice-breaker" which can help balance any hierarchy or group diversity. We often observe inherent resistance to role-play and group simulation due to its exposing nature, so facilitating an open discussion on the group's goals and prior experiences with role-play or simulated patient encounters may help to establish buy-in to the experience. As with individual coaching, we also find it helpful to review the logistics of the session such as ground rules, overview of roles and how the session will run, as well as if the session's purpose is evaluative or formative.

Group learning sessions may include predefined or learner-defined cases, either of which, using situated learning theory (see above), should invoke relevant aspects of the learners' practices.[10] Hence, educators can maximize learning by using case material that feels familiar and relates to the learners' roles, prior experience, and level of expertise. Alternatively, a facilitator might prompt learners to select and describe their own case relevant to the learning goal of the session. For instance, a learner might identify a time in which they saw a patient show sadness in response to a new diagnosis, in which they could apply the skills of recognizing and responding to emotion. Generally, we find that cases, whether predesigned or learner-designed, achieve highest impact when encouraging an individual or group to address a learning goal while maintaining it within the realm of achievable success. According to the learning ladder theory (see above), the elusive goal of balancing psychological safety while providing appropriately challenging learning will maximally benefit learning. We generally use elements of effective change management in our small groups: we initially engage learners around their prior experiences, start with voluntary participation as much as possible, and set the expectation that everyone will eventually practice and contribute to the discussion.[25]

Our review of high-quality feedback from individual coaching applies in the group setting as well, with a focus on reinforcing positive behaviors, facilitating opportunities for modifying feedback, and focusing on learner-directed opportunities for improvement. Some approaches may also include rerunning a role-play or simulation if desired for application of such group discussions.

Observation of Learner and Educator Emotions

Purposefully positioning learners in an emotionally charged experience can make them feel vulnerable and exposed. Responding to patient emotions may also open the door to more authentic, and often stronger, emotional discussions. We firmly believe that an educator must recognize and provide strong support to learners when they approach the limit of their psychological safety or capabilities. Since personal awareness and perspective-taking are central to both patient care and teaching emotional responses, we encourage educators to observe and assess both the patient's and learner's emotions simultaneously. For instance, in a real-time patient encounter, an educator may need to interject or relieve the learner when a patient's emotions escalate without adequate recognition, or if the learner shows signs of difficulty managing their own emotional response (such as feeling angry, despondent, or defensive). Interventions may include redirecting a patient encounter or pausing an individual or group simulation with judicious debriefing. For example, if an educator notices increasing anger in a learner during a simulated patient encounter in a small group setting, they can pause the encounter and utilize skills of perspective-taking and personal awareness to determine the extent of the learner's emotional vulnerability. During the debrief, the educator may decide to focus on universal skills of managing one's emotions during a patient encounter rather than further exploring that specific learner's response, particularly if there are concerns that it might place the learner's vulnerability on display for the group and exacerbate their discomfort. The educator may then choose to approach the learner after the session to more personally address the experience.

■ ONLINE LEARNING

In the era of the COVID pandemic, the world of communication skill education has rapidly changed, as with most other healthcare education. This has forced a transition to online learning and adapting the previously discussed methods to a virtual environment. Though there is great opportunity for further empirical study, we have found that, given that robust educational theory informs our methods, our approach to facilitating learning translates very effectively. Clear technical ground rules for engagement, participation, and limited audio and visual distractions are just as necessary as those ground rules established when meeting face to face. Additionally, we have found it helpful to provide explicit guidance for camera setup and navigation, such as looking into the camera while talking, and minimizing all distractions both on the computer and in users' physical backgrounds. Encouraging participants to turn on their video and directing toward use of "gallery view" for small group discussions maximizes engagement. When running a role-play, we invite observers (and ourselves as educators) to stop video (turning all observers' video cameras off) during role-play to offer a reasonably authentic facsimile of a telehealth encounter. This practice also lessens the sensation of an onstage performance, which appears to support more introverted learners. We invite observers to turn their videos back on and reestablish gallery view for the debriefing phase. To mitigate the risk of disengagement related to "Zoom fatigue," educators should offer shorter sessions and consider supplemental asynchronous learning.

■ SPECIAL CONSIDERATIONS

Special areas of consideration include novice learners and burnt-out practicing clinicians. Some learners may not have sufficient situated clinical experience yet to fully relate to the content or apply the skills used in facilitation. As such, educators should design the curriculum to meet the needs and experience of the target group. This may mean that learners must observe strong patient emotions and understand the skills to recognize and name such emotions before they can effectively practice.

Meanwhile, even the most practiced clinicians have opportunity to improve on their response to patient emotions, but some show resistance to such formal learning experiences. Some might feel that they have nothing more to learn, and others may feel "burnt out" by the heavy burden of their other tasks and cannot manage others' emotions in addition to their own emotional state. Whether the experience is voluntary or made mandatory by a workplace, we find the same steps detailed above, emphasizing positive situated learning experiences, to be most critical to establishing buy-in. Providing ample opportunity for open discussion and individual goals often can bridge even the most resistant learner to participate. We recommend formal teaching programs to become an expert in such facilitation, as this skill can be challenging and nuanced.[3,26–34]

■ CONCLUSION

Although critical to patient care, clinicians often do not innately possess expertise or skills to recognize and respond to emotion. As with most effective medical education activities, educators must adopt theory-driven and evidence-based practices for teaching in order for learners to successfully adopt and improve skills. Here, we have described teaching approaches that develop personal awareness, emotion recognition, perspective-taking, behaviors to show concern, and cognitive frameworks to express verbal empathy. With structured training that incorporates the methods described in this chapter, we find that most educators who value attention to patient emotion and a mission to improve learners' skills can achieve success.

REFERENCES

1. Woods B, Byrne A, Bodger O. The effect of multitasking on the communication skill and clinical skills of medical students. *BMC Med Educ.* 2018;18(1):76.

2. Knowles MS. *The Modern Practice of Adult Education: From Pedagogy to Andragogy.* Wilton, CT; Chicago, IL: Association Press; Follett Pub. Co.; 1980.

3. Berkhof M, van Rijssen HJ, Schellart AJ, Anema JR, van der Beek AJ. Effective training strategies for teaching communication skills to physicians: an overview of systematic reviews. *Patient Educ Couns.* 2011;84(2):152-162.

4. Libert Y, Conradt S, Reynaert C, et al. Improving doctor's communication skills in oncology: review and future perspectives. *Bulletin du cancer.* 2001;88(12):1167-1176.

5. Dewey J. *Experience and Education.* New York, NY: Macmillan; 1938.

6. Palis AG, Quiros PA. Adult learning principles and presentation *pearls. Middle East Afr J Ophthalmol.* 2014;21(2):114-122.

7. Beard C, Wilson JP. *Experiential Learning: A Best Parctice Handbook for Educators and Trainers.* 2nd ed. London: Kogan Page; 2002.

8. Lave J, Wenger E. *Situated Learning: Legitimate Peripheral Participation.* Cambridge, UK: Cambridge University Press; 1991.

9. Bandura A. *Social Foundations of Thought and Action: A Social Cognitive Theory.* Englewood Cliffs, NJ: Prentice-Hall, Inc; 1986.

10. Merriam SB, Caffarella RS, Baumgartner L. *Learning in Adulthood: A Comprehensive Guide.* 3rd ed. San Francisco, CA: Jossey-Bass; 2007.

11. Lipscomb L, Swanson J, West A. Emerging perspectives on learning, teaching, and technology. In: Orey M, ed. *Scaffolding.* 2004. http://epltt.coe.uga.edu/.

12. Designing Technology for Adult Learners: Support and Scaffolding. http://digitalpromise.org/wp-content/uploads/2016/09/designing_-technology.pdf. 2016.

13. Weber RA, Aretz HT. Climbing the ladder from novice to expert plastic surgeon. *Plast Reconstr Surg.* 2012;130(1):241-247.

14. Croskerry P, Abbass A, Wu AW. Emotional influences in patient safety. *J Patient Safety.* 2010;6(4):199-205.

15. Silva JV, Carvalho I. Physicians experiencing intense emotions while seeing their patients: what happens? *Perm J.* 2016;20(3):15-229.

16. Arao B, Clemens K. From safe spaces to brave spaces: a new way to frame dialogue around diversity and social justice. In: Landreman L, ed. *The Art of Effective Facilitation: Reflections from Social Justice Educators.* Sterling, VA: Stylus Publishing; 2013:135-150.

17. Goleman D. *Emotional Intelligence.* New York, NY: Bantam Books; 1995.

18. Levinson W, Gorawara-Bhat R, Lamb J. A study of patient clues and physician responses in primary care and surgical settings. *JAMA.* 2000;284(8):1021-1027.

19. Suchman AL, Markakis K, Beckman HB, Frankel R. A model of empathic communication in the medical interview. *JAMA.* 1997;277(8):678-682.

20. Sternlieb JL. Demystifying Balint culture and its impact: an autoethnographic analysis. *Int J Psychiatr Med.* 2018;53(1-2):39-46.

21. Taylor C, Xyrichis A, Leamy MC, Reynolds E, Maben J. Can Schwartz Center Rounds support healthcare staff with emotional challenges at work, and how do they compare

with other interventions aimed at providing similar support? a systematic review and scoping reviews. *BMJ Open*. 2018;8(10):e024254.

22. Yazdankhahfard M, Haghani F, Omid A. The Balint group and its application in medical education: a systematic review. *J Educ Health Promot*. 2019;8:124.

23. Ericsson KA. An expert-performance perspective of research on medical expertise: the study of clinical performance. *Med Educ*. 2007;41(12):1124-1130.

24. Westberg J, Jason H. *Fostering Learning in Small Groups: A Practical Guide*. New York, NY: Springer; 1996.

25. Kotter JP. Leading change: why transformation efforts fail. *Harv Bus Rev*. 2007:92-107.

26. Back AL, Arnold RM, Baile WF, et al. Faculty development to change the paradigm of communication skills teaching in oncology. *J Clin Oncol*. 2009;27(7):1137-1141.

27. Back AL, Arnold RM, Tulsky JA, Baile WF, Edwards K. "Could I add something?": teaching communication by intervening in real time during a clinical encounter. *Acad Med*. 2010;85(6):1048-1051.

28. Jackson VA, Back AL. Teaching communication skills using role-play: an experience-based guide for educators. *J Palliat Med*. 2011;14(6):775-780.

29. Spagnoletti CL, Merriam S, Milberg L, Cohen WI, Arnold RM. Teaching medical educators how to teach communication skills: more than a decade of experience. *South Med J*. 2018;111(5):246-253.

30. Boissy A, Windover AK, Bokar D, et al. Communication skills training for physicians improves patient satisfaction. *J Gen Intern Med*. 2016;31(7):755-761.

31. Chou CL, Cooley L, Pearlman E, White MK. Enhancing patient experience by training local trainers in fundamental communication skills. *Patient Exp J*. 2014;1(2):36-45.

32. Grome LJ, Banuelos RC, Lopez MA, Nicome RK, Leaming-Van Zandt KJ. communication course for pediatric providers improves self-efficacy. *Plast Reconstr Surg Glob Open*. 2018;6(10):e1964.

33. Kennedy DM, Fasolino JP, Gullen DJ. Improving the patient experience through provider communication skills building. *Patient Exp J*. 2014;1(1):56-60.

34. Saslaw M, Sirota DR, Jones DP, Rosenbaum M, Kaplan S. Effects of a hospital-wide physician communication skills training workshop on self-efficacy, attitudes and behavior. *Patient Exp J*. 2017;4(3):48-54.

Changing Medical Education to Support Emotional Wellness

CHAPTER 15

Stuart Slavin

■ INTRODUCTION

For clinicians to deal effectively with emotions—their patients' and their own—it is critically important to preserve student and trainee wellness across the education continuum. Unfortunately, substantial evidence exists that, at least for physicians, this goal is not being met. This chapter will focus on the educational path for doctors-in-training, but many of the problems and challenges found in medical school and residency also likely exist in the educational paths for nurses and allied health professionals. In describing the problems, challenges, and potential solutions in this chapter, evidence will be drawn when possible from the medical education literature. When evidence is not available, I will base my assertions drawn from experience over the past several years of my career in which I have been invited to and visited more than 25 academic medical centers. The primary purpose of these visits was to give talks and workshops, but they allowed me, in committee meetings, in one-on-one conversations, at lunches and dinners, to hear from countless medical students, residents, and faculty about the challenges they faced in their professional and personal lives. Those conversations, and those that preceded them when I was Associate Dean for Curriculum at Saint Louis University School of Medicine, have informed and guided my work and I am immensely grateful to those who have shared so openly with me.

Unfortunately, significant numbers of medical students and residents suffer from mental health problems during their training. Meta-analyses have found that 27.2% of medical students and 28.8% of residents are clinically depressed.[1,2] (Notably, a meta-analysis found an even higher rate, 34%, in nursing students.[3]) The anxiety rate in medical students globally is 33.8%, and 35.1% of residents are estimated to meet criteria for burnout.[4,5] Burnout is somewhat dependent on medical specialty; a national study of surgical residents found a burnout rate of 69%.[6] Suicidal ideation is commonplace in medical school, with 11% of medical students reporting suicidal ideation in the previous year.[1] In a recent study, suicidal ideation was reported by 4.5% of surgical residents.[7] The suicide rate for residents is lower than the national average for age-matched peers in the general population, but it is the second leading cause of death in residency.[8] And the impact of a community member's suicide is often profoundly traumatic for that community, both for their loved ones and for the broader community. Unfortunately, the rate of medical student suicide is not known as no national database of medical student deaths currently exists.

In response to this substantial and growing evidence of distress, medical schools, hospitals, and residency programs have made substantial investments in the well-being of their learners. In white coat ceremonies at the beginning of medical school across the country, administrators pledge each year that students' mental health is their top priority. Despite these investments and commitments, the mental health of medical students is not improving. In the Association of American Medical Colleges (AAMC) Graduation Questionnaire (GQ) given to all graduating U.S. medical students, two components of burnout—disengagement and exhaustion—have remained unchanged between 2016 and 2020.[9] Graduating students' satisfaction with wellness programming actually fell during those years. Perhaps even more concerningly, the AAMC Year 2 Questionnaire (given to all second-year students) showed that perceived stress, disengagement, and exhaustion all *rose* between 2017 and 2019.[10] While research has proliferated on the prevalence and drivers of burnout and depression in residency, far fewer studies have been published that demonstrate efficacy of various interventions.

The reasons for the apparent ineffectiveness of these efforts are not entirely clear, but some factors are likely. Despite strong evidence that the environment is the primary driver of distress in learners, most medical schools and residency programs have approached the problem with well-being initiatives that focus largely on the individual. Meditation, yoga, nutrition education, and exercise advice are all of value—but if the toxicity of the experience is great enough, then self-care activities will not suffice.

Unfortunately, the environment holds even more toxicity for many groups of learners. Students who are marginalized in medical education—including Black, Latinx, Native American, female, LGBTQ+, first-to college, Muslim, International Medical Graduates—now represent a sizable majority of medical students. A survey of medical students conducted by the AAMC found that Underrepresented in Medicine (URiM) and Asian students reported higher stress than White students, LGBTQ+ students experienced higher stress than heterosexual students, and first-generation college students experienced higher stress compared to others.[11] A study of students at five medical schools found that minority medical students had *lower* burnout rates than their White classmates, indicating that minority students may have higher resilience than their classmates.[12] A concerning finding of the study, however, is that students who said that their race had adversely impacted their medical school experience had greater burnout, depression scores, and lower quality of life than nonminority students. A systematic review of depression and anxiety in medical students found mixed results relating to gender and mental health, with studies suggesting that psychological distress may be higher in female students than their male classmates.[13]

Another problem with well-being initiatives to date is that they have tended to direct more resources to the *treatment* of mental illness rather than the *prevention* of it. While having adequate mental health resources is vital, there will not be significant strides in addressing the mental health crisis until a more preventive approach is taken—not just in addressing environmental drivers of distress, but also by supporting learners in developing and honing resilience skills that can help prevent depression and anxiety.

Finally, the most widely implemented individual-focused programs—these programs emphasizing mindfulness, self-compassion, and physical health—often do not include metacognitive techniques to help learners recognize and better manage cognitive distortions; mindsets such as maladaptive perfectionism and impostor phenomenon; and negative emotions of inadequacy, embarrassment, and shame that are correlated with depression and anxiety in medical students.

In this chapter, we will explore the array of environmental and individual stressors that contribute to medical student and resident distress, many of which likely afflict other health professions students. Furthermore, we will explore potential avenues for change that are evidence-based, theoretically grounded, and resource-conscious.

THE ENVIRONMENT IN UNDERGRADUATE MEDICAL EDUCATION

Stressors in Undergraduate Medical Education

Significant joys can be found in medical school and residency: the acquisition of a vast new knowledge base, the development and honing of clinical skills, the opportunity to work with bright and accomplished classmates and faculty, and the growth into a competent healthcare professional who is positioned to make a difference in the lives of current and future patients. Unfortunately, the educational path has significant stressors that contribute to the poor mental health outcomes previously described. These stressors will be the focus of this chapter section.

Despite curricular variation across schools and recent structural changes at many medical schools, undergraduate medical education can be divided into three phases: (1) the largely classroom-based pre-clerkship phase lasting 1–2 years; (2) the clerkship year (the core clinical year) in which students typically rotate through a variety of specialty-based core clinical courses (though some schools have longitudinally structured curricula); and (3) the fourth year in which students engage in subinternship and elective rotations, and apply to, and hopefully match into, a residency program.

All three phases pose substantial stress, and mental health outcomes across these phases are similar: depression and anxiety begin early in medical school and they continue unabated to graduation. The nature of the stressors across the phases, however, varies substantially and they each call for different remedies.

The Pre-Clerkship Period

The pre-clerkship period, no matter the curricular format, remains largely classroom based. What students are doing in those classrooms varies by curricular type, whether traditional lecture-based, problem/case-based learning (PBL/CBL) or flipped classroom. But students, no matter the curriculum, are in relatively controlled learning environments, in contrast to the later phases where clinical learning predominates. Each pre-clerkship curricular type has associated stressors. For those in lecture-dominant curricula, students may feel isolated and may crave more social interaction. In PBL, CBL, or flipped classroom curricula, introverted students may feel inherent anxiety with the group interaction. Yet, no matter the curriculum, the biggest driver of distress at most, if not all, medical schools is the sheer volume of information and the level of detail that must be memorized. That was the finding in surveys of first- and second-year students in 2008 at Saint Louis University (SLU) School of Medicine.[14] The same holds true in conversations I've had with students across the country since that time: information overload remains an enormous driver of distress. This distress may be compounded by a recent trend to shorten the pre-clerkship period. Many schools have moved to 18 or 20-month pre-clerkship curricula, but some have reduced the pre-clerkship phase to 1 year. These schools risk raising stress on students even more if they have not cut the curricular content proportionately. For, it is not the total volume of the material that actually is the direct source of stress. Rather, it is the volume of material over time—the intensity and rapidity of delivery of the curricular content—that is of most importance and impact.

The third highest rated stressor by SLU students was competition for grades.[14] This is also likely a significant source of distress for students in medical schools that have pre-clerkship grades.[15] In pass/fail schools, student performance may still provide significant stress if class rank is used to determine eligibility for Alpha Omega Alpha (AOA) Honor Society membership or if quartile of performance is provided to residency programs. In those schools that are pass/fail, students who are not performing up to their own expectations may still feel significant distress simply because of their own perfectionism colliding with the firm reality that half of medical students will fall below the median academically.

The United States Medical Licensing series of examinations, particularly the Step 1 exam, has become an enormous source of stress for students.[16] The stress of Step 1 can be placed in several categories. First is the direct stress and distress associated with the herculean effort to prepare for the exam—a relentless review of flashcards and an endless completion of practice questions—in what has become a parallel curriculum to medical school coursework.[17] The second stress is the anticipatory worry and fear caused by the fact that a lower score can close the door to the most desirable specialties or the most prestigious institutions for residency training, or that a failing score can threaten prospects of matching to a program at all. The third category of stress is experienced weeks after the exam when some students receive low or failing scores, which may feel like a life-altering event.

The National Board of Medical Examiners (NBME) has taken a significant step to mitigate the distress associated with the Step 1 exam by announcing a shift to pass/fail score reporting. This will undoubtedly decrease the stress associated with the exam for many students. However, it is imperative to recognize that Step 1 is not the primary source of stress; it is simply a vehicle for it. The primary driver remains the stress associated with the residency matching process, and that stress will not be diminished by this change. We can expect the stress to transfer to other metrics, most likely to the Step 2 exam, but also potentially to the clinical clerkships and their associated grades.

The Clerkship Year

The clerkship year represents the first immersive experience in the clinical setting for most students and it presents emotional challenges of dealing intimately with illness, death, and loss. In a survey of third-year medical students at SLU, however, students did not identify these patient factors as the greatest sources of personal distress. Instead, working with unhappy residents, working with unhappy faculty, and subjectivity and unfairness of grading in the clerkships were the factors students felt to be most distressing and disheartening.[18]

Mistreatment in clerkships is widespread and it comes from a variety of sources including faculty, residents, nurses, other hospital employees, and patients and families. In the AAMC GQ in 2020, 39.6% of students reported experiencing behaviors such as being subject to offensive remarks, receiving lower evaluations or grades, or being denied opportunities for training or rewards based on gender, race/ethnicity, or sexual orientation.[9] 21.8% of students reported being publicly humiliated. The most common perpetrators were clerkship faculty, with 15.1% of students reporting being publicly humiliated by clerkship faculty as compared to just 1% for pre-clerkship faculty. The second highest ranked source was residents at 9.1%.

Another contributing factor to student stress is time pressure during the clerkship years. On inpatient rotations, 12- to 16-hour days, 6 days a week are not uncommon. Combined with studying time required for end-of-clerkship examinations, students may find inadequate time for self-care, family, or friends, or even sleep. This time pressure, and the fact that students are often sent to geographically disparate clinical sites, can contribute to significant feelings of isolation, even with the social nature of the clinical setting.

Competition for grades in the clerkship year is a major stressor for students. Unlike the pre-clerkship period, the vast majority of medical schools assign grades to students in courses in the clerkship year. With the change to pass/fail scoring of the Step 1 exam, the stress of clerkship grades may well intensify as the Step 1 score, which has historically been an incredibly important factor in the residency application process, is eliminated. Evaluations and grading systems in the clerkship remain notoriously flawed, inequitable, and embedded with bias.[19] Given the importance of clinical grades and evaluations, and the capricious nature of the system, student anxiety, frustration, and at times, outright anger are commonplace and, in many cases, justified.

Many schools have moved in recent years to use NBME subject examinations for their end-of-clerkship exams. These exams, because of the wide range of scores as compared to the much narrower range of scores on clinical evaluations, have an outsized impact on students' final grades. This fact is not lost on students and, understandably, behavior often follows—namely, a desire to select clinical services with the fewest clinical hours and to exit the clinical setting as quickly as possible so that more time can be devoted to studying for their subject exam.

For some students, the clinical environment is even more inhospitable. Microaggressions and overt racism alike remain far too commonplace. The experience of impostor phenomenon that many medical students feel disproportionately impacts women and students of color who are repeatedly made to feel they do not belong.[20]

Final Year Stresses

The final phase of medical school is characterized by a new set of stressors. In a very short time, students must decide on a specialty, arrange for away rotations, prepare their application materials, gather letters of recommendation, apply to what is often dozens of programs, travel the country to interview at the ones that they have been invited to, mourn the ones that they haven't been invited to, and add $10,000 or even more in application and travel costs to an average medical school debt of close to $200,000. They then endure the day when they are informed if they did not match to a program, followed a few days later by opening letters that tell them where they will be spending the next 3 to 7 years of their lives. Soon thereafter, most have to prepare to move to another city and medical center, say goodbye to their friends, and begin what will arguably be the most challenging professional transition of their lives: the first months of residency training. Combined with the USMLE Step 2 Clinical Knowledge exam and, until recently, the Step 2 Clinical Skills Examination (which was placed on indefinite suspension during the COVID-19 pandemic), it becomes clear how this phase can be an emotionally taxing experience for students.

Culture and Emotion across the Four Years

The culture in medical school has a significant impact—for better or for worse—on medical student well-being. The cultural factor with the greatest potential impact is that created by administration, course chairs, and the faculty populating the various curricular and student-facing committees. Unfortunately, medical school culture remains deeply hierarchical, paternalistic, and inflexible at far too many schools. In the AAMC GQ, only 70.6% of students were satisfied with their deans' offices' (student affairs and curricula affairs) awareness of student concerns, and only 67.9% were satisfied with the offices' responsiveness to student problems.[9] Conversations with students from across the country have revealed too many schools with rigid policies and inflexibility in accommodating needs of students facing life crises such as the illness or death of a family member. The result, too often, is a lack of trust that is bidirectional.[21]

This culture can act as a chronic weight on students and their well-being. To be sure, in the midst of this less than ideal environment, some administrators—particularly student affairs deans—and some faculty are sympathetic to student perspectives and concerns, but their voices rarely hold sway in improving the forces of cultural inertia.

Medical school curricula have been described as having a formal, an informal, and a hidden curriculum.[22,23] Hafferty described these interrelated spheres as: "(1) The stated, intended, and formally offered and endorsed curriculum (e.g., the 'this is what we do' curriculum); (2) An unscripted, predominantly ad hoc, and highly interpersonal form of teaching and learning that takes place among and between faculty and students (the informal curriculum); and (3) a set of influences that function at the level of the organizational structure and culture (the hidden curriculum)."[23] While emotions are a subject of the formal curriculum, the more powerful messages in medical school likely come from the informal and hidden curricula. The formal curriculum dominates in the pre-clerkship phase with clinical skills courses focusing on empathy, exploring the patient's experience of illness, and providing compassionate care to those in distress. The informal and hidden curricula take over in the clerkship year and they do not release their grip through the rest of training and into practice. The message frequently conveyed in the informal and hidden curricula is for students to distance themselves from patients, striving toward emotional detachment. This is one factor that likely contributes to declines in empathy seen in medical students and residents.[24] Students may also be subject to even stronger messages, as illustrated by a story told to me by a third-year student on her surgery clerkship. She had been on morning rounds with her team and was reporting on her patient's status over the past 24 hours. In the subjective portion of the presentation, she shared that the patient had been sobbing that morning when she went in to examine her. The resident replied, "We don't care about that," and told her to move on with her presentation. While not always so aggressively discounted and devalued, patients' emotions remain an afterthought on many clinical teams with patients' emotional well-being a distant second to all of the numbers—vital signs and lab results—that are tracked, recorded, and corrected.

Patients are not the only ones whose emotions are subject to the informal and hidden curricula. Medical students have been noted to experience a range of emotions including anxiety, guilt, sadness, anger, and shame.[25] They are also discouraged from expressing these emotions.[26] The following messages from supervising faculty and residents relating to student emotions remain all too common: Do not show weakness or discomfort. Hide any feelings of inadequacy, embarrassment, or shame that you may have. If you have personal crises, you need to suppress and compartmentalize your feelings so that they don't interfere with your work. Don't cry—but if you do, do it privately.[27]

Potential Solutions

The stressors in medical school vary across the three phases as do the potential interventions to promote emotional well-being. In the pre-clerkship phase, a model for change that one medical school instituted can serve as a cost- and time-efficient model for any medical school in the country.[11,14] The curricular and policy changes included the following: reduction of core curricular time by 10%; efforts to reduce curricular content by 10% or more; creating time for elective opportunities and for self; theme-based learning communities such as Community Health, Research, Global Health, and Well-being; and efforts to reduce the toxicity of some courses (with excessive content, harsh grading practices, and/or disrespectful behavior by course directors and faculty). These changes, when combined with a brief resilience curriculum, produced marked decreases in rates of depression and anxiety in students compared to a historical control group prior to implementation. Depression rates, as compared to a historical control group before changes were implemented, fell from 27 to 4% for first-year students, and from 31 to 6% for second-year students. Anxiety rates also fell, from 55 to 14% for first-year students, and from 60 to 31% for second-years. At the same time, despite the substantial decrease in curricular content and pressure, academic performance improved.

Unfortunately, improving medical student mental health in the clerkship year will be significantly more difficult. How can we expect students to be happy and well when they are working with so many unhappy, stressed, burned out, and depressed residents and faculty? The most valuable and most promising programs for medical student well-being in the clerkship year may well be ones that support resident and faculty well-being. In addition, efforts can and should be made to improve the evaluation and grading system in the clerkship year.

Decreasing the stress of the fourth year will, unfortunately, also be difficult to achieve if the intense competition for residency positions continues. Some hope may be found in helping students manage mindsets, described later in this chapter, that can contribute to the distress that they feel.

■ THE ENVIRONMENT IN GRADUATE MEDICAL EDUCATION

Systems and Culture

A great deal of attention has been placed in recent years on the problem of burnout in physicians and, by extension, medical residents. A number of organizations have mobilized to address this problem and the efforts have coalesced in the National Academy of Medicine (NAM) Action Collaborative on Clinician Well-being and Resilience that is addressing the mental health crisis, not just in physicians, but in all healthcare providers. A report from NAM "Taking Action Against Clinician Burnout: A Systems Approach to Professional Well-Being" used a systems engineering lens to view the problem and offer solutions.[28] A major focus of a systems approach is on the work itself and the job demands faced. As such, issues such as excessive workload, inadequate staffing, administrative burden, inefficient workflow, cumbersome electronic record systems, time pressure, and productivity pressure are high-lighted. These factors undoubtedly have an impact on resident well-being, but some may be less acutely felt by residents than by practicing physicians, and importantly they are not likely to be the only driver of resident distress. Another potential lens through which to view the problem is one that focuses more on culture. Work by Christina Maslach and Michael Leiter, and principles from the book *Drive* by Daniel Pink, have a more cultural focus that can be used to understand critical stressors and inform potential intervention.[29-31] (Clinician wellness is further discussed in Chapter 16, Striving and Thriving: Challenges and Opportunities for Clinician Emotional Wellness.)

Maslach and Leiter
Maslach and Leiter identified six potential drivers of burnout: Workload, Control, Reward, Community, Fairness, and Values.

Workload Residency is a time that is known for long hours and grueling schedules. Residents can work up to 80 hours per week, and up to 88 hours a week in some programs. Individual shifts can stretch to 28 hours. Residents in recent years have been afforded some protections that faculty may not have: an average of at least 1 day off in 7 and caps on numbers of admissions and patient loads. Administrative burden is significant for residents and many have lamented the amount of time that residents spend away from the bedside. One study found that only 12% of resident time on inpatient services was spent in direct patient care.[32] The electronic health record system is a source of great frustration for faculty, but in conversations with many residents, who are more facile with technology than their more senior faculty supervisors, this does not seem to be as substantial a driver of frustration as it is for faculty.

Tension exists in balancing different roles: balance between service and education, and between work and outside life. Workload can compromise residents' ability to attend educational conferences such as morning report, didactic series for residents, and Grand Rounds lectures.[33] Too often, work responsibilities bleed over into personal time as residents are expected to engage in quality improvement projects, scholarly activity, board exam study, reading about their patients' diseases, and online training modules often without sufficient protected time in the workday.

Some efforts have been made to address the workload problem. As stated earlier, caps on numbers of admissions and patient census have been instituted at some programs. Nonteaching hospitalist services have also been instituted at some medical centers to relieve the patient load for residents.[34] Some programs that I have visited take residents' pagers during educational conferences so that they are not interrupted while learning. Some programs have hired staff to help resident teams with administrative tasks such as discharge planning and contacting insurance companies for authorizations, while other programs have instituted schedules that afford residents more protected educational time. In Internal Medicine, 4 plus 1 schedules have become more common, meaning that residents have 4 weeks on service followed by a week that is devoted to more educationally focused activities.[35]

Parental/family leave has received increased attention recently with housestaff pushing for more expansive leave policies. In response to a report from the Accreditation Council for Graduate Medical Education Council of Review Committee Residents, the American Board of Medical Specialties instituted a policy effective July 2021 that allows residents to take a minimum of 6 weeks for parental, caregiver, or medical leave during their training without having to use vacation or sick leave and without having to extend their training.[36] While this is an important step, many housestaff remain concerned that fellow residents will need to provide coverage for the residents on leave in many cases, creating greater service burdens and potential resentment for some.

Control Residents have notoriously little control in their lives. They are told what clinical rotations they will be on and in which order, when their call nights will be, what days off they will have, and who their patients are. The result can be that residents feel little sense of agency and this can contribute to a sense of powerlessness that can be dispiriting. Some residency programs that I visited have worked to address this problem by involving residents themselves in helping to create schedules. In addition, some programs have active resident councils that can serve as a voice for change. Administrative decision making must be transparent and residents' voices must be integral to this process. The issue of control can also be addressed by reminding residents that they do have ultimate control over one thing—what Viktor Frankl called the last of the "human freedoms": "to choose one's attitude in any given set of circumstances, to choose one's own way."[37]

Reward In viewing reward, Maslach and Leiter did not focus just on financial reward, but also on a personal sense of reward and appreciation. Resident salaries have risen consistently over the years, with average yearly compensation standing at approximately $63,000 annually.[38] When calculated as an hourly rate, however, some residents may feel grossly underpaid. A form of reward less addressed, however, is the more personal sense of reward. Do residents feel appreciated and valued by their institution and the faculty? In my travels around the country, residents routinely expressed feeling taken for granted, unappreciated, and undervalued (and faculty reported their own feelings of lack of appreciation for their own work). Institutions need to move beyond interventions like resident appreciation day to infuse the wider culture with a sense of appreciation and gratitude. Administration in the C-suite, department chairs, and program directors can model this behavior, but residents and faculty need to recognize that they are cocreators of the culture and that they can work to show appreciation for their fellow healthcare workers.

Community Medical care is more reliant on teams now than ever before, but inpatient teams have become increasingly fractured and fragmented in the academic medical center setting. In the not too distant past, faculty would often rotate on a ward service for a month. Faculty, residents, and students had the opportunity to work closely together and bond. At the end of the month, it was fairly common for the faculty member to take the team out for lunch or have them over for dinner. Community developed in ways that are much more difficult to facilitate today. The typical rotation for faculty at medical centers that I have visited are 1 week in length—periods of time that are so brief that true connection and community are difficult to achieve. Add to that the productivity pressures, documentation requirements, and administrative burden that faculty face, and this can lead to weakened relationships between faculty and learners.

Some hospital services continue to have 2-week rotations for faculty, but many faculty whom I spoke with who have 1-week blocks on service felt like they would not be able to lengthen the time on service. Given that reality, more needs to be done in the way of faculty and resident development to help maximize their time together, making sure that time is allotted at the start of rotations to make expectations clear, as well as time during rotations for teaching and to provision of feedback.

Fairness Fairness is difficult to quantify and factors that may influence residents' feelings of program fairness vary. One important way that fairness can play out is in the treatment of disruptive faculty and residents. Too often, disruptive staff are given free rein to behave with relative impunity and few academic medical centers appear to manage problematic staff in ways that curb their behavior. As mentioned earlier, the clinical learning environment may be more hostile to many marginalized groups who may feel mistreated without opportunity for recourse.[39]

Programs and institutions can and should institute programs modeled after those, such as Vanderbilt and the Brigham and Women's Hospital in Boston, that have introduced effective stepwise, graduated approaches for managing disruptive staff.[40,41]

Values Medical centers often have aspirational messages in their marketing campaigns and outward-facing messaging to patients that espouse the compassionate nature of their care. This may not match the reality on the wards and in the clinics. Individuals in leadership roles do not necessarily exemplify the institutional values and this can contribute to cynicism, pessimism, and negativity on the part of the of faculty and residents.

Leaders and supervisors need to be held to high ethical standards. Opportunities to evaluate individual behavior relating to values should be included in annual reviews of performance and should inform change or have real consequences.

Daniel Pink

In his book, *Drive,* Daniel Pink postulated that three areas were critical in motivating and boosting productivity of employees: autonomy, mastery, and purpose.[31] Autonomy is subsumed under Maslach and Leiter's model, so mastery and meaning will be discussed here.

Mastery Promotion of mastery, which is a sense of growth and confidence in professional skill development, is an essential aspect of an effective educational program. To help promote mastery, three components are critically important: making expectations clear; building in time for observation of clinical skills; and provision of regular, specific, and actionable feedback. Because of the rapid turnover of faculty on ward services and the often-heavy service demands seen on these services, time to set expectations is often felt to be inadequate. Some faculty do a good job in setting expectations, but this simple step is sometimes skipped. This means that residents and students are left to figure out what the attending physician wants from them with little in the way of guidance, expectations, and proactive feedback. The milestones program promulgated as part of the Accreditation Council for Graduate Medical Education (ACGME) Common Program Requirements have pushed programs to improve the specificity and regularity of performance feedback for residents, though it is not entirely clear how seriously programs have taken these requirements.

Faculty should be provided with development sessions on effective observation and feedback. Residents should also receive training on how to give, and also how to receive, feedback.

Meaning Maslow developed a hierarchical model for human needs that had five levels: physiological (including food, water, warmth, and rest), safety, belongingness and love, esteem needs, and self-actualization.[42] He later added transcendence to the model. Maslow postulated that needs lower down in the hierarchy must be satisfied before individuals can attend to higher needs on the scale. This hypothesis has never been validated by research however, and Viktor Frankl's observations of prisoners enduring the horrific conditions in the concentration camps would argue otherwise. Frankl stated, "There is nothing in the world, I venture to say, that would so effectively help one to survive even the worst conditions as the knowledge that there is a meaning in one's life. There is much wisdom in the words of Nietzsche: 'He who has a why to live for can bear almost any how.'"[43] While attention to the lower levels of Maslow's hierarchy is critically important, helping residents and faculty find purpose and meaning in their clinical work not only contributes to motivation, but also to well-being and resilience.

Two programs have been created to help clinicians and trainees find meaning in their work. Healer's Art courses, developed by Dr. Rachel Naomi Remen, have been instituted at more than 90 medical schools across the country.[44,45] One potential limitation to their long-term efficacy, however, may be that they are most often offered as electives in the pre-clerkship period before the informal and hidden curricula really begin. As such, these may not be ideally situated to counteract the corrosive influences that students may face in their clinical years. Schwartz Rounds is another approach aimed at clinicians, where "in contrast to traditional medical rounds, the focus is on the human dimension of medicine."[46] Self-evaluations for the program have been very positive, but evidence of impact on clinician well-being remains linited.[47]

■ INDIVIDUAL FACTORS

Problematic Mindsets, Automatic Thoughts, and Mental Health History

Environmental factors are not the only ones that can impact student and resident mental health and emotional well-being. Students bring to medical school and residency long-standing patterns of thinking—mindsets and automatic thoughts—acquired on the long and arduous education continuum before medical school that can contribute to negative emotions and potentially to adverse mental health outcomes. These mindsets are not the only risk factors for mental health problems that students may bring to medical school or residency. Students may also have past histories of depression and/ or anxiety that can make the demanding journey through medical training even more challenging.

Mindsets

An array of *mindsets* (mental filters through which students view themselves and their environment) appear prevalent in medical students and residents. Viewing *performance as identity* appears widespread, and medical students can experience it in the following way: "I *am* my Step 1 score," rather than "I *got* this Step 1 score." Given the relentless measuring, sorting, and ranking along the educational continuum, comparison to peers is almost inevitable. When combined with performance as identity, scoring below average, and for some, not being at the top of the class, can contribute significantly to distress. *Maladaptive perfectionism (MP)* involves setting the bar so high for yourself that you are repeatedly disappointed with yourself. Residents who have MP may suffer inordinately when they make an error, forget to check a lab, or stumble on rounds. *Impostor phenomenon (IP)* describes feeling like a fraud or an impostor despite objective evidence to the contrary. Students typically feel IP more intensely in transitions in medicine: from pre-clerkship to clerkship, from fourth year to internship, and from residency to fellowship or practice. Both MP and IP may contribute to distressing feelings of shame and guilt. A study of first-year medical students found significant correlations between MP and IP with feelings of inadequacy, embarrassment, and shame about academic performance.[48] Those with these negative feelings had a significantly higher rate of depression and anxiety, supporting a cognitive behavioral model for mental illness with thoughts driving feelings and feelings contributing to mental illness.

Putting on the mask is a mindset and behavior in which learners take great pains to hide their struggles and negative emotions from others. This behavior, when widely practiced, can contribute to distress because it may lead to individual thoughts of being the only one struggling, and by corollary, that there is something wrong with *themselves* rather than something wrong with the *environment*. Finally, many students have been conditioned over the educational continuum before medical school to *chase success* rather than *find meaning*. For some students, this plays out as a relentless pursuit of matching into one of the "dream" or "holy grail" specialties—dermatology, neurosurgery, ophthalmology, orthopedic surgery, plastic surgery—that all have the shared attribute of high compensation. Students may also be consumed by the desire to match at a prestigious institution or in a desirable geographic area. If these goals are not achieved, some may feel like their life is forever compromised—a common cognitive distortion of predicting the future with certainty. I describe the process of chasing success without personal judgment. Students are products of the educational culture and system they have experienced. They have competed academically their entire lives. It is understandable that those who have succeeded in this long and demanding path—particularly those who have wanted to be (for whatever reason) a neurosurgeon since the age of 5—may feel completely devastated by having that dream crushed so near the finish line by a mediocre score on Step 1.

Another cluster of mindsets, characterized by negative mood and outlook, are more likely to arise under the stresses and demands of residency. These include *cynicism, negativity bias,* and *pessimistic explanatory style.* These individual mindsets, if affecting enough residents (and faculty), can contribute to the toxicity of the environment, as evidenced by the findings in one study of clerkship medical students that found that working with unhappy residents and faculty were the most disheartening factors in the clerkship year.[21]

Shame and Guilt

The experiences of shame and guilt across the medical education continuum has received greater attention in recent years. Work by William Bynum has explored the intersection of these feelings with decreased empathy and impaired self-forgiveness.[49] In a study of medical residents, Bynum found that feelings of shame contributed to social isolation, disengagement from learning, impaired wellness, unprofessional behavior, and impaired empathy.[50]

Automatic Thoughts

Automatic thoughts, or cognitive distortions, have long been a focus of mental health researchers and clinicians. They are part of the human condition, but they may play out with particular intensity in the competitive environment in medical school and under the demands of residency. Automatic thoughts are the primary target of cognitive behavioral therapy, which remains the gold standard treatment for anxiety. It is also helpful in treating depression and in managing maladaptive perfectionism and impostor phenomenon. Automatic thoughts are often unrecognized to the self as distortions, and they can produce a reality for learners that is significantly darker than the actual situation. Some of the distortions that appear commonplace in medical students and residents include the following:

- Magnification: taking a relatively small event like a poor score on a quiz or forgetting to check on a lab and blowing it up into a major problem.
- All-or-none thinking: if you do not achieve the outcome you hoped for, you consider yourself a failure. For example, if you hoped for at least a 90 on an exam, but only got an 85, the tendency to view this as a failure rather than saying to yourself that you did pretty well.
- Personalization and self-blame: when facing an adverse personal outcome, laying *all* of the blame on yourself.
- Overgeneralization: taking a relatively small event and feeling like it is part of a pattern of bad things that you do or that always happen to you.
- Tunnel vision: focusing on a single negative event and discounting all of the positive things in your life.
- Catastrophizing: taking a relatively small event and blowing it up to catastrophic portions, believing the event will lead to certain adverse personal outcomes.
- Mind-reading: the belief that you know what someone is thinking. For example, a colleague walks by you in the hallway and avoids eye contact, frowns, and doesn't say hello and you believe with some certainty that the

person is angry with you even though there are numerous other potential causes for the behavior.

- Fortune-telling: predicting the future with certainty. For example, believing with certainty that you are going to fail an exam or not match into a program rather than being concerned that this might be a possibility.

Collectively, these thoughts can contribute to a sense of distress. Unfortunately, if a person has not previously seen a therapist, they are unlikely to be familiar with these distortions or have any idea how to combat them.

Mental Health History

Mental health history can also have an impact on mental health in medical school and residency. A number of studies have shown that medical students and residents begin their respective programs with mental health equal to, or better than, their age-matched peers in the general population.[51-53] The comparison may be problematic however, as medical students and residents are generally surveyed at orientation: a period of time where they are not subject to the demands and psychological pressure of the measurement, sorting, and ranking that have characterized their lives. In a longitudinal study of first-year residents at orientation, 3.9% met criteria for major depression, but a striking 55.9% reported a history of depression.[54] While not depressed at orientation, students and residents are very susceptible to it when immersed in the demands of medical school or residency.

Individual-Focused Approaches

Many medical schools and residency programs have expanded their mental health services to better meet the needs of students with mental illness, and this includes efforts to reduce stigma and other barriers to care. These efforts are critically important and laudable, but they are not sufficient. More preventive mental health measures must be implemented. Many medical schools have offered training in mindfulness, meditation, and yoga. Again, this is laudable, but these programs are not likely to be sufficient for many students or residents and relatively few may take up these practices. In my talks across the country over the past several years, I would routinely ask audience members to raise their hands if they had a meditation practice of 15 minutes or more per day. No more than 3% raised their hands in any audience. Meditation works, but it also requires the desire and ability to meditate regularly to be effective. Structural barriers in medicine stand in the way of many students' and residents' ability to commit a time-consuming meditative practice into their daily lives.

A resilience curriculum implemented at Saint Louis University contributed to positive mental health outcomes in pre-clerkship students.[14] Only 4 hours in length across all 4 years of the curriculum, the resilience training primarily focused on cognitive behavioral techniques and informal mindfulness techniques to help students with the automatic thoughts and mindsets described previously. In addition, the curriculum included a toolbox of strategies to help in dealing with other threats to well-being: counteracting pessimism, enhancing emotional self-regulation, dealing with difficult people, cultivating positive emotions, investing in personal health, and finding meaning in work and life. The curriculum was adapted for use in residency training as an initial 2-hour workshop followed by discussions every 6 to 8 weeks about life challenges and stressors. In a pilot study, this curriculum led to significant reductions in rates of depression and anxiety in first-year pediatric residents compared to a historical control group.[55] The curriculum has been further adapted and is available for free as a video workshop, series of podcasts, and an app on the ACGME website.[56]

■ CONCLUSION

Significant stressors remain across the medical educational continuum that threaten the mental health and well-being of medical students and residents. Leaders in medical education can and must expand upon current well-being efforts, adopting a more preventive approach and gearing more of their efforts to reducing the toxicity of the learning experience, particularly in the clinical learning environment. Similarly, it is imperative to give attention to faculty mental health because medical students and residents are less likely to be well if their direct supervisors are not (see Chapter 16, Striving and Thriving: Challenges and Opportunities for Clinician Emotional Wellness for more on this topic). While we address systems factors that influence mental health, we also need to focus more on improving the culture so that students, residents, and faculty feel valued, appreciated, listened to, and respected. Not only our physicians' well-being hangs in the balance, that of our patients does as well.

REFERENCES

1. Rotenstein LS, Ramos MA, Torre M, et al. Prevalence of depression, depressive symptoms, and suicidal ideation among medical students: a systematic review and meta-analysis. *JAMA*. 2016;316(21):2214-2236.

2. Mata DA, Ramos MA, Bansal N, et al. Prevalence of depression and depressive symptoms among resident physicians: a systematic review and meta-analysis. *JAMA*. 2015;314(22):2373-2383.

3. Tung YJ, Lo KK, Ho RC, Tam WS. Prevalence of depression among nursing students: a systematic review and meta-analysis. *Nurse Educ Today*. 2018;63:119-129.

4. Tian-Ci Quek T, Tam WS, Tran BX, et al. The global prevalence of anxiety among medical students: a meta-analysis. *Int J Environ Res Public Health*. 2019;16(15):2735.

5. Rodrigues H, Cobucci R, Oliveira A, et al. Burnout syndrome among medical residents: a systematic review and meta-analysis. *PLoS One*. 2018;13(11):e0206840.

6. Lebares CC, Guvva EV, Ascher NL, O'Sullivan PS, Harris HW, Epel ES. Burnout and stress among US surgery residents: psychological distress and resilience. *J Am Coll Surg*. 2018;226(1):80-90.

7. Hu YY, Ellis RJ, Hewitt DB, et al. Discrimination, abuse, harassment, and burnout in surgical residency training. *New Engl J Med*. 2019;381(18):1741-1752.

8. Yaghmour NA, Brigham TP, Richter T, et al. Causes of death of residents in ACGME-accredited programs 2000 through 2014: implications for the learning environment. *Acad Med*. 2017;92(7):976-983.

9. Association of American Medical Colleges. Medical school graduation questionnaire: 2020 all schools summary report. https://www.aamc.org/system/files/202007/2020%20GQ%20All%20Schools%20Summary.pdf. Published July 2020. Accessed August 10, 2020.

10. Association of American Medical Colleges. Year two questionnaire: 2019 all schools summary report. https://www.aamc.org/system/files/202004/2019%20Y2Q%20All%20Schools%20Summary%20Report.pdf. Published March 2020. Accessed August 10, 2020.

11. Personal well-being among medical students: findings from an AAMC pilot survey. https://www.aamc.org/system/files/reports/1/april2014aib_personalwell-beingamong-medicalstudents.pdf. Published April 2014. Accessed September 15, 2020.

12. Dyrbye LN, Thomas MR, Eacker A, et al. Race, ethnicity, and medical student well-being in the United States. *Arch Intern Med*. 2007;167(19):2103-2109.

13. Dyrbye LN, Thomas MR, Shanafelt TD. Systematic review of depression, anxiety, and other indicators of psychological distress among US and Canadian medical students. *Acad Med*. 2006;81(4):354-373.

14. Slavin SJ, Schindler DL, Chibnall JT. Medical student mental health 3.0: improving student wellness through curricular changes. *Acad Med*. 2014;89(4):573-577.

15. Reed DA, Shanafelt TD, Satele DW, et al Relationship of pass/fail grading and curriculum structure with well-being among preclinical medical students: a multi-institutional study. *Acad Med*. 2011; 86(11):1367-1373.

16. Chen DR, Priest KC, Batten JN, et al. Student perspectives on the "Step 1 climate" in preclinical medical education. *Acad Med*. 2019;9(3):302-304.

17. Burk-Rafel J, Santen SA, Purkiss J. Study behaviors and USMLE Step 1 performance: implications of a student self-directed parallel curriculum. *Acad Med*. 2017;92(11S):S67-S74.

18. Slavin S. Reflections on a decade leading a medical student well-being initiative. *Acad Med*. 2019;94(6):771-774.

19. Hauer KE, Lucey CR. Core clerkship grading: the illusion of objectivity. *Acad Med*. 2019;94(4):469-472.

20. Villwock JA, Sobin LB, Koester LA, Harris TM. Impostor syndrome and burnout among American medical students: a pilot study. *Int J Med Educ*. 2016;7:364-369.

21. Slavin S, Smith G. Taking students as they should be: restoring trust in undergraduate medical education. *Acad Med*. 2019;94(12):1847-1850.

22. Hafferty FW. Beyond curriculum reform: confronting medicine's hidden curriculum. *Acad Med.* 1998;73(4):403-407.

23. Hafferty FW, Hafler JP. The hidden curriculum, structural disconnects, and the socialization of new professionals. In: *Extraordinary Learning in the Workplace.* Dordrecht: Springer; 2011:17-35.

24. Neumann M, Edelhäuser F, Tauschel D, et al. Empathy decline and its reasons: a systematic review of studies with medical students and residents. *Acad Med.* 2011;86(8):996-1009.

25. Kasman DL, Fryer-Edwards K, Braddock CH III. Educating for professionalism: emotional experiences on medical and pediatric inpatient wards. *Acad Med.* 2003;78:730-741.

26. Karnieli-Miller O, Vu TR, Holtman MC, Clyman SG, Inui TS. Medical students' professionalism narratives: a window on the informal and hidden curriculum. *Acad Med.* 2010;85:124-133.

27. Angoff NR. Crying in the curriculum. *JAMA.* 2001; 286(9):1017-1018.

28. National Academies of Sciences, Engineering, and Medicine. Taking action against clinician burnout: a systems approach to professional well-being. National Academies Press; 2020.

29. Leiter MP, Maslach C. *Banishing Burnout: Six Strategies for Improving Your Relationship with Work.* San Francisco, CA: John Wiley & Sons; 2005.

30. Leiter MP, Maslach C. A mediation model of job burnout. In: Antoniou ASG, Cooper CL, eds. *Research Companion to Organizational Health Psychology.* Cheltenham: Edward Elgar; 2005:544-564.

31. Pink DH. *Drive: The Surprising Truth about What Motivates Us.* New York City, NY: Penguin; 2011.

32. Block L, Habicht R, Wu AW, et al. In the wake of the 2003 and 2011 duty hours regulations, how do internal medicine interns spend their time? *J Gen Intern Med.* 2013;28(8):1042-1047.

33. Wayne DB, Arora V. Resident duty hours and the delicate balance between education and patient care. *J Gen Intern Med.* 2008; 23(7):1120-1121

34. Sehgal NL, Shah HM, Parekh VI, Roy CL, Williams MV. Non–housestaff medicine services in academic centers: models and challenges. *J Hosp Med.* 2008;3(3):247-255.

35. Mariotti JL, Shalaby M, Fitzgibbons JP. The 4–1 schedule: a novel template for internal medicine residencies. *J Grad Med Educ.* 2010;2(4):541-547.

36. American Board of Medical Specialties Policy on Parental, Caregiver and Medical Leave During Training. https://www.abms.org/media/258004/parental-caregiver-and-medical-leave-during-training-policy.pdf. Accessed September 13, 2020.

37. Frankl VE. *Man's Search for Ultimate Meaning.* Cambridge, MA: Perseus Publishing; 2000.

38. Medscape Residents Salary & Debt Report 2020. https://www.medscape.com/slideshow/2020-residents-salary-debt-report-6013072. Published August 7, 2020. Accessed September 10, 2020.

39. Hu YY, Ellis RJ, Hewitt DB, et al. Discrimination, abuse, harassment, and burnout in surgical residency training. *New Engl J Med.* 2019;381(18):1741-1752.

40. Hickson GB, Pichert JW, Webb LE, Gabbe SG. A complementary approach to promoting professionalism: identifying, measuring, and addressing unprofessional behaviors. *Acad Med.* 2007;82(11):1040-1048.

41. Shapiro J, Whittemore A, Tsen LC. Instituting a culture of professionalism: the establishment of a center for professionalism and peer support. *The Joint Commission Journal on Quality and Patient Safety.* 2014;40(4):168-177.

42. Maslow A, Lewis KJ. Maslow's hierarchy of needs. Salenger Incorporated. 1987;14:987.

43. Frankl VE. *Man's Search for Meaning.* Simon & Schuster; 1985.

44. Healer's Art Overview. http://www.rishiprograms.org/healers-art/#:~:text=The%20 Healer's%20Art%20course%20utilizes,rarely%20discussed%20in%20medical%20training. Accessed September 17, 2020.

45. Remen RN, Rabow MW. The healer's art: professionalism, service and mission. *Med Educ.* 2005;39:1167-1168.

46. https://www.theschwartzcenter.org/programs/schwartz-rounds/. Accessed September 17, 2020.

47. Taylor C, Xyrichis A, Leamy MC, Reynolds E, Maben J. Can Schwartz Center Rounds support healthcare staff with emotional challenges at work, and how do they compare with other interventions aimed at providing similar support? a systematic review and scoping reviews. *BMJ Open.* 2018;8(10):e024254.

48. Hu KS, Chibnall JT, Slavin SJ. Maladaptive perfectionism, impostorism, and cognitive distortions: threats to the mental health of pre-clinical medical students. *Acad Psychiatry.* 2019;43(4):381-385.

49. Bynum WE IV, Goodie JL. Shame, guilt, and the medical learner: ignored connections and why we should care. *Med Educ.* 2014;48(11):1045-1054.

50. Bynum WEIV, Artino AR Jr, Uijtdehaage S, Webb AM, Varpio L. Sentinel emotional events: the nature, triggers, and effects of shame experiences in medical residents. *Acad Med.* 2019;94(1):85-93.

51. Brazeau CM, Shanafelt T, Durning SJ, et al. Distress among matriculating medical students relative to the general population. *Acad Med.* 2014;89(11):1520-1525.

52. Sen S, Kranzler HR, Krystal JH, et al. A prospective cohort study investigating factors associated with depression during medical internship. *Arch Gen Psychiatry.* 2010;67(6):557-565.

53. Pereira-Lima K, Gupta RR, Guille C, Sen S. Residency program factors associated with depressive symptoms in internal medicine interns: a prospective cohort study. *Acad Med.* 2019;94(6):869-875.

54. Ridout KK, Ridout SJ, Guille C, Mata DA, Akil H, Sen S. Physician-training stress and accelerated cellular aging. *Biol Psych.* 2019;86(9):725-730.

55. Slavin S, Shoss M, Broom MA. A program to prevent burnout, depression, and anxiety in first-year pediatric residents. *Acad Pediatr.* 2017;17(4):456-458.

56. AWARE Well-Being Resources. https://acgme.org/What-We-Do/Initiatives/Physician-Well-Being/AWARE-Well-Being-Resources. Accessed September 17, 2020.

Striving and Thriving: Challenges and Opportunities for Clinician Emotional Wellness

CHAPTER 16

Julie W. Childers, Robert M. Arnold, and Elise C. Carey

■ INTRODUCTION

As clinicians, our work is focused on achieving patients' health. A chapter on clinician wellness may feel extraneous, narcissistic even. Why is maintaining our well-being important? First, there is evidence that clinician well-being affects patient care.[1] Physicians and other healthcare professionals who are experiencing burnout are more likely to report making medical errors,[2] and less likely to be perceived as compassionate and caring by patients and families.[3] Second, clinicians who are burned out are more likely to leave the practice of medicine or reduce the hours that they devote to medicine; similar results have been found for nurses.[4,5] This loss of clinicians is costly for society. For physicians alone, in the United States we spend $15 billion per year to train residents to become practicing physicians.[6] Finally, as community leaders promoting well-being it feels hypocritical to urge our patients to make difficult changes to promote their well-being, if we are unwilling to make the same changes.

In addition, contrary to the historical view of physicians in particular as sacrificing themselves and their families for the sake of patients, in our view we can better promote values of wellness and caring for patients and their families if we manifest the same values toward ourselves and our colleagues. As clinicians ourselves, we recognize that physicians, nurses, and other professionals working in the medical field form a community of individuals that is worthy of care. We care about the physicians, nurses, and other clinicians with whom we work and want to promote their well-being, just as we promote the well-being of patients.

In this chapter, we start by describing the concept of wellness, and how emotions play a part in maintaining, developing, or at times, destroying wellness. We will focus on the special challenges that healthcare providers face that may either detract from or support their well-being. We then describe emotional intelligence and other skills that clinicians need to develop to ensure they can manage the challenges inherent to clinical work.

Two introductory remarks. First, while much of the research focuses on physicians, this chapter includes all professionals who work in clinical settings. Physicians face some challenges that may be unique; however, nurses and other healthcare professionals work in the same clinical environment. For the purposes of this chapter, we will talk about clinician wellness. We acknowledge that as physicians ourselves, we are able to speak from our experiences more truly when writing about the physician experience.

Second, wellness has been traditionally defined by what is not present: distress or disease. *Burnout* is one such phenomenon of unwellness. Other studies assess stress as well as clinical depression and unhealthy coping behaviors such as substance use. More recently, there has been a movement to define wellness in terms of positive qualities: having meaning in life, strong social connections, and integrating work with the rest of life.[5] There are many different definitions of wellness (or well-being, which we use synonymously). The World Health Organization (WHO) defines wellness as "a state of complete physical, mental, and social well-being, and not merely the absence of disease or infirmity."[7] One systematic review of studies of physician wellness gave the following definition:

> Physician wellness (well-being) is defined by quality of life, which includes the absence of ill-being and the presence of positive physical, mental, social, and integrated well-being experienced in connection with activities and environments that allow physicians to develop their full potentials across personal and work-life domains (p. 103).[8]

In our discussion we will use this definition, while applying it more broadly to all clinicians, and also acknowledging that many of the studies measure disease rather than true wellness.

■ THE EMOTIONAL LANDSCAPE OF CLINICAL MEDICINE

Clinicians' life experiences and emotions, outside of their professional lives, are similar to those of any individual. Physicians, nurses, and other health professionals such as ourselves and our colleagues experience grief, joy, anger, and other emotions based on life events such as death, illness, birth, and divorce. Health professionals are also vulnerable to mental health conditions such as depression and anxiety. When events occur in our personal lives, this can increase the emotional valence of issues that arise at work. For example, when caring for a dying patient, a physician whose own parent is dying may feel grief that is out of proportion to what she might feel caring for the same patient under different personal circumstances. Clinicians in these settings may struggle with preserving boundaries between their work and personal life.

Even without those personal factors, clinical experience can bring up emotional responses in professionals. Emotions we experience as clinicians include sadness when a patient dies, and anger toward patients with whom we are experiencing conflict. We may also experience emotions in our workplace that are not related to patients: for example, frustration or anxiety when the amount of work expected of us exceeds our capacity. Many clinicians also describe positive emotions at work, including a sense of meaning, connection, and gratitude.

Emotions at work are not necessarily a drawback. Having an emotional response points to our values, and shows that we care about our patients and our work. In addition, research shows that emotions are crucial to cognitive processing, and may aid us in making clinical decisions (as discussed further in Chapter 13, Emotion and Decision Making in the Clinical Encounter). However, the culture and professional norms of medicine may make it more difficult to acknowledge and express emotions. Studies of medical training have found a marked decline in empathy over the course of medical school.[9,10] A "hidden curriculum" in medical education drives the formation of professional identity and norms, and may include a prohibition against the acknowledgment or expression of emotions in professional settings.[11,12] Medical training focuses on learning facts and clinical reasoning, and may disregard the role of emotions in health, both in patients and in ourselves. Physicians, in particular, are trained to be highly cognitive in their approach to their work, and may suffer a kind of professional alexithymia—an inability to see or name their own emotions. This suboptimal ability to acknowledge emotions may decrease the resources that medical professionals have to manage their emotional reactions to difficult situations at work.

Clinicians, thus, enter into their work with a normal range of human emotions, are frequently exposed to suffering and death in the patients for whom they care, and operate in a high-stress environment. At the same time, their training may not have included education that helps them recognize and manage their emotions. Later in this section, we use clinical vignettes to elicit your reflection on emotion in medicine, and describe some of the unique emotional challenges which clinical medicine can present. Our hope is that after learning more about the evidence for an emotional side to our clinical lives, you will be better prepared to reflect upon and respond to your own emotions as part of your work.

Threats to Clinician Wellness

A lack of training in identifying our own emotions and responding to them, combined with our work environment, constitute threats to clinician wellness. Measurable identifiers of clinician unwellness that have been studied include rates of mental illnesses such as depression, rates of suicide and suicide attempts, and the prevalence of substance use.

Mental health issues such as depression in medical professionals and trainees are at least as common as in the general population. For example, in medicine, students beginning medical school have been found to have rates of major depression similar to others in the same age group, but by their later years of training, up to one-third of medical students have experienced clinical depression.[13,14] Medical residents have been found to have an average prevalence of depression of 28.8%,[15] while the lifetime prevalence of depression in male physicians is 12% and 19.5% in female physicians.[13,16] Studies of nurses have found that rates of depression similarly are at least as high as the general population, if not higher.[17]

Physicians, particularly female physicians, are more likely to complete suicide than nonhealthcare professionals. In 2004, Schernhammer analyzed 25 studies of physician suicide and found that male physicians were about 40% more likely to complete suicide than male nonphysicians, while female physicians were more than twice as likely as their nonphysician counterparts to complete suicide.[18] A later meta-analysis replicated these findings and again showed that female physicians had a higher rate of suicide than male physicians.[19] Other health professions may also face elevated suicide risk. For example, one analysis of data in the nursing profession found that female nurses were significantly more likely to complete suicide than female non-nurses, and male nurses slightly more likely to complete suicide.[20] Other health professionals, such as veterinarians, are also at high risk.[21]

Why the gender gap? No clear answers exist, but we can speculate that part of the reason may be due to the increased stresses on female healthcare professionals, as detailed later in this chapter. In addition, in the general population, women are more likely to be diagnosed with depression and to attempt suicide than men. However, women who are not health professionals tend to choose less lethal means than men. Perhaps greater access to prescription drugs and more knowledge of what is likely to be lethal contribute to a greater likelihood of "successful" suicide attempts in female healthcare professionals. Suicide in both nurses and physicians correlates with both untreated mental health issues and the degree of job stress.[22]

Closely tied to the issue of mental health disorders is the use of substances. Substance use by clinicians is a maladaptive strategy for coping with work stress. Alcohol is the most common substance used by health professionals. In one large survey of U.S. physicians, 12.9% of male physicians and 21.4% of female physicians met diagnostic criteria for an alcohol use disorder.[23] Higher rates of substance use have been found within certain specialties, including anesthesiology, emergency medicine, and psychiatry.[24,25] The rates of substance use disorders among nurses have been described as similar to the general population; however, as with physicians, certain populations of nurses, such as nurse anesthetists, are noted to be at higher risk.[26,27]

While the rates of clinician mental illness are similar to the general population, they face more barriers to treatment. For example, whether due to lack of time or to failure to prioritize their own personal health, about one-third of physicians do not have a primary care physician, which may limit their access to routine healthcare.[28] In addition, physicians often cite concern for professional licensing and the ability to continue in their field as barriers to seeking treatment for any mental health or substance use concern. Some states ask about mental health conditions as part of licensing application, though there is an increasing move to ask only about impairment of job performance rather than the presence of a condition.[29]

System factors often also contribute to emotional challenges for clinicians. With changes in the healthcare landscape over the past 30 years, clinicians experience pressure to provide more patient care in less time. They often function in an environment that places more emphasis on documentation and billing than on connecting with patients. Physicians describe spending several hours a day calling insurance companies to obtain authorization for medications, tests, and procedures, and often take their work home with them, completing chart notes in the evening.[30] Nurses are often assigned more patients to care for than is optimal, with decreased time for breaks. All of these factors may cause frustration, stress, and a loss of meaning, which may contribute to negative coping with substances and mental health issues in clinicians.

Stress, burnout, and mental health issues are some of the consequences that can occur when clinicians' well-being is threatened. However, the presence of emotion is normal for all human beings, including physicians, nurses, and other healthcare professionals. Healthcare professionals face situations which at times are more extreme than what nonclinicians experience in their daily lives: intense trauma, death, birth, and conflict. Below we describe unique aspects of working in healthcare that give rise to emotions in clinicians. While we focus for most of this section on negative emotion, we also describe some positive emotions that are engendered by our work. We start with a case.

> ### Vignette 1, part 1
>
> Tom is a registered nurse in a busy medical ICU. He is caring for Dana, a 20-year-old woman with spinal meningitis, Gary, an 80-year-old patient with advanced cancer who is suffering from sepsis, and multisystem organ failure, and Rick, a 52-year-old man with liver failure related to alcohol. During one of Tom's weeks at work, Dana becomes acutely worse and suffers what the doctors believe to be severe brain damage from the progression of her meningitis. Tom participates in the family meeting in which her parents and 13-year-old sister are given the news. Dana dies the next day, and Tom comforts her family at the bedside while supporting Dana through the dying process. Gary has worsening kidney failure, and cannot be weaned from the ventilator. Tom feels that Gary is suffering, but the oncologist who has been discussing further chemotherapy is reluctant to have anyone address the family's end-of-life concerns. And Rick's estranged wife has come to the ICU and is now assuming the responsibility for decisions regarding his care. She is frequently asking the medical team to make changes in the medications they are using to treat him, based on things she has read on the Internet. Their adult children, meanwhile, are also there, and frequently get into loud arguments with their mother about long-standing family issues and with her approach to his care.
>
> Questions for reflection:
>
> - How might each of these clinical situations—a young woman dying unexpectedly, feeling powerless to help an elderly, dying man, and dealing with family conflict—affect Tom differently?
>
> - What are some positive things Tom could do on his own to respond to these challenges at work?
>
> - What are some resources a nurse such as Tom might be able to call upon in a difficult week such as this?

    Clinicians' lives at work are different than those of many lay people in several ways. For those in healthcare, death and serious illness can become a part of their everyday life. An average person may encounter death once or twice per year; many medical professionals, particularly those who work in fields such as geriatrics, oncology, critical care, or palliative care, may experience a death on a weekly or even more frequent basis. Additionally, the clinical environment usually lacks rituals to acknowledge death. When there is a loss due to death in the family or community, having a funeral and acknowledgment of the loss helps people to grieve. Such rituals are lacking in the medical setting for professionals who experience loss of their patients. In the vignette above, Tom experiences the death of a young patient, someone who in the normal order of things should not die, and her death is fairly sudden. He comforts the parents and her sister during a time of unimaginable loss. Tom may then go home from work still thinking about Dana and her family.

Of course, daily experience of intense grief at the loss of any patient would make one's job as a healthcare professional unsustainable. Studies show that grief and other emotional responses are more likely in certain situations. First, when healthcare providers are earlier in their career, they are likely to be emotionally affected by death.[31,32] Connections to the patient, perhaps based in shared characteristics, such as age, gender, or background, or having a long-standing relationship over time, often lead to a more intense emotional reaction upon patient death.[33] Finally, an unexpected death, such as one without a clear medical explanation, or caused by violence such as suicide, often leads to more intense emotion. For example, oncology nurses who cared regularly for seriously ill patients reported heightened emotional reactions when a patient declined rapidly or when death was unexpected.[34]

Patient care may evoke other types of negative emotions in us. Every experienced clinician has interacted with a patient who is perceived as "difficult" or "unreasonable." In 1978, Dr. Groves' article described "the hateful patient," stating that "a few patients kindle aversion, fear, despair, or even downright malice in their doctors" (p. 883).[35] He describes patient behavior that can evoke this reaction in their providers: those who are excessively needy ("clingers"); those who are "entitled," demanding certain tests, procedures, or medications and threatening their providers if they do not get them; those who repeatedly complain but reject solutions and help; patients who engage in self-destructive behavior such as uncontrolled addiction that repeatedly causes hospitalization. The patient's family members are often included among these conflictual reactions. In the vignette above, Tom may be experiencing an emotional reaction to Rick's wife, including frustration and anger.

The literature describes a "heartsink patient," one who evokes "an overwhelming mixture of exasperation, defeat, and sometimes plain dislike" when we see them on our schedule for the day.[36] These patients are often those who are labeled "frequent flyers," with repeated hospital admissions, or "high utilizers," who repeatedly present to their doctors' offices with symptoms that may be medically unexplained. In recent years, patients with chronic pain, substance use disorder, or anxiety, who have both difficult-to-treat symptoms and may request prescriptions for opioids, benzodiazepines, or other controlled substances, often evoke similar feelings. The first step in providing good care for patients who evoke dislike or dread in us as clinicians is acknowledging these feelings. If Tom recognizes the emotions he is experiencing when interacting with his patient's family member, he may be able to find ways to deal with his emotions and not let them interfere with his care of the patient.

While interactions with patients and their families can cause conflict, other types of conflict are also common in the medical setting. Clinicians function as members of a team of professionals and may not agree with the decisions of other team members, or with patients or family members. This can give rise to *moral distress*, a concept first described in the nursing literature but common to many domains of medicine.[37] When a clinician perceives that there is a moral dilemma or wrong in the care being provided, and they lack power to resolve this conflict, they may feel moral distress.[38,39] Moral distress often includes a mix of emotions, including frustration, anger, and sadness. Tom may be experiencing moral distress in the above vignette: he perceives that Gary is likely to die soon and is suffering in the ICU, but he feels powerless to bring up end-of-life issues when the oncologist is still offering chemotherapy. The literature describes a variety of styles of conflict management, including some that may be less healthy for individuals and organizations, such as avoiding and obliging.[40,41] The choice of which conflict management style an individual uses is related to a variety of factors, including personality, experience of conflict in family of origin, age, rank, profession, gender, and organizational culture. If Tom is unable to manage interpersonal conflict in a constructive way, it may affect his emotional wellness.

Many, if not all, clinicians experience trauma related to their work. The U.S. Substance Abuse and Mental Health Administration defines trauma as "an event, series of events, or set of circumstances that is experienced by an individual as physically or emotionally harmful or life threatening and that has lasting adverse effects on the individual's functioning and mental, physical, social, emotional, or spiritual well-being." As clinicians, we care for patients who are traumatized, when they are confined to a hospital for prolonged periods, having uncontrolled symptoms, and experiencing the loss of former roles, among other things. Individuals who experience trauma are vulnerable to posttraumatic stress disorder (PTSD). PTSD is defined as greater than 1 month of symptoms of avoidance, hypervigilance, and impaired functioning or significant distress after experiencing a traumatic event.[42] Nurses have been described as experiencing *secondary posttraumatic stress* or secondary PTSD, when, over time, they have felt emotional attachment and empathy toward patients who have experienced trauma. Symptoms of secondary posttraumatic stress may be similar to PTSD itself, including intrusive thoughts about patients, sense of a foreshortened future, and irritability.[43] One study of oncology clinicians, primarily nurses, found that 38% of them met criteria for secondary posttraumatic stress.[43] Nurses working in the emergency department also reported high levels of symptoms of posttraumatic stress.[44]

System factors both contribute to and intensify clinicians' emotional challenges, including time pressures as described above. Larger scale issues such as pandemics or other disasters that overload the healthcare system also add to difficulty coping and mental health consequences for clinicians.[45] Recently, COVID has intensified the workload while also raising clinicians' fears regarding their health and the possibility they may infect their family. Healthcare professionals have also been exposed to increased patient and family suffering, as hospitalized patients have died in isolation due to pandemic visiting restrictions.[46]

A high level of secondary trauma at work, along with system factors such as time pressure and inadequate resources to meet the needs of patients, is thought to be contributors to *compassion fatigue*, which was first described in the nursing literature in the 1990s. Coetzee and Laschinger define compassion fatigue as "disengagement of caregivers from their patients, which culminates in a reduction or inability to feel empathy and compassion toward patients and an inability to provide the patient care that is deemed appropriate" (p. 4).[47] One study of compassion fatigue in nurses found a rate of 52%.[48] Of course, compassion fatigue is an element of the phenomenon of burnout. One of the three elements of burnout is depersonalization, where healthcare providers feel cynical and emotionally detached from their patients. In the same study, about half of the nurses included also experienced burnout.[48]

We explore some other clinician experiences in Vignette #2:

Vignette 2, part 1

Dr. R is a 40-year-old surgical oncologist. She enjoys her work, which includes both operating and teaching medical students and residents. She finds it satisfying to complete an operation and see a patient through the post-operative period with their cancer effectively cured or controlled. However, there are cases with which she struggles Like her fellow surgeons, she feels a strong bond with her patients, and a responsibility to them. For example, she recently operated on Ms. J, a 35-year-old woman with an aggressive form of colon cancer. During the surgery, the patient was found to have metastatic disease throughout her abdomen. Postoperatively, the patient did not do well, and 30 days later she remained in the ICU after suffering from respiratory and renal failure. The nurses and the critical care team were urging discussions about end of life, but Dr. R found herself avoiding the patient's room; when she thought about Ms. J, she repeatedly wondered what she did wrong. In addition, as the only female surgeon within her practice group, she felt like she had something to prove in terms of her capabilities.

Questions for reflection:

- What factors in this situation could be contributing to emotional distress for Dr. R?

- What are some wellness strategies which Dr. R could practice which might help her manage her reaction to this case?

- What are some external resources that Dr. R might access?

There are a number of factors that may cause emotional reactions to Ms. J's case for Dr. R. First, Dr. R shares some commonalities with her patient, who also is female and not too far apart in age from Dr. R. Studies show that our emotional reactions to patient suffering and death may be stronger when there is a reason for us to identify with the patient. Grief is also intensified when patients die young or unexpectedly. In this case, Dr. R might have been expecting to cure her patient's disease, and the finding of metastatic disease now means that a cure is not possible. Ms. J also suffered a number of adverse events after her surgery, including infections and respiratory failure. While these events may not have been preventable, Dr. R feels responsible, and repeatedly reviews the case in her mind, wondering if there is anything she might have done differently. Below we describe some common issues in clinical care, some of which may be affecting Dr. R, including medical errors and adverse events, emotional labor, and minority stress.

Adverse Events and Medical Errors

Both adverse events and medical errors are common, and often cause emotional distress for healthcare providers. Adverse events are those in which patients experience harm as a result of medical or surgical interventions. Some of these consequences are expected to occur in a small number of patients, even with the best care. For example, a small percentage of hospitalized patients will suffer from a deep venous thrombosis (DVT), even if prophylaxis is carried out perfectly. Medical errors are involuntary deviations from the standard of care; a medical error may or may not cause harm to the patient or even be noticed. If a patient was not appropriately prescribed DVT prophylaxis and suffered a DVT, that would be a medical error that resulted in an adverse event.

Medical errors and adverse events can also cause emotional harm to healthcare providers, who have been described in the literature as "second victims."[49] Physicians and other clinicians tend to have high standards for themselves, and often take on excessive blame for adverse events, experiencing guilt, shame, anxiety, depression, and even suicidality. One study of 265 physicians and nurses in the United Kingdom and the United States found that clinicians experienced a range of emotions in response to a medical error, with nurses reporting more intense negative emotions, including being upset, worried, distressed, scared, or nervous. The study also suggested that medical errors can result in more positive and neutral reactions, such as feeling more alert, determined, and attentive, when reflection on an error allowed clinicians to make changes in their practice. Interestingly, the degree of patient harm was not correlated with the extent of the emotional response in this study.[50,51] Clinicians whose patients have experienced a medical error or adverse event that has caused harm might benefit from employing some specific wellness strategies, such as debriefing with supportive colleagues and reflecting on what they have learned from the event.

Emotional Labor

Physicians, nurses, and other clinicians encounter patient emotion regularly, from sadness to anger to anxiety. At times, as with giving bad news, medical professionals even are the instigators of emotion. Recommendations and training have taught clinicians how to respond to these patient emotions with expressions of empathy, such as naming or exploring the patient's emotional reaction rather than providing facts or seeking to distance from them. However, this requires us to open ourselves to patient emotion and perhaps echo it with our own. This task of clinicians is a kind of *emotional labor*, which is defined as the "process of regulating experienced and displayed emotions to present a professionally desired image during interpersonal transactions at work" (p. 1103).[52] Skilled clinicians engage actively with patient emotions to respond empathically, not necessarily with their own personal emotion, but they may reflect and explore the emotion that they encounter. Larson differentiates between "surface acting," in which the clinician is faking the appearance of emotional congruence with the patient, versus "deep acting," in which the professional actually alters their own internal experience to match the encounter.[52] This deeper effort toward emotional congruence may be more reflective of genuine empathy. Regardless of the level at which we mirror the emotions that patients or families are experiencing, the practice of repeatedly engaging with the emotion of others may affect our own emotional state. We may find ourselves actually experiencing the emotions of others—or, perhaps, we will become numb from feeling our own emotions at all when we must engage with emotion so actively as part of our work life.[53] It takes practice to be able to genuinely connect with patients' suffering and be able to take a break from it at the end of the day. Practices such as mindfulness, as well as healthy habits such as exercise and maintaining close personal relationships, may help. Even simply cognitively reminding oneself that these emotions are not yours to own or imagining them passing through you as you leave the room may help a clinician not carry others' pain and suffering.[54]

Specific Challenges

Specific groups within medicine face unique challenges. This may be related to discipline or area of clinical practice. For example, surgery is one subculture within medicine with values that are distinct. Elements within surgical training value independence, strength, technical skill, perseverance, and pride in success. Surgeons have a strong sense of responsibility for patients on whom they are operating, seeing it as their job to get them through the postoperative period, and they may be highly self-critical if they are not successful. Studies of surgeons' emotional responses to adverse patient outcomes show a variety of negative emotions, including anger, frustration, and guilt—at times culminating in posttraumatic stress, burnout, or clinical depression.[55] Few surgeons access formal counseling services after adverse patient outcomes—and institutional support for emotional exploration of surgeons' responses to these events is often minimal.[55,56] Changing this culture will require senior physicians and surgeons to promote wellness in their colleagues and role model healthy coping by being transparent about their own emotional struggles. Additionally, institutions must create more programs to support healthcare professionals who have experienced adverse events—some of which have already begun.[57]

Nonphysicians, such as nurses, face different challenges. Nurses typically have less control over the medical or surgical decisions that are made for their patients—leading to a higher propensity for moral distress, frustration, and anger. At the same time, in a hospital setting, it is the nurse who is at the patient's bedside for an entire shift and bears the brunt of any patient–provider or patient–family conflict. Nurses typically also have less autonomy than their physician colleagues, and nurses are subject to greater physical demands in meeting patient care needs.

Beyond specialty or domain of practice, other aspects of our identities influence our experience of our work. Individuals who are underrepresented in the medical field face unique challenges. This includes women in fields in medicine in which they are underrepresented within medicine (such as Dr. R in surgery), and African Americans and other people of color within clinical practice. In U.S. medical schools, only 24% of full professors are female, while only 3% of medical school faculty are African American.[58] Challenges that members of these groups may face include being steered toward certain specialties, and, when they enter into clinical or academic practice, they may feel an added degree of burden that their skills as a physician represent their entire group.

A study of first-year medical students found that African-American students had less social support, less confidence in their intellectual abilities, and a higher incidence of depression and anxiety than their white peers. Students from these groups, as well as female students in some academic contexts, face *stereotype threat*—the fear that they will confirm a negative stereotype, which in turn impairs performance.[59,60]

Women in medicine often face different challenges than those encountered by their male colleagues. Even in two career households, in heterosexual couples, the female partner typically takes on the lion's share of childcare and household management.[61,62] Women in medicine are more likely to opt to work part time after a couple has children, and women are more likely tasked with responsibilities such as staying home from work to care for a sick child. Female physicians in particular describe working in an environment that is not family-friendly, when they are expected to balance 12-hour days or 80-hour work weeks with home responsibilities. This contributes to the stress and burnout of females working in the medical profession.[62–64]

Research on lesbian, gay, bisexual, transgender, and other gender/sexual minority groups within clinicians is just beginning. Limited studies suggest that these individuals experience significant discrimination in the workplace related to their orientation or identity, both from colleagues and patients, including being denied jobs, tenure, or promotions, as well as witnessing discrimination or derogatory language toward LGBTQ+ patients.[65] LGBTQ+ individuals also face the stress and uncertainty of whether to reveal their orientation or identity to both patients and colleagues. In one study, most individuals reported positive coping strategies such as advocacy and education of their colleagues, but some reported depression or burnout as a consequence of workplace stress related to their sexual orientation or gender identity.[66]

In general, experiencing overt prejudice is more common in caring for patients than in interacting with colleagues—for example, as when a clinician not from the United States hears patients ask for an "American doctor." Even more common are *microaggressions*, which have been defined as "indirect expressions of prejudice that contribute to the maintenance of existing power structures."[58] Microaggressions are small actions or statements that show unconscious prejudice or implicit bias. Some examples of microaggressions in the U.S. medical setting are as follows:

- A female physician who is addressed as "nurse" despite introducing herself as "doctor."
- An African American nurse is assumed by the patient's family member to be with the housekeeping department when she enters a patient's room at the beginning of her shift.
- A Latina medical resident whose attending physician comments to her: "Wow, you speak really good English."
- An Asian American physical therapist is evaluating a patient who asks her, "Where are you from?" and when she replies "New Jersey," he asks: "No, where are you *really* from?"
- A pharmacist who has a spouse of the same sex; however, when colleagues notice his wedding ring, they commonly ask him about his wife.

Those who enact microaggressions generally do not intend harm. Rather, they are expressions contributed by unconscious bias. However, both overt prejudice and the repeated exposure to microaggressions have been shown to engender stress and other negative emotional responses, even impacting the mental health, of those toward whom they are directed.[67]

■ POSITIVE EMOTIONS IN CLINICAL MEDICINE

Of course, working in healthcare is also rewarding, and contributes positively toward our emotional lives and level of happiness. Many of us choose our work because we find meaning in helping others, and doing so gives us a sense of satisfaction and purpose. We thrive on connections with patients and their families, and those relationships may sustain us through difficulties in our practice.[68] Positive emotions engendered by patient care can include affection and caring for our patients, and the joy we experience when we feel we have made a positive contribution to patients' lives or health. Studies of medical professionals who care for patients near the end of their lives have found that they frequently experience joy in their work and a sense of hope.[69-71] The experience of caring for dying patients encourages us to reflect on the important things in our lives, and leads us to feel gratitude for the life we have. Dying, when individuals are able to achieve closure and say important things to their family, can be a life-affirming and spiritual experience.[33,69]

Clinicians also have the opportunity to share other positive moments with patients and their families. These include those who work in obstetrics, helping to bring new life into the world, and clinicians who rehabilitate patients from injury and illness and can see improvement and return of function. Family medicine clinicians often comment on the fulfillment they get caring for children as they grow up and have their own children. Clinicians in these and other domains of medicine experience deep satisfaction and meaning in their work, contributing to their overall sense of meaning and joy.

Connection to others contributes to positive emotions in medical professionals. Studies show that the number of connections individuals have impacts their satisfaction with life, their mental health and emotional state, and even their physical health.[72,73] In primary care, especially in small towns and rural communities, healthcare professionals are privileged to have long-term relationships with families and communities, often caring for several generations.

These clinicians may have especially deep relationships with members of their community who are also their patients.

Clinicians experience this connection not only with their patients, but also with the interdisciplinary teams with whom they work in hospitals or other settings. Working as a functioning team toward a common goal gives us a sense of purpose—and, even beyond patient care, our work families may become important communities in our lives, celebrating major life events together. For many of us, our work relationships provide a sense of belonging, being known and cared for as well as caring for others, and many of us find it difficult to leave these work communities upon retirement.

In addition, our status as healthcare professionals gives us societal advantages that affect our well-being. Whatever our healthcare profession, we have spent years getting an education, and our income is higher than the average American who does not work in healthcare. We also have a degree of job security that is unusual in the United States—there are few unemployed doctors or nurses. Job satisfaction is also highly correlated to the degree of autonomy we have in our work—the ability to choose what we will focus on at any specific time, and our hours. Some healthcare professionals, particularly physicians, may enjoy a high degree of autonomy in their work life. Finally, working as a healthcare provider, we enjoy a high degree of status in society. Most people with whom we interact view our job as important and meaningful, and in fact may turn to us for advice about their own or a family member's medical problems. All of these factors generate positive emotions in many of us, including pride, a sense of purpose and meaning, and general satisfaction.

Our work in healthcare also gives us opportunities for inner growth and learning. We start as students, and then become apprentices—finally we complete training and become clinicians, though our learning is not done, as our clinical skills improve constantly as we grow in experience. We take advantage of continuing education to improve our clinical knowledge and skills and may enter further degree programs. As we advance in our careers, we may grow into roles: we may become a manager, and then a leader; we may develop our abilities in research, and then mentor others in research; we may become an educator, and eventually develop new curricula. We may do all three. Our profession continues to offer the ability to learn and grow. For many of us, learning and improving provide inner rewards, including rekindling excitement and passion for our work.

> **Exercise**
>
> Below we list common emotional experiences that clinicians can have related to their work. Try to recollect which ones you have experienced yourself so far in your clinical work, and those which you have seen in colleagues or clinical supervisors.
>
> Joy
> Grief
> Anger
> Gratitude
> Connectedness/belonging
> Pride
> A sense of meaning
> Guilt
> Worry

All of these emotions are a normal part of our lives, and, for the authors, all of these have manifested at work for us. As we will see in the next section, identifying our emotions, responding to them skillfully, and allowing them to exist peacefully within us as an intrinsic part of who we are helps us be more effective clinicians. The following exercises will help you begin this journey:

> **Exercise**
>
> 1. Pick an emotion from the list above, or another one that you feel is relevant, that you have experienced yourself related to your clinical work.
>   a. What was the situation that led to the emotion?
>   b. How did you respond to the experience of having that emotion?
>   c. Looking back, what might you want to do next time you have that emotional reaction?
> 2. Think of a colleague or clinical supervisor who is a role model for you. If you can remember a time when you observed that person having an emotional reaction, ask yourself the following questions. (If you cannot remember observing this, move on to exercise #3.)
>   a. What was the situation that led to the emotion?
>   b. How did they respond to the experience of having that emotion?
>   c. What can you learn from your role model's response?
> 3. Find a colleague or clinical supervisor with whom you feel comfortable, and ask them if they can recall a time when they experienced a strong emotion at work, and ask them the questions above.

■ CULTIVATING WELLNESS IN WORK AND IN LIFE

Clinicians are not simply people who provide care. Clinicians themselves are an instrument in the care they provide, and, like any other instrument, they need to stay calibrated. Thus, striving for well-being for clinicians is not simply a nicety or ancillary pursuit; it is a professional responsibility. As we have seen so far in this chapter, our emotional responses are an inextricable part of our work life, and both difficult and positive emotions contribute to our wellness. In the remainder of this chapter we describe strategies for improving our wellness as clinicians. Some of these strategies involve the direct cultivation of emotional regulation, while others indirectly cultivate the space and prepare the ground for an improved emotional life.

In this section, we focus on individual factors one can modulate and skills one can develop to increase one's well-being and foster emotional endurance. In emphasizing personal skills, we do not mean to imply that wellness is solely your responsibility. Quite the contrary, organizational structures and leadership choices are critical to creating and sustaining a high-functioning work environment that allows individuals to stay engaged, successfully integrate their work and life, and succeed both professionally and personally. Systems issues such as the nurse-to-patient ratio or the choice of electronic health record have a large impact on clinicians' wellness. Indeed, our greatest sources of conflict occur when individual beliefs collide with systems and team issues and cause personal distress. (For example, consider a physician who feels her care is suboptimal because of external system constraints.) Excellent resources are available for those who are interested in working toward organizational change to promote wellness.[74]

We have focused on the skills and tools that clinicians can use to promote their own well-being because all change starts with individuals. Indeed, research extending from neuroscience to positive psychology teaches us that our worldview, including where we choose to focus our attention and energy and how we interpret our world,[1,75–77] not only influences our happiness but also determines it. As such, we will start by looking at workplace factors that are known to influence one's ability to thrive in a given workplace and then use the bulk of the discussion to describe a robust set of tools individual clinicians can use to cultivate and sustain emotional hardiness.

Workplace Attributes Associated with Wellness

Engagement has been described as the "positive antithesis to burnout" and is "characterized by vigor, dedication, and absorption in work."[74] At a systems level, increasing productivity requirements, excessive workload, time pressures, inefficient practice models, loss of control over aspects of work, and clerical and documentation burden all contribute to burnout. Conversely, studies of physicians have demonstrated that physicians are more likely to be engaged and less likely to be burned out when their leaders actively include them in problem solving for the betterment of the practice, inform them of changes and updates, have career development conversations with them to promote career growth, and recognize them for a job well done.[74,78,79] When one considers that independent thinking, proactive problem solving, and even a healthy skepticism are characteristics deliberately honed through years of physician training and practice, this should come as no surprise. Indeed, all employees wish to be known and valued for their unique contributions and skills and thus are most satisfied with leaders who deliberately work to harness their strengths.[80]

The question is: how can you be more engaged in your work, regardless of the environment? While there are no data, these two simple behaviors may help. First, you can let others know that you see and appreciate them. By praising your colleagues and appreciating their work, you are building a more pleasant work environment. The data suggest that your colleagues, feeling supported, will be more likely to support you. Second, even small behaviors have large impacts. Thus, while you may not be able to control how your hospital or clinic sets policy, you can change the way your team works. You can ensure that your team is informed of changes and updates and work to involve everyone in decision making about the tasks under your control.

■ DEVELOPING SKILLS TO FOSTER WELLNESS AND EMOTIONAL HARDINESS

Staying healthy, building resilience, and creating an adaptive reserve require careful attention to self-care. Moreover, this repertoire requires self-awareness and capacity for growth. We must not only be aware of our own emotions, we must also be open to them and be able to respond to them skillfully, recognizing that, with insight, they can serve as a compass pointing to what we value. Below, we describe a range of personal skills that individual clinicians can use to foster wellness and engagement, highlighting several of the most well-studied and impactful tools from the medical, psychological, and business literature. These tools are variously demonstrated to promote resiliency, increase self-awareness and emotional intelligence, expand one's capacity for empathy, and more—all of which we consider to be fundamental building blocks of emotional hardiness.

Wellness Essentials: Clinician Heal Thyself

At a bare minimum, self-care requires eating well, exercising, getting sufficient rest, and attending to one's own medical needs. This includes going to the doctor and the dentist, taking prescribed medication, following through with recommended preventative care measures, and staying home to recover when ill. Optimal self-care also includes basic (but still challenging!) daily wellness endeavors, such as meeting minimal standards for exercise (150 minutes of moderate-intensity aerobic activity per week plus strength training twice weekly)[81] and sleep (at least 7 hours per day).[82] Of course, all of this is easier said than done for clinicians with demanding work and personal lives and what often seems like infinite competing imperatives and an ever-growing list of unachievable tasks. Clinicians, particularly physicians, avoid seeking routine medical care[83] and may not feel they are able to meet recommended sleep[84-86] and exercise[87,88] guidelines. Not only that, many of us specifically neglect these activities when we are stressed and need them the most. (There is abundant literature on how difficult it is to make lifestyle changes—and the challenges we face motivating patients to make these changes apply to clinician–patients as well!)

For many clinicians, maintaining emotional wellness also includes seeking professional counseling and, for those with mental health conditions such as depression or anxiety, may also include taking prescribed medications such as antidepressants. For clinicians for whom mental health or substance use interferes with their work, physician and nurse health programs provide a structured program of recovery and supervision for clinicians who are impaired. These programs are confidential resources for licensed healthcare professionals and are available in nearly every state.[89] Those who seek help have a good prognosis for recovery and return to work.[90]

Integrating one's personal and professional life is another essential, as it allows one's skills, lessons learned, and even relationships to transfer across life domains. Work–life integration rejects the notion that "work" and "life" must compete with one another or be "balanced." Instead, work–life integration recognizes that "life" occurs at the very point at which the various domains of our life (e.g., work, home, community, and self) overlap and interact.[91] Because they are integral to one another, they cannot be "balanced" but must be accepted as parts of a whole. Yet working toward work–life integration is a challenge unto itself, so how do we do it? Friedman suggests that we harness the skills and strengths we have in different parts of our lives (the four major life domains listed above) and turn them into "four-way wins," which he defines as "actions that result in life being better in all four domains."[91] To give a concrete example of a "four-way win," several years ago, one of us (ECC) learned to bring the coaching skills she uses while teaching to help a preadolescent family member who had been newly diagnosed with attention deficit disorder and was consequently struggling with confidence and schoolwork. To do this, she used specific teaching skills, including helping him identify what he did well and where he was succeeding first before moving onto problem-solving. Subsequently, she encouraged him to identify one incremental step to work on at a time. In this way, he was able to shift toward a positive, action-oriented, and stepwise approach to improvement, instead of being overwhelmed by negativity and the seeming vastness of the problem. Bringing these work skills to her personal life not only helped her family member gain confidence and skills to achieve academic success, but it also strengthened the adult–teen relationship under circumstances that commonly lead to rifts. She subsequently helped friends facing similar challenges support their own struggling loved ones, enhancing friendships and community relationships.

Other essentials include finding meaning in one's work and cultivating personal relationships, as well as investing in activities that train attention and mindfulness, enhance self-awareness, and build resilience, each of which promotes engagement and reduces burnout.[92] Taken together, these habits of wellness help clinicians to be more responsive to patients, team members, and colleagues and to function more effectively in their personal lives.

Finding Meaning in Work

Work is integrally linked to our dignity and our sense of being valued and contributing positively to the world. Participating in work that one finds meaningful has been found to improve satisfaction and protect against burnout. And, it takes less than one might think—Shanafelt and colleagues identified that physicians who spent at least 20% of their professional effort focused on aspects of work they find most meaningful were significantly less likely to be burned out.[93] Having happy, engaged clinicians is better for patients and organizations too: Research has found that doctors who were put in a positive state prior to making a diagnosis demonstrated more intelligence and creativity than doctors in a neutral state and made accurate diagnoses 19% faster.[94,95]

Clinicians are fortunate: most find their work, which centers on helping others, inherently meaningful. Yet we would be hard-pressed to find any clinicians who had not faced exhaustion or a sense of being overwhelmed at work at some point in their careers. So, what can we do when that sense of inherent meaning has paled or been misplaced? The good news is that, for all comers, finding meaning in one's work is a multidimensional construct, such that meaning and purpose can be cultivated regardless of the nature of the work itself. Indeed, work can be experienced as meaningful whenever one is positively contributing to the lives of others; able to learn, grow, and develop; recognized for a job well done; accomplishing something of value; or building community and relationships.[96,97] Still, we have found that this search for meaning requires intentional focus. For example, when one of us (RMA) is having a bad day, he looks for visitors in the hospitals who are having trouble finding their way. Spending two minutes giving them directions gives him a sense of satisfaction and often praise.

Fostering Self-Awareness and Capacity for Growth

Self-awareness, empathy for others, and capacity for growth are key components of Emotional Intelligence (EI), a concept that has been defined as "the capacity for recognizing our own feelings and those of others, for motivating ourselves, and for managing emotions well in ourselves and in our relationships"[98] in order that we may "pilot through the emotional undercurrents always at play rather than being pulled under by them."[98] EI is associated with abundant positive outcomes, including improved job satisfaction as well as stronger performance, leadership ability, and relationships.[98,99] Among clinicians, higher EI is associated with stronger relationships with patients,[100] higher patient satisfaction,[100] and improved health outcomes,[101] as well as with higher job satisfaction, improved stress management, and reduced anxiety and burnout.[102] EI is a necessary pillar of wellness and resilience—without it, the roof may just collapse.

Importantly, EI is a capacity that we can grow and develop over time, through personal efforts at self-improvement, deliberate practice and reflection, coaching, and lived experiences. Goleman has defined five characteristics of EI at work[103]:

- *Self-awareness*: the ability to recognize and understand one's own emotions and moods and their effect on others
- *Self-regulation*: the will and ability to control or redirect disruptive thoughts, moods, and inclinations
- *Motivation*: the wherewithal to pursue goals with passion, energy, and persistence
- *Empathy*: the capacity to understand other people's feelings and respond to them productively
- *Social skill*: facility with creating and sustaining relationships

The first three, self-awareness, self-regulation, and motivation, encompass skills such as emotional self-awareness and self-control, accurate self-assessment, adaptability, stress management, perseverance, and task completion. The latter two, empathy and social skill, include things like relationship management, social awareness, teamwork, collaboration, and conflict resolution.[98,103]

There are myriad tools that are helpful in developing the component skills of EI. Critical self-reflection and mindfulness, discussed in detail below, help nurture self-awareness. Self-management skills can be fostered through tools that aid in accurate self-assessment and allow individuals to develop insight into the impact of their behavior on others, such as peer and colleague feedback. Self-management is also bolstered by behavior management tools, such as techniques that aid in relaxation and the management of stress, anxiety, and even anger. Social awareness and relationship management can be strengthened through expanding one's capacity for empathy and cultural humility and by improving active listening and communication skills.

You may recall Tom's story from earlier in the chapter. Here is the second part of it:

Vignette 1, part 2: Tom, RN

Tom is an ICU nurse who cared for a 20-year-old patient who died of meningitis (Dana), an older adult with advanced cancer who was suffering from multisystem organ failure (Gary), a man dying of liver failure (Rick), whose family members were experiencing conflict with each other and the medical staff—all in the same week. Some emotional reactions Tom experienced during and after that week were sadness at the loss of Dana in particular (due to her age and how sudden her death was), anger at Rick's family members, and frustration at the oncologist who was reluctant to discuss prognosis with Gary's family. Tom also felt pride in a job well done, particularly in having been able to comfort Dana's family during her loss, encouraging the family to share anecdotes and memories. For Gary and Rick, he was able to get support from ICU team members in dealing with the conflict. Tom also used specific strategies to manage his own experience during these long days. He made sure to pack a healthy lunch to bring with him, and went for a walk after work a couple of days that week. During his workday, he was able to take a minute or two during his break time to sit quietly and focus on his breathing, consciously letting go of stressful thoughts. He intentionally focused on the positive interactions he had with his new patient and how he helped the student nurse learn how to calibrate the patient's arterial line.

Reflection questions:

1. What skills did Tom use that helped him approach these patient challenges with equanimity? List two adaptive strategies and reflect on the role each played.
2. What other strategies might have been helpful for Tom or someone in his circumstance?

Manage Your Attention and Improve Your World

"The real voyage of discovery consists not in seeking new landscapes, but in having new eyes."
    Marcel Proust, *Remembrance of Things Past*

Research has shown us that choosing where we place our focus and energy is integrally linked to happiness. In her book, *Rapt*, science writer Winifred Gallagher describes the benefits of choosing where we place our focus, emphasizing that our focus is a limited resource that defines our personal worldview. By focusing on positive emotions and things that bring us joy, we can expand our worldview, improve our attitude, and accumulate positive experiences that nourish us in the present and serve as an ongoing foundation for our well-being.[76,104] Indeed, psychologists teach us that skillful use of emotional leverage points can result in significantly more positive outcomes following negative events, offering us a chance to reset and restart more productively.[104]

This has been backed up by functional MRI data.[75,77] Mather, Carstensen, and colleagues studied both young and elderly adults, providing each with positive, negative, and neutral visual imagery. The researchers checked participants' functional MRI response at the amygdala and hippocampus while asking both groups to rate their response to the different images. The researchers found that, while both groups showed greater activation to emotionally laden images over neutral images, young people had amygdala firing (and thus an emotional response) to both types of imagery, while the elderly subjects had the largest amygdala responses to the positive stimuli. Their conclusion was that the elderly patients had trained their prefrontal cortex to inhibit the amygdala in the presence of negative stimuli.[77] In other words, the elderly subjects had trained their attention to focus on the positive, a well-founded psychological phenomenon that is termed the "age-related positivity effect."[105,106] Below we discuss a number of strategies for training one's attention, including mindfulness and cultivating positive emotions.

Mindfulness—Train Your Attention and Change Your Brain

Mindfulness is a method of training one's attention to focus on the present moment in a purposeful yet nonjudgmental manner, nurturing attention, self-awareness and focus in the moment, and learning to accept sensations and feelings as they are and without judgment.[107,108] Mindfulness expands the present moment allowing one to focus on the here and now instead of functioning on autopilot, ruminating about the past, or fixating on future hazards and rewards.[109] Mindfulness is practiced through various forms of contemplative practices, including meditation and yoga, designed to cultivate peaceful self-awareness and insight while boosting energy and focus.

Mindfulness has been found to positively influence several health, relational, and productivity outcomes[110] and has even been found to change several areas of the brain for the healthier.[111,112] Mindfulness programs have been found to improve immune responses and reduce pain, anxiety, stress, and burnout while creating an adaptive reserve and promoting resiliency, self-compassion, and improved quality of life.[107,112] These findings have even been identified among medical students and practicing physicians.[113,114] In the business world, mindfulness has been embraced as a means of enhancing leadership, interpersonal skills, and even performance.[108,110] Mindfulness makes one more accepting of oneself and others and less evaluative overall, thus enhancing one's ability to reframe mistakes as learning opportunities,[108] even if the mistakes themselves and their impact remain painful.

What are some of the specific changes we see in performance, function, and brain plasticity? Neuroscientists have revealed that practicing mindfulness affects brain areas related to perception, emotion regulation, complex thinking and introspection, memory, pain tolerance, and body awareness.[112] A systematic review and meta-analysis published in 2014 looked at more than 20 brain mapping studies and found that after 8 weeks of daily mindfulness practice, meditators had increased neuronal activity in the anterior cingulate cortex (ACC) as compared to nonmeditators, with resulting superior performance on tests of self-regulation and self-control.[112] Meditators are better able to resist distractions, inhibit impulsivity, and provide accurate answers. They are also better than nonmeditators at modulating their emotions and learning from past experiences, both of which are hallmarks of effective decision making.[110-112] Brain mapping studies show that mindfulness increases grey matter density in areas of the brain associated with memory, learning, and regulation of emotions.[111] Mindfulness decreases reactivity in the amygdala (the home of the "fight or flight" response) and increases activity in the prefrontal cortex, which helps the mindful regulate emotion more effectively, rebound from acute stressors more quickly, and experience less stress overall. [111,115] Putting all of this together, proponents ranging from neuroscientists to business leaders to wellness experts endorse mindfulness as a "must" for brain health, stress reduction, self-management, decision making, and even leadership.

The Nitty Gritty—Practicing Mindfulness for Everyone

Initiating a mindfulness practice is without question challenging—so challenging in fact that, for many people, it simply feels like one more thing to feel bad about. But the strategies for approaching mindfulness are so wide-ranging and customizable that there really can be a "good fit" for everyone, though finding that fit may take some work. By way of example, one of the present authors (ECC) informed her team chaplain many years ago that she wanted to start meditating, to which the chaplain serenely responded, "I think, for you, yoga," proceeding to note that this physician's particular energy level might be incompatible with long periods of stillness. And, indeed, after experimenting with multiple modalities, mindfulness in motion was ultimately the best solution for this physician (thank goodness we have a team!), with the occasional addition of brief, guided meditations through an app. The Harvard Business Review book, *Mindfulness*, advises us to "Take a seat, take a breath, and commit to being mindful,"[110] as a way of encouraging simply starting even before finding one's perfect path. Below, we describe a few of the many potential "hows" of approaching a mindfulness practice:

- As a part of either a secular or spiritual practice.
- Through a seated or lying meditation practice or through mindfulness integrated into movement—be it yoga, walking, running or swimming—any practice that allows one to focus on the breath and the present moment.
- Through longer periods of daily meditation, similar to those taught for thousands of years and honed and modernized through programs such as the program in *Mindfulness Based Stress Reduction*,[107] which promotes 30–45 minutes of daily meditation of various forms, including traditional sitting meditations, body scans (paying attention to parts of one's body), and walking meditation.
- By integrating small, regular points of practice throughout one's day. This can be done in multiple ways, including app reminders to spend a minute focusing on the breath every hour or deliberately pausing to focus on the breath prior to meetings or while walking or driving. Some examples include:
  - Utilizing mindfulness applications, such as Headspace (www.headspace.com) or Calm (www.calm.com), either for regular daily meditation or focused, as needed, meditation interventions to use to address specific stressors.
  - Incorporating a mindfulness practice throughout the workday[116]: Begin the day with 1–2 minutes of attending to the breath upon awakening while still in bed. Once at work, begin the day with 10 minutes spent in seated meditation. Then, interspersed throughout the day, take regular

1- to 2-minute pauses to attend to the breath, such as at the beginning and end of every meeting and once an hour. Finally, practice 10 minutes of meditation at the conclusion of the workday, such as before leaving one's desk or while walking to the parking lot.

o Cultivating kindness, gratitude, and intentional attention in 1- to 2-minute increments at multiple, well-chosen points in the day.[117] This modern mindfulness program specifically recommends: (1) beginning and ending the day with a reflection of gratitude upon first awakening and just prior to sleep; (2) sending silent good wishes to others whenever crossing their path throughout the day; and (3) deliberately focusing gratitude and attention on loved ones at the end of the day without trying to improve them for at least 3 minutes.

Cultivating Positive Emotion—Investing in Social Relationships and Accumulating Positive Currency

There is ample evidence that social relationships are not only the greatest predictor of happiness and high performance, but they are also integrally connected with health, well-being, and ability to recover from setbacks. In his book, *The Happiness Advantage*, Sean Achor refers to one's inner circle of friends and family as a personal "offensive line"—no matter what is coming at us, they can block for us and protect us, improve our play, and help us recover when we have lost our footing.[1] Beyond friendships and family connections, even more casual ties can contribute to well-being, positivity, and productivity, such as warm interactions with colleagues and expressions of gratitude and appreciation. This may be particularly important for clinicians who are members of groups that have experienced discrimination within medicine—for example, women, LGBTQ+ individuals, or people of color. Informal support networks of other individuals with similar experiences, as well as allies, are crucial to coping with microaggressions and implicit bias in the medical setting. Involvement in formal organizations and groups may also provide support and an outlet for positive action.[66,118]

Work in resiliency universally refers to the importance of positivity and gratitude as paths to wellness.[119] What is more, research has taught that emotions are contagious, and thus the ability to generate positivity for others and ourselves can dramatically impact our interactions and relationships with others and with ourselves.[1] So how do we go about cultivating positivity?

Practice Gratitude

Studies have shown that regularly practicing gratitude enhances well-being, lifts the spirit, and provides a sense of calm, while causing the release of happiness-inducing chemicals like serotonin.[120] Gratitude helps us focus on the positive aspect of events and people around us. As such, it has been shown to reduce anxiety and depression and lower the risk of disease. There are multiple ways to integrate a gratitude practice into one's day:

- Deliberately reflect on the good things and people in your life at specific points in the day, such as upon awakening and just before going to sleep. Writing in a journal or tracking in an app can help you keep track of these positive thoughts in ways that may serve to boost your spirits again and again. One of my (ECC) favorite versions of the above journaling exercise comes from Rachel Naomi Remen's book, *My Grandfather's Blessings*, in which she promotes gratitude as a way of "finding new eyes." Building on the work of Angeles Arrien, she suggests setting aside 15 minutes each evening to reflect on the following three questions: "What surprised me today? What moved me or touched me today? What inspired me today?"[121]
- Set aside time each week to write notes of gratitude to friends, family, and coworkers. Sharing gratitude in this way spreads the wealth, generating positivity and goodwill to both of you.
- Support a cause about which you are passionate, either by volunteering or through a financial commitment.

Commit Random Acts of Kindness

Look for ways to offer kindness to others. Whether it is bringing a meal to a friend in need, digging someone's car out of the snow, putting a colleague up for an award, or pitching in to help a neighbor without being asked, small acts of kindness not only generate positivity but also build relationships. It shows you are paying attention to the needs of others and that you care.

Deliberately Accumulate Positivity—and Celebrate It

In the Harvard Business Review book, *Resilience*, Kopans refers to positivity as "creating a bull market"—the more you create, the more there is, and the more everyone wants in. The authors recommend deliberately reflecting on and celebrating the positivity one generates on a regular basis, comparing this "bank of positivity" to an investment portfolio that will grow best if one makes regular contributions. And, continuing the investment metaphor, the authors recommend "diversifying your positivity portfolio," investing most heavily in areas that have the "highest returns," which almost universally means deliberately focusing on one's personal life—on family, friends, and hobbies.[119]

Now we return to Dr. R, our surgical oncologist who had been struggling the fact that her 35-year-old patient, Ms. J, had not done well after surgery.

Vignette 2, part 2: Dr. R, 40-year-old surgical oncologist

Dr. R in fact was so distraught by Ms. J's condition that she was not only avoiding the patient, she was avoiding her colleagues as well. One of her mentors caught her in the hallway to check in on her, prompting Dr. R to share her recent experience with Ms. J and her distress. Her mentor empathized with Dr. R and pointed out that she had done well by her patient. After all, Dr. R couldn't change the path of the cancer; she could only treat what was there to the best of her ability. And now, the mentor noted, Ms. J and her family needed her differently—they needed her to come and stand with them as they faced what was ahead with the disease. The mentor encouraged Dr. R to reach out to her mentors and other colleagues during tough cases in the future, noting that every surgeon struggles with unanticipated complications and undesirable outcomes from time to time. She was not alone and, as colleagues, they all needed to support each other. The mentor also gently asked Dr. R what she was doing to care for herself.

Dr. R went home that evening feeling more peaceful and reflected on things that had helped her be resilient in the past. When she got home, instead of pouring a glass of wine, she went for a walk with her dog and called a friend. When she got home from her walk, she focused her attention on her spouse and kids, enjoying their time together. And that night, she did a written gratitude exercise in her journal. She realized that she was grateful for her relationship with Ms. J and her family and eager to help see them through the next phase. She also reflected on the things she had learned and how this experience would help her going forward. She went to bed resolved to be there for Ms. J and, like her mentor, to watch for and reach out to colleagues in need of support.

Reflection questions:

- Name three adaptive strategies Dr. R uses to boost her resilience. Which do you think helped her most (or most quickly)?

- In this scenario, the mentor showed up as Dr. R's "offensive line." What can Dr. R do in the future to enhance her social support and community independently, including her community at work? Using the mentor in this vignette as a model, name one thing you can do next week to support a colleague's well-being, making it clear that you are a resource for them?

- What daily wellness commitments do you hope Dr. R makes for herself going forward? Pick 2 she can do every day and 1 she can use every week. Which of these could you use in a similar situation?

> **Closing self-reflection questions**
>
> 1. Reflect on the strategies for cultivating positivity. Choose one new skill that you would like to develop in the next year (e.g., practicing gra titude, focusing your attention, investing in your social support network). What steps can you take to develop this skill? What is one thing you can do next week to get closer to this goal?
> 2. Describe two strategies for approaching mindfulness, focusing on those you would find most effective for yourself. Which strategy can you begin to integrate into your daily routine tomorrow? Which might you consider a longer-term goal?
> 3. Name one self-care strategy that you can incorporate daily and one you can incorporate weekly.

■ CONCLUSION

In this chapter we have described a variety of emotional challenges that are inherent for clinicians in their work—as well as positive emotions that many of us experience in caring for patients and in our roles as physicians, nurses, and other healthcare professionals. Taking care of our emotions and attending to our general wellness helps us be better at our jobs and attain longevity in our careers. We have described a few techniques for doing this, including practices such as mindfulness and expressions of gratitude, as well as fostering emotional intelligence. We encourage you to consider these practices, and others that you may find suitable for you, as an essential part of your clinical work.

REFERENCES

1. Achor S. *The Happiness Advantage: How a Positive Brain Fuels Success in Work and Life.* New York, NY: Crown Publishing Group, a division of Penguin Random House LLC; 2010.

2. Shanafelt TD, Balch CM, Bechamps G, et al. Burnout and medical errors among American surgeons. *Ann Surg.* 2010;251(6):995-1000.

3. Anagnostopoulos F, Liolios E, Persefonis G, Slater J, Kafetsios K, Niakas D. Physician burnout and patient satisfaction with consultation in primary health care settings: evidence of relationships from a one-with-many design. *J Clin Psychol Med Settings.* 2012;19(4):401-410.

4. Heinen MM, van Achterberg T, Schwendimann R, et al. Nurses' intention to leave their profession: a cross sectional observational study in 10 European countries. *Int J Nurs Stud.* 2013;50(2):174-184.

5. Shanafelt TD, Mungo M, Schmitgen J, et al. Longitudinal study evaluating the association between physician burnout and changes in professional work effort. *Mayo Clin Proc.* 2016;91(4):422-431.

6. Salsberg ES. Is the physician shortage real? implications for the recommendations of the institute of medicine committee on the governance and financing of graduate medical education. *Acad Med.* 2015;90(9):1210-1214.

7. World Health Organization. World Health Organization Constitution. https://www. who.int/about/who-we-are/constitution. Accessed September 10, 2020.

8. Brady KJS, Trockel MT, Khan CT, et al. What do we mean by physician wellness? a systematic review of its definition and measurement. *Acad Psychiatry.* 2018; 42(1):94-108.

9. Hojat M, Vergare MJ, Maxwell K, et al. The devil is in the third year: a longitudinal study of erosion of empathy in medical school. *Acad Med.* 2009;84(9):1182-1191.

10. Neumann M, Edelhäuser F, Tauschel D, et al. Empathy decline and its reasons: a systematic review of studies with medical students and residents. *Acad Med.* 2011;86(8):996-1009.

11. Gaufberg EH, Batalden M, Sands R, Bell SK. The hidden curriculum: what can we learn from third-year medical student narrative reflections? *Acad Med.* 2010; 85(11):1709-1716.

12. Lawrence C, Mhlaba T, Stewart KA, Moletsane R, Gaede B, Moshabela M. The hidden curricula of medical education: a scoping review. *Acad Med.* 2018;93(4):648-656.

13. Center C, Davis M, Detre T, et al. Confronting depression and suicide in physicians: a consensus statement. *JAMA.* 2003;289(23):3161-3166.

14. Dyrbye LN, Thomas MR, Shanafelt TD. Systematic review of depression, anxiety, and other indicators of psychological distress among U.S. and Canadian medical students. *Acad Med.* 2006;81(4):354-373.

15. Mata DA, Ramos MA, Bansal N, et al. Prevalence of depression and depressive symptoms among resident physicians: a systematic review and meta-analysis. *JAMA.* 2015;314(22):2373-2383.

16. Frank E, Dingle AD. Self-reported depression and suicide attempts among U.S. women physicians. *Am J Psychiatry.* 1999;156(12):1887-1894.

17. Welsh D. Predictors of depressive symptoms in female medical-surgical hospital nurses. *Issues Ment Health Nurs.* 2009;30(5):320-326.

18. Schernhammer ES, Colditz GA. Suicide rates among physicians: a quantitative and gender assessment (meta-analysis). *Am J Psychiatry.* 2004;161(12):2295-2302.

19. Dutheil F, Aubert C, Pereira B, et al. Suicide among physicians and health-care workers: a systematic review and meta-analysis. *PLoS One.* 2019;14(12):e0226361.

20. Davidson JE, Proudfoot J, Lee K, Terterian G, Zisook S. A longitudinal analysis of nurse suicide in the United States (2005-2016) with recommendations for action. *Worldviews Evid Based Nurs.* 2020;17(1):6-15.

21. Platt B, Hawton K, Simkin S, Mellanby RJ. Suicidal behaviour and psychosocial problems in veterinary surgeons: a systematic review. *Soc Psychiatry Psychiatr Epidemiol.* 2012;47(2):223-240.

22. Gold KJ, Sen A, Schwenk TL. Details on suicide among US physicians: data from the National Violent Death Reporting System. *Gen Hosp Psychiatry*. 2013;35(1):45-49.

23. Oreskovich MR, Shanafelt T, Dyrbye LN, et al. The prevalence of substance use disorders in American physicians. *Am J Addict*. 2015;24(1):30-38.

24. Baldisseri MR. Impaired healthcare professional. *Crit Care Med*. 2007;35(2 Suppl): S106-16.

25. Bryson EO. The opioid epidemic and the current prevalence of substance use disorder in anesthesiologists. *Curr Opin Anaesthesiol*. 2018;31(3):388-392.

26. Kunyk D. Substance use disorders among registered nurses: prevalence, risks and perceptions in a disciplinary jurisdiction. *J Nurs Manag*. 2015;23(1):54-64.

27. Bell DM, McDonough JP, Ellison JS, Fitzhugh EC. Controlled drug misuse by Certified Registered Nurse Anesthetists. *AANA J*. 1999;67(2):133-140.

28. Gross CP, Mead LA, Ford DE, Klag MJ. Physician, heal thyself? Regular source of care and use of preventive health services among physicians. *Arch Intern Med*. 2000;160(21):3209-3214.

29. Dyrbye LN, West CP, Sinsky CA, Goeders LE, Satele DV, Shanafelt TD. Medical licensure questions and physician reluctance to seek care for mental health conditions. *Mayo Clin Proc*. 2017;92(10):1486-1493.

30. Saag HS, Shah K, Jones SA, Testa PA, Horwitz LI. Pajama time: working after work in the electronic health record. *J Gen Intern Med*. 2019;34(9):1695-1696.

31. Rhodes-Kropf J, Carmody SS, Seltzer D, et al. "This is just too awful; I just can't believe I experienced that...": medical students' reactions to their "most memorable" patient death. *Acad Med*. 2005;80(7):634-640.

32. Redinbaugh EM, Sullivan AM, Block SD, et al. Doctors' emotional reactions to recent death of a patient: cross sectional study of hospital doctors. *BMJ*. 2003;327(7408):185.

33. Jackson VA, Sullivan AM, Gadmer NM, et al. "It was haunting...": physicians' descriptions of emotionally powerful patient deaths. *Acad Med*. 2005;80(7):648-656.

34. Wenzel J, Shaha M, Klimmek R, Krumm S. Working through grief and loss: oncology nurses' perspectives on professional bereavement. *Oncol Nurs Forum*. 2011;38(4):E272-82.

35. Groves JE. Taking care of the hateful patient. *New Engl J Med*. 1978;298(16):883-887.

36. O'Dowd TC. Five years of heartsink patients in general practice. *BMJ*. 1988;297 (6647):528-530.

37. McAndrew NS, Leske J, Schroeter K. Moral distress in critical care nursing: the state of the science. *Nurs Ethics*. 2018;25(5):552-570.

38. Sajjadi S, Norena M, Wong H, Dodek P. Moral distress and burnout in internal medicine residents. *Can Med Educ J*. 2017;8(1):e36-e43.

39. Lamiani G, Borghi L, Argentero P. When healthcare professionals cannot do the right thing: a systematic review of moral distress and its correlates. *J Health Psychol*. 2017;22(1):51-67.

40. Sportsman S, Hamilton P. Conflict management styles in the health professions. *J Prof Nurs*. 2007;23(3):157-166.

41. Labrague LJ, Al Hamdan Z, McEnroe-Petitte DM. An integrative review on conflict management styles among nursing professionals: implications for nursing management. *J Nurs Manag.* 2018;26(8):902-917.

42. American Psychiatric Association. *Diagnostic and Statistical Manual of Mental Disorders.* 5th ed. Arlington, VA: American Psychiatric Association; 2013.

43. Quinal L, Harford S, Rutledge DN. Secondary traumatic stress in oncology staff. *Cancer Nurs.* 2009;32(4):E1-7.

44. Dominguez-Gomez E, Rutledge DN. Prevalence of secondary traumatic stress among emergency nurses. *J Emerg Nurs.* 2009;35(3):199-204; quiz 273.

45. Schwartz R, Sinskey JL, Anand U, Margolis RD. Addressing postpandemic clinician mental health: a narrative review and conceptual framework. *Ann Intern Med.* 2020.

46. Wakam GK, Montgomery JR, Biesterveld BE, Brown CS. Not dying alone—modern compassionate care in the Covid-19 pandemic. *New Engl J Med.* 2020;382(24):e88.

47. Coetzee SK, Laschinger HKS. Toward a comprehensive, theoretical model of compassion fatigue: an integrative literature review. *Nurs Health Sci.* 2018;20(1):4-15.

48. Zhang Y-Y, Han W-L, Qin W, et al. Extent of compassion satisfaction, compassion fatigue and burnout in nursing: a meta-analysis. *J Nurs Manag.* 2018;26(7):810-819.

49. Marmon LM, Heiss K. Improving surgeon wellness: the second victim syndrome and quality of care. *Semin Pediatr Surg.* 2015;24(6):315-318.

50. Harrison R, Lawton R, Perlo J, Gardner P, Armitage G, Shapiro J. Emotion and coping in the aftermath of medical error: a cross-country exploration. *J Patient Saf.* 2015;11(1):28-35.

51. Robertson JJ, Long B. Suffering in silence: medical error and its impact on health care providers. *J Emerg Med.* 2018;54(4):402-409.

52. Larson EB, Yao X. Clinical empathy as emotional labor in the patient-physician relationship. *JAMA.* 2005;293(9):1100-1106.

53. Psilopanagioti A, Anagnostopoulos F, Mourtou E, Niakas D. Emotional intelligence, emotional labor, and job satisfaction among physicians in Greece. *BMC Health Serv Res.* 2012;12:463.

54. Schwartz R, Haverfield MC, Brown-Johnson C, et al. Transdisciplinary strategies for physician wellness: qualitative insights from diverse fields. *J Gen Intern Med.* 2019;34(7):1251-1257.

55. Srinivasa S, Gurney J, Koea J. Potential consequences of patient complications for surgeon well-being: a systematic review. *JAMA Surg.* 2019;154(5):451-457.

56. Orri M, Farges O, Clavien P-A, Barkun J, Revah-Lévy A. Being a surgeon—the myth and the reality: a meta-synthesis of surgeons' perspectives about factors affecting their practice and well-being. *Ann Surg.* 2014;260(5):721-8; discussion 728.

57. Shanafelt TD, Schein E, Minor LB, Trockel M, Schein P, Kirch D. Healing the professional culture of medicine. *Mayo Clin Proc.* 2019;94(8):1556-1566.

58. Torres MB, Salles A, Cochran A. Recognizing and reacting to microaggressions in medicine and surgery. *JAMA Surg.* 2019.

59. Bullock JL, Lockspeiser T, Del Pino-Jones A, Richards R, Teherani A, Hauer KE. They don't see a lot of people my color: a mixed methods study of racial/ethnic stereotype threat among medical students on core clerkships. *Acad Med.* 2020.

60. Hardeman RR, Przedworski JM, Burke SE, et al. Mental well-being in first year medical students: a comparison by race and gender: a report from the Medical Student CHANGE Study. *J Racial Ethn Health Disparities.* 2015;2(3):403-413.

61. Guille C, Frank E, Zhao Z, et al. Work-family conflict and the sex difference in depression among training physicians. *JAMA Intern Med.* 2017;177(12):1766-1772.

62. Jolly S, Griffith KA, DeCastro R, Stewart A, Ubel P, Jagsi R. Gender differences in time spent on parenting and domestic responsibilities by high-achieving young physician-researchers. *Ann Intern Med.* 2014;160(5):344-353.

63. Adamson R, Brady AK, Aitken ML. Gender equality in academic medicine requires changes for both men and women. *Acad Med.* 2017;92(8):1067.

64. Rochon PA, Davidoff F, Levinson W. Women in academic medicine leadership: has anything changed in 25 years? *Acad Med.* 2016;91(8):1053-1056.

65. Dimant OE, Cook TE, Greene RE, Radix AE. Experiences of transgender and gender nonbinary medical students and physicians. *Transgend Health.* 2019;4(1):209-216.

66. Eliason MJ, Streed C, Henne M. Coping with stress as an LGBTQ+ health care professional. *J Homosex.* 2018;65(5):561-578.

67. Torres L, Driscoll MW, Burrow AL. Racial microaggressions and psychological functioning among highly achieving African-Americans: a mixed-methods approach. *J Soc Clin Psychol.* 2010;29(10):1074-1099.

68. O'Riordan M, Skelton J, de la Croix A. Heartlift patients? An interview-based study of GP trainers and the impact of "patients they like". *Fam Pract.* 2008;25(5):349-354.

69. Zambrano SC, Chur-Hansen A, Crawford GB. The experiences, coping mechanisms, and impact of death and dying on palliative medicine specialists. *Palliat Support Care.* 2014;12(4):309-316.

70. Steinmetz D, Walsh M, Gabel LL, Williams PT. Family physicians' involvement with dying patients and their families: attitudes, difficulties, and strategies. *Arch Fam Med.* 1993;2(7):753-60; discussion 761.

71. Kaplan LI. The greatest gift: how a patient's death taught me to be a physician. *JAMA.* 2017;318(18):1761-1762.

72. Yanguas J, Pinazo-Henandis S, Tarazona-Santabalbina FJ. The complexity of loneliness. *Acta Biomed.* 2018;89(2):302-314.

73. Thoits PA. Mechanisms linking social ties and support to physical and mental health. *J Health Soc Behav.* 2011;52(2):145-161.

74. Shanafelt TD, Noseworthy JH. Executive leadership and physician well-being: nine organizational strategies to promote engagement and reduce burnout. *Mayo Clin Proc.* 2017;92(1):129-146.

75. Carstensen LL, DeLiema M. The positivity effect: a negativity bias in youth fades with age. *Curr Opin Behav Sci.* 2018;19:7-12.

76. Gallagher W. *Rapt: Attention and the Focused Life.* New York, NY: The Penguin Press; 2009.

77. Mather M, Canli T, English T, et al. Amygdala responses to emotionally valenced stimuli in older and younger adults. *Psychol Sci.* 2004;15(4):259-263.

78. Shanafelt TD, Hasan O, Dyrbye LN, et al. Changes in burnout and satisfaction with work-life balance in physicians and the general US working population between 2011 and 2014. *Mayo Clin Proc.* 2015;90(12):1600-1613.

79. Wohlever AS. "Burnout" in the workplace: strategies, omissions, and lessons from wounded healers. *Am J Health Promot.* 2020;34(5):568-571.

80. Amabile TM, Kramer SJ. The power of small wins—improve inner work life. In: *Happiness.* HBR Emotional Intelligence Series. Boston, MA: Harvard Business Review Press; 2017.

81. The Mayo Clinic. Exercise: how much do I need every day? https://www.mayoclinic.org/healthy-lifestyle/fitness/expert-answers/exercise/faq-20057916. Accessed September 13, 2020.

82. The Mayo Clinic. How many hours of sleep are enough? https://www.mayoclinic.org/healthy-lifestyle/adult-health/expert-answers/how-many-hours-of-sleep-are-enough/faq-20057898. Accessed September 13, 2020.

83. Kay M, Mitchell G, Clavarino A, Doust J. Doctors as patients: a systematic review of doctors' health access and the barriers they experience. *Br J Gen Pract.* 2008;58(552):501-508.

84. Howard SK, Gaba DM, Rosekind MR, Zarcone VP. The risks and implications of excessive daytime sleepiness in resident physicians. *Acad Med.* 2002;77(10):1019-1025.

85. Howard SK. Sleep deprivation and physician performance: why should I care? *Proc (Bayl. Univ. Med. Cent).* 2005;18(2):108-12; discussion 112.

86. Wali SO, Qutah K, Abushanab L, Basamh R, Abushanab J, Krayem A. Effect of on-call-related sleep deprivation on physicians' mood and alertness. *Ann Thorac Med.* 2013;8(1):22-27.

87. Dyrbye LN, Satele D, Shanafelt TD. Healthy exercise habits are associated with lower risk of burnout and higher quality of life among U.S. medical students. *Acad Med.* 2017;92(7):1006-1011.

88. Shanafelt TD, Oreskovich MR, Dyrbye LN, et al. Avoiding burnout: the personal health habits and wellness practices of US surgeons. *Ann Surg.* 2012;255(4):625-633.

89. Federation of State Physician Health Programs. 2018. https://www.fsphp.org/state-programs. Accessed October 15, 2020.

90. Rose JS, Campbell M, Skipper G. Prognosis for emergency physician with substance abuse recovery: 5-year outcome study. *West J Emerg Med.* 2014;15(1):20-25.

91. Friedman SD. What successful work and life integration looks like. *Harv Bus Rev.* 2014.

92. Shanafelt TD, Dyrbye LN, West CP. Addressing physician burnout: the way forward. *JAMA.* 2017;317(9):901-902.

93. Shanafelt TD, West CP, Sloan JA, et al. Career fit and burnout among academic faculty. *Arch Intern Med.* 2009;169(10):990-995.

94. Anchor S. The happiness advantage: the seven principles of positive psychology that fuel success and performance at work. *Choice Reviews Online.* 2011;48(07):48-4166-48-4166.

95. Lyubomirsky S, King L, Diener E. The benefits of frequent positive affect: does happiness lead to success? *Psychol Bull.* 2005;131(6):803-855.

96. Hansen M, Keltner D. Finding meaning at work, even when your job is dull. In: *Purpose, Meaning, and Passion.* HBR Emotional Intelligence Series. Boston, MA: Harvard Business Review Press; 2018.

97. Coleman J. You don't find your purpose—you build it. In: *Purpose, Meaning, and Passion.* HBR Emotional Intelligence Series. Boston, MA: Harvard Business Review Press; 2018.

98. Goleman D. *Working with Emotional Intelligence.* New York, NY: Bantam Dell; 1998.

99. Wong C-S, Law KS. The effects of leader and follower emotional intelligence on performance and attitude. *Leadersh Q.* 2002;13(3):243-274.

100. Weng H-C, Chen H-C, Chen H-J, Lu K, Hung S-Y. Doctors' emotional intelligence and the patient-doctor relationship. *Med Educ.* 2008;42(7):703-711.

101. Hojat M, Louis DZ, Markham FW, Wender R, Rabinowitz C, Gonnella JS. Physicians' empathy and clinical outcomes for diabetic patients. *Acad Med.* 2011;86(3):359-364.

102. Weng H-C, Hung C-M, Liu Y-T, et al. Associations between emotional intelligence and doctor burnout, job satisfaction and patient satisfaction. *Med Educ.* 2011;45(8):835-842.

103. Goleman D. What makes a leader? *Harv Bus Rev.* 1998;76(6):93-102.

104. Fredrickson B. *Positivity.* New York, NY: Crown Publishing Group, a division of Penguin Random House LLC; 2009.

105. Carstensen L, Mikels JA. At the intersection of emotion and cognition. *Curr Dir Psychol Sci.* 2005;14(3):117-121.

106. Mather M. The affective neuroscience of aging. *Annu Rev Psychol.* 2016;67:213-238.

107. Kabat-Zinn J. *Full Catastrophe Living: Using the Wisdom of Your Body and Mind to Face Stress, Pain, and Illness.* 2nd ed. New York, NY: Bantam Books; 2013.

108. Beard A. 1. Mindfulness in the age of complexity—an interview with Ellen Langer. In: *Mindfulness.* HBR Emotional Intelligence Series. Boston, MA: Harvard Business School Publishing Corporation; 2017.

109. Sood A, Jones DT. On mind wandering, attention, brain networks, and meditation. *Explore (N.Y.).* 2013;9(3):136-141.

110. Congleton C, Hölzel BK, Lazar SW. Mindfulness can literally change your brain. In: *Mindfulness.* HBR Emotional Intelligence Series. Boston, MA: Harvard Business Review Press; 2017.

111. Hölzel BK, Carmody J, Vangel M, et al. Mindfulness practice leads to increases in regional brain gray matter density. *Psychiatry Res.* 2011;191(1):36-43.

112. Fox KCR, Nijeboer S, Dixon ML, et al. Is meditation associated with altered brain structure? A systematic review and meta-analysis of morphometric neuroimaging in meditation practitioners. *Neurosci Biobehav Rev.* 2014;43:48-73.

113. Epstein RM. Mindful practice. *JAMA.* 1999;282(9):833-839.

114. Sood A, Sharma V, Schroeder DR, Gorman B. Stress Management and Resiliency Training (SMART) program among Department of Radiology faculty: a pilot randomized clinical trial. *Explore (N.Y.).* 2014;10(6):358-363.

115. Goldin PR, Gross JJ. Effects of mindfulness-based stress reduction (MBSR) on emotion regulation in social anxiety disorder. *Emotion.* 2010;10(1):83-91.

116. Hougaard R, Carter J. How to practice mindfulness throughout your work day. In: *Mindfulness.* HBR Emotional Intelligence Series. Boston, MA: Harvard Business Review Press; 2017.

117. Sood A. *Mindfulness Redesigned for the Twenty-First Century: Let's Not Cage the Hummingbird.* Rochester, MN: Global Center for Resiliency and Wellbeing; 2018.

118. Nunez-Smith M, Curry LA, Berg D, Krumholz HM, Bradley EH. Healthcare workplace conversations on race and the perspectives of physicians of African descent. *J Gen Intern Med.* 2008;23(9):1471-1476.

119. Kopans D. How to evaluate, manage, and strengthen your resilience. In: *Resilience.* HBR Emotional Intelligence Series. Boston, MA: Harvard Business Review Press; 2017.

120. Wood AM, Froh JJ, Geraghty AWA. Gratitude and well-being: a review and theoretical integration. *Clin Psychol Rev.* 2010;30(7):890-905.

121. Remen RN. *My Grandfather's Blessings.* New York, NY: Riverhead Books; 2000.

Afterword: Future Directions

Lars G. Osterberg, Judith A. Hall, and Rachel Schwartz

The authors of this book come from a broad diversity of fields and have covered an equally wide range of topics on the impact of emotion in healthcare: both the impact it has on patients, and its impact on healthcare providers. We have highlighted the functions of emotions, the interaction of illness and emotion, and addressed the nuances of emotion in a variety of patient populations, in addition to covering many aspects of emotional intelligence. We have sought to address emotions in the culture of medicine, including the challenges of teaching emotion-relevant skills and the importance of achieving emotional wellness in trainees and practicing healthcare providers. We have described the many emotion-related interactions in healthcare, highlighted the numerous problems, obstacles, and benefits in addressing emotions, and have offered guidance and advice. The remaining question is: how will clinicians and trainees navigate tomorrow's healthcare landscape while effectively addressing their patients' emotions and managing their own?

In recent years, the delivery of healthcare has changed significantly and will continue to change as technology allows for the care of patients to occur more frequently within patients' homes. Telehealth in the form of telephone visits, video visits, and other remote methods of communication and care (text, email, and remote monitoring devices) is enhancing the convenience of healthcare and giving patients more options. However, the lack of physical presence adds challenges in understanding and dealing with emotions. Telehealth visits challenge both how providers and patients perceive the emotions of the other person and limit the ways providers have to address patients' emotions. In a telehealth visit, the provider is required to have a heightened awareness in picking up emotional clues remotely, and if the visit is a phone visit, this is even more challenging since visual clues are not available. Best practices in care and education on how to perceive emotion and address emotion in the telehealth visit are evolving and more research is needed to respond to this challenge.

Artificial intelligence approaches to detecting emotional cues, both in voice and face, have been developed over the past decade, and may offer new tools for emotional training. While this type of technology may prove useful in patient care and education, relying too heavily on technology to detect the nuanced and complex facets of emotion comes with its own risks, and should not replace the training required to hone clinicians' emotional perception and intelligence.

We advocate for making training in, and assessment of, emotional intelligence a standard part of medical education in order to improve patient care and provider wellness. This training should be as central to developing a well-educated clinician as teaching anatomy and physiology is, since emotion is intimately tied to health and the appropriate handling of emotion can make all the difference in whether a patient is able to engage with the recommended treatment. While the abundance of content in the medical education curriculum is overwhelming, it is clear that *not* educating clinicians around emotion is too costly. Requiring a level of competency in emotional intelligence is critically important for healthcare trainees, and assessments in emotional intelligence should be required prior to graduation, with remediation programs available for those who need targeted support in various aspects.

Attending to the patient's emotions has implications far beyond the successful response to an emotion in the moment. Attending to the patient's emotions has a reinforcing effect on many other aspects of healthcare that are central to the goals of patient-centered and relationship-centered practice. The patient's emotions reflect the person and their background; thus, emotional cues become beacons for delivering effectively tailored care and further support the biopsychosocial model of treating the patient as a whole person rather than just a collection of body parts and disease processes. The patient's emotions inform the provider about how to discuss and proceed with treatment decisions—serving the goal of increasing participatory decision making. The patient's emotions have a well-documented impact on outcomes including adherence to treatment regimen, appointment keeping, and the success of both diagnosis and treatment. Patient satisfaction—itself an emotion-laden construct—depends on how well the provider can grasp and respond to the patient's emotional experience. Thus, the whole panoply of desired humanistic care practices is served by the provider's adequacy in effectively recognizing and responding to patients' emotions.

An important question lies at the intersection of effort and intention on one hand, and formalized skill development on the other. Stated differently, does a healthcare provider actually need formal training in emotion recognition and other discrete skills in order to be more effective in this domain? The answer is that, of course, training is needed but in truth the appropriate pedagogy has not been fully developed and trainings that do exist are not yet a standard part of medical curricula. This does not mean, however, that trainees and experienced clinicians are helpless to be more effective in the emotion domain.

We say this because education and consciousness raising—such as provided in the present book—promote philosophical buy-in, encouraging clinicians to *want* to notice, identify, and respond to patient emotions. This is surely the first step to better patient care. Blanch-Hartigan showed that a physician's effort to acknowledge and name a patient's emotion is valued, even if the physician's guess is wrong.[1] A patient needs to see that their provider is *trying*.

Furthermore, healthcare providers probably have a better toolkit of emotion skills than they think they have. Not long ago, one of us was observing a coaching session of medical students with pediatric emergency room patients. The students were understandably nervous, but what stood out was how formal and stilted they were, seeming to forget that they already *knew* a lot about how to interact comfortably with little children—they had siblings or younger cousins and they were children themselves not long in the past. They seemed to be substituting a "doctor performance" for the people skills they already had. This observation in no way subtracts from the urgent need for more professional education on emotion; it merely underscores that if they try, most providers already have a set of skills to draw upon.

Finally, as we look toward the future of healthcare delivery, it becomes increasingly clear that clinician wellness must become a priority, and this is intertwined with serving patients well. Indeed, the ability of a clinician to be fully present and capable of delivering attentive, responsive care that is tailored to the individual needs of each patient depends on the clinician being able to maintain their own resilience, motivation, and mental health. Thus, the provision of outstanding care requires a professional context that allows clinicians to develop and maintain optimal functioning; then they can engage with patients in a manner that honors both parties' complexity and humanity. This necessitates providing clinicians with a set of tools, and a practice and training environment, that allows them to manage emotion in themselves and others. There is still much work to be done.

We hope that this book may be a useful resource for supporting the cultural change that is already underway; while more work is needed to acknowledge, integrate, and respond to emotion in the medical setting, the first step toward effecting this change is to understand the utility of emotion, then provide new tools for training what is a learnable skill set. Finally, effecting cultural change will require a community of thought leaders, medical educators, and clinicians to join together in sharing new best practices, modeling vulnerability, and collectively developing new methods for training the next generation of healers. We hope this book may lead to new conversations for how to better protect our clinicians, trainees, and the patients they serve.

William Osler once said, *"He who studies medicine without textbooks sails on uncharted seas, but he who studies medicine without patients does not go to sea at all."*[2]

We would add to Osler's famous advice: *A clinician who cares for patients without tending to the patients' emotions sails on uncharted seas, but without also tending to their own emotions they cannot go to sea at all.*

REFERENCES

1. Blanch-Hartigan D. Patient satisfaction with physician errors in detecting and identifying patient emotion cues. *Patient Educ Couns.* 2013;93(1):56-62.

2. Osler W. Address on the dedication of the new building. *Boston Med Surg J.* 1901: 144:60-61.

Index

Note: Page number followed by f and t indicates figure and table respectively.